PSYCHODYNAMIC THERAPY

FOR PERSONALITY PATHOLOGY

TREATING SELF AND INTERPERSONAL FUNCTIONING

PSYCHODYNAMIC THERAPY

FOR PERSONALITY PATHOLOGY

TREATING SELF AND INTERPERSONAL FUNCTIONING

Eve Caligor, M.D.
Otto F. Kernberg, M.D.
John F. Clarkin, Ph.D.
Frank E. Yeomans, M.D., Ph.D.

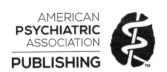

AMERICAN
PSYCHIATRIC
ASSOCIATION
PUBLISHING

If you wish to buy 50 or more copies of the same title, please go to www.appi.org/specialdiscounts for more information.

Copyright © 2018 American Psychiatric Association Publishing

ALL RIGHTS RESERVED

First Edition

Manufactured in the United States of America on acid-free paper
22   5   4

American Psychiatric Association Publishing
800 Maine Ave. SW, Suite 900
Washington, DC 20024-2812
www.appi.org

Library of Congress Cataloging-in-Publication Data
Names: Caligor, Eve, 1956- author. | Kernberg, Otto F., 1928- author. |
    Clarkin, John F., author. | Yeomans, Frank E., 1949- author. | American
    Psychiatric Association Publishing, issuing body.
Title: Psychodynamic therapy for personality pathology : treating self and
    interpersonal functioning / Eve Caligor, Otto F. Kernberg, John F. Clarkin,
    Frank E. Yeomans.
Description: First edition. | Washington, DC : American Psychiatric Association
    Publishing, [2018] | Includes bibliographical references and index.
Identifiers: LCCN 2018008140 (print) | LCCN 2018008873 (ebook) | ISBN
    9781615371815 (ebook) | ISBN 9781585624591 (alk. paper)
Subjects: | MESH: Psychotherapy, Psychodynamic | Personality Disorders—
    therapy | Transference (Psychology) | Psychotherapy—methods
Classification: LCC RC489.P72 (ebook) | LCC RC489.P72 (print) | NLM WM
    420.5.P75 | DDC 616.89/14—dc23
LC record available at https://lccn.loc.gov/2018008140

British Library Cataloguing in Publication Data
A CIP record is available from the British Library.

To Mike

Contents

Section I

Personality and Personality Disorders
Through the Lens of Object Relations Theory

Section II

Overview of TFP-E
BASIC TASKS, THE THERAPEUTIC RELATIONSHIP, AND STRATEGIES OF TREATMENT

Section III

The Skillful Consultation

Section IV

Establishing the Treatment Frame

Section V

Techniques and Tactics of TFP-E

Section VI
Phases of Treatment and Trajectories of Change

About the Authors

Eve Caligor, M.D., is Clinical Professor of Psychiatry at Columbia University College of Physicians and Surgeons, and Director of Psychotherapy Division and Training and Supervising Analyst at the Columbia University Center for Psychoanalytic Training and Research, New York, New York.

Otto F. Kernberg, M.D., is Director of the Personality Disorders Institute at Weill Cornell Medical College, Professor of Psychiatry at Weill Cornell Medical College, and Training and Supervising Analyst at the Columbia University Center for Psychoanalytic Training and Research, New York, New York.

John F. Clarkin, Ph.D., is Codirector of the Personality Disorders Institute at Weill Cornell Medical College and Clinical Professor of Psychology in Psychiatry at Weill Cornell Medical College, New York, New York.

Frank E. Yeomans, M.D., Ph.D., is Clinical Associate Professor of Psychiatry at Weill Cornell Medical College, and Director of Training at the Personality Disorders Institute at Weill Cornell Medical College. He is also Adjunct Associate Professor of Psychiatry at the Columbia University Center for Psychoanalytic Training and Research, New York, New York.

Disclosures of Interest

The authors have indicated that they have no financial interests or other affiliations that represent or could appear to represent a competing interest with their contributions to this book.

Foreword

WRITING A BOOK THAT COMBINES BOTH contemporary theory and clinical practice is an enormous feat. Eve Caligor and her coauthors accomplish this feat in *Psychodynamic Therapy for Personality Pathology: Treating Self and Interpersonal Functioning*. In this book (which grew out of and is a companion volume to the authors' *Transference-Focused Psychotherapy for Borderline Personality Disorder: A Clinical Guide* [Yeomans et al. 2015] and *Handbook of Dynamic Psychotherapy for Higher Level Personality Pathology* [Caligor et al. 2007]), the authors attempt to do many things and succeed at all of them. In fact, this book is a gift to anyone who wants to understand or to treat patients.

This is an exciting time for personality disorders. We are on the verge of having a model of personality pathology associated both with a model of the normal personality and with a model of treatment. This new model includes all points of view such as genetics, the brain, and, of course, psychology. This model includes an understanding of the development of each factor and the interactions between these factors. Eve Caligor and her coauthors explain it all.

First of all, in Section I of this book, the authors demonstrate in detail how the object relations model of the mind (developed by Otto Kernberg, a coauthor of this book) works for an understanding of personality, both normal and pathological. In the course of presenting this model, the authors focus on self experience and interpersonal functioning, both of which are brought together by identity consolidation. In so doing, they show how this object relations model fits with new findings from other fields, including neuroscience, attachment theory, developmental theory, and even relational psychoanalysis. They also discuss, among many other topics, how object relations theory interacts with other kinds of psychodynamics, how neurotic personality organization can be understood in contrast to borderline personality organization, and how Kernberg's theory differs from Kleinian theory. In addition, the reader is also treated to a guide for reading this book, to a concise definition of many terms, to many clinical examples, to numerous charts and tables providing a wide variety of information (for example, a clear hierarchy of defenses), and to many relevant references.

Most important, Caligor and coauthors demonstrate how the object relations model of personality fits with the Alternative Model for Personality Disorders in DSM-5, which also focuses on self experience and interpersonal relationships as the hallmarks of personality. The authors' construct is an important development that invites readers to bring together contemporary psychiatry and contemporary psychoanalysis, as these two fields merge to develop an integrated theory of personality. Such an integration has been a long time in coming and is one of the authors' greatest achievements.

In Section II, the authors turn to treatment. They outline the basics of transference-focused psychotherapy—extended (TFP-E), both at the highest theoretical level and at the most experience-near, "how-to" level. Throughout, Caligor and coauthors explain that the aim of TFP-E is always to promote identity consolidation, with the goal of improving self experience and interpersonal functioning; TFP-E always involves an active, supportive, and positive attitude toward each patient. The authors explore the use of the therapeutic relationship, and how to understand and use transference and countertransference. They also outline the strategies of the treatment itself in a logical fashion. They explore how to understand and engage in treatment for narcissistic personality disorder and borderline personality disorder. Finally, they explore issues around tailoring the treatment for the individual patient, so that TFP-E is both principle driven and flexible. As a result, the reader comes away with both a theoretical understanding of the relationship among the patient's personality organization, the therapeutic relationship, and treatment strategies—and a well-organized and humane guide for how to do dynamic psychotherapy.

In Section III, the reader gets a hands-on approach to evaluation of the patient. This evaluation includes an assessment of both personality functioning and level of personality organization. In the course of showing how to do these things, Caligor and coauthors illustrate how this evaluation fits with the theoretical model of personality disorders outlined in Section I. They also explore the rationale behind such an evaluation. Finally, they show in detail how to use evaluation tools such as the Structured Interview of Personality Organization—Revised (STIPO-R; an interview developed by Clarkin et al. [2016] for diagnosis of personality along relevant dimensions) and the Structural Interview developed by

Kernberg (1984). The reader learns how to use specific evaluation techniques while always building and maintaining the therapeutic alliance. The reader also learns how to share diagnostic impressions with the patient, how to set treatment goals, and how to discuss treatment options, risks, and benefits.

The remaining sections of the book provide the reader with thorough practical approaches in the practice of TFP-E. Section IV continues to explore and outline a guide to building and maintaining a treatment frame (including issues such as negotiating a contract with the patient, describing respective roles of the therapist and the patient, and handling special situations such as poor motivation for treatment, eating disorders, substance abuse, and suicidality, to mention only a few). Section V discusses the techniques and strategies of TFP-E in greater detail, including the principles behind interventions; this section includes many useful details about how to set priorities and set limits, and about the role of supportive interventions— again to mention only a few. The final section of the book, Section VI, provides an exploration of the phases of treatment. In addition, online videos and an appendix of helpful resources provide further guidance to the reader.

This book has much to offer students from all disciplines, including the many disciplines of mental health. It has much to offer both the novice and the expert. It has much to offer both the researcher who seeks to understand patients and the clinician who seeks to treat patients. It has much to offer both clinicians interested in the treatment of personality disorders and clinicians less interested in these specific disorders. Finally, it has much to offer to those clinicians working in psychotherapy in an outpatient setting and those working in more acute, inpatient, consultation-liaison and medical settings. In short, this book is a tour de force. I am sure it will become a classic, referred to often, and for many years to come. I cannot wait to recommend it to my colleagues and my students!

Elizabeth L. Auchincloss, M.D.

Vice-Chair for Education, Director of the Institute for Psychodynamic Medicine, DeWitt Wallace Senior Scholar, and Professor of Clinical Psychiatry at Weill Cornell Medical College in New York City; Senior Associate Director and Training and Supervising Analyst, Columbia University Center for Psychoanalytic Training and Research

References

Caligor E, Kernberg OF, Clarkin JF: Handbook of Dynamic Psychotherapy for Higher Level Personality Pathology. Washington, DC, American Psychiatric Publishing, 2007

Clarkin JF, Caligor E, Stern BL, Kernberg OF: Structured Interview of Personality Organization—Revised (STIPO-R), 2016. Available at: www.borderlinedisorders.com. Accessed September 20, 2017.

Kernberg OF: Structural diagnosis, in Severe Personality Disorders: Psychotherapeutic Strategies. New Haven, CT, Yale University Press, 1984, pp 3–26

Yeomans F, Clarkin JF, Kernberg OF: Transference-Focused Psychotherapy for Borderline Personality Disorder: A Clinical Guide. Washington, DC, American Psychiatric Publishing, 2015

Preface

IN THIS BOOK, WE INTRODUCE TRANSFER-
ence-focused psychotherapy—extended (TFP-E), a specialized, theory-
driven approach to the treatment of personality pathology. TFP-E offers
clinicians at all levels of experience an accessible framework to guide evaluation and treatment of personality disorders in a broad variety of clinical
and research settings. This volume provides our readers with 1) a coherent
model of personality functioning and disorder based in psychodynamic
object relations theory; 2) a clinically near approach to classification of
personality disorders, coupled with a coherent approach to assessment;
3) an integrated treatment model based on general clinical principles that
apply across the spectrum of personality disorders as well as to subsyndromal personality pathology; and 4) an understanding of specific modifications of technique that tailor intervention to the individual patient's
personality pathology, based on the severity of his pathology and clinical
presentation, and his moment-to-moment psychological functioning.

History and Development of the Treatment

The model of treatment we describe is an outgrowth of *transference-
focused psychotherapy* (TFP). TFP is an evidence-based specialized treatment for borderline personality disorder and other severe personality disorders that was developed at the Personality Disorders Institute of Weill
Cornell Medical College. The strategies, tactics, and techniques of TFP
are clearly described in a treatment manual (Yeomans et al. 2015). TFP
has been empirically studied in randomized controlled trials in the United
States and Europe. One year of TFP has been shown to result in symptomatic improvement, decreased suicidality and hospitalization, and decreased internal and external expressions of aggression, as well as unique

changes in levels of personality organization, reflective functioning, attachment status, and narrative coherence in patients with borderline personality disorder (Clarkin et al. 2007; Doering et al. 2010; Fischer-Kern et al. 2015; Levy et al. 2006).

As a result of our clinical and research experience with TFP, it became evident that embedded in the strategies, tactics, and techniques of TFP is a more general approach to the psychotherapeutic treatment of personality pathology. Clinical discussion and supervision of videotaped treatments of patients with personality disorders at different levels of severity enabled us to identify core clinical principles as well as modifications of techniques based on the specific nature of pathology; we used these clinical principles and techniques to build a general theory of dynamic therapy of personality pathology. Our first formal modification of TFP as part of this project was the development of *dynamic psychotherapy for higher level personality pathology* (DPHP), a treatment approach for patients with less severe personality disorders and subsyndromal personality pathology (Caligor et al. 2007). The interest generated by this first extension of TFP prompted us to develop the current volume. This book, the third in our trilogy, provides an extension and amplification of the two previously published manuals (see Caligor et al. 2007 and Yeomans et al. 2015), while presenting an overarching and comprehensive description of an object relations theory–based approach to the conceptualization and treatment of the entire range of personality pathology.

Why Is the Treatment Called Transference-Focused Psychotherapy—Extended?

TFP was originally developed to address the clinical needs of patients with borderline personality disorder, and the first TFP treatment manual was published in 1999 (Clarkin et al. 1999). TFP combines a psychodynamic approach with a highly structured treatment frame introduced in the form of a treatment contract and supported by limit setting as needed. In TFP the therapist focuses on the patient's moment-to-moment experience in the therapy, helping the patient to attend to, elaborate, and explore what he is thinking, feeling, and doing in the session. In the treatments of patients with borderline personality disorder (BPD), patients' experience in therapy is very often actively focused on the relationship with the therapist, which tends to become grossly distorted, affectively charged, and highly emotionally invested. Although these transferences can become highly disruptive, when successfully managed they offer an immediate and real-time point of entry into the patient's internal and interpersonal difficulties. In the TFP treatments of patients with BPD, exploration of transference is often the clinical focus, and transference-focused interventions are considered to be a central vehicle of change.

TFP has evolved considerably since the publication of the first TFP manual. Accumulated experience treating patients with BPD and related severe personality disorders, coupled with empirical research studies of TFP treatment of BPD patients, led to significant modification of clinical technique, including greater emphasis on the patient's functioning outside the treatment, greater focus on treatment goals, greater value on the patient's positive attachment to the therapist, and greater attention to the role of fluctuations in the patient's reflective capacities in the clinical process. Meanwhile, experience using TFP and TFP principles to study the treatment of patients with milder personality disorders as well as those with subsyndromal personality pathology led to the development of a more complex understanding of the role of transference exploration in the treatment of personality pathology; it became clear that the optimal emphasis on transference is highly variable, across patients and across phases of treatment. As a rule, the more severe the patient's personality pathology, the more consistently the relationship with the therapist tends to take on emotional salience for the patient; the healthier the patient, the more likely the patient's interpersonal relationships and life outside the treatment are likely to assume affective dominance. Across the range of pathology, the patient's moment-to-moment experience, especially experience marked by affect investment, is the focus of intervention; as a result, intervention may be focused on the transference, or it may be focused elsewhere. However, even when intervention does not focus on the transference, the therapist remains, in his or her own internal focus, consistently mindful of the transference. The therapist's attention to the transference-countertransference is a steady source of information for the TFP-E therapist, contributing to his or her understanding of the patient's current internal situation, of the state of the therapeutic alliance, and of the extent of the patient's reflective capacities in the moment.

Underlying Model of Personality Functioning, Pathology, and Structural Change

The TFP-E approach to the treatment of personality disorders is embedded in psychodynamic object relations theory as it has been developed by

Otto Kernberg and his collaborators (Kernberg 1984, 2004; Kernberg and Caligor 2005). This model of personality disorders adopts a dimensional perspective on personality pathology. Rather than simply viewing each personality disorder as a discrete entity, this model 1) identifies core pathological features of psychological functioning shared by the personality disorders as a group, focusing on self and interpersonal functioning; 2) characterizes how pathological features of self and interpersonal functioning differ according to severity of personality pathology; and 3) conceptualizes self and interpersonal functioning as expressions of the nature and organization of underlying psychological structures, focusing on identity formation, with 4) pathology of self and interpersonal functioning reflecting, to a greater or lesser degree, failure of identity consolidation. This approach is consistent with a growing consensus among personality disorder researchers that pathology of self and other functioning is central to the personality disorders (Bender and Skodol 2007; Gunderson and Lyons-Ruth 2008; Horowitz 2004; Livesley 2001; Meyer and Pilkonis 2005; Pincus 2005).

Self and Interpersonal Functioning and DSM-5

Our work has proven timely. Concurrent with the development of this volume, there has been a shift in the general psychiatric nosology away from categorical diagnoses of personality disorders based on specified diagnostic criteria—and toward a dimensional approach to personality disorders based on severity of impairment of personality functioning, with a focus on the domains of self and interpersonal functioning. This shift resulted in the introduction in DSM-5 (American Psychiatric Association 2013) of an alternative model for personality disorders (AMPD), which corresponds very closely to our own model. The AMPD, included in DSM-5 Section III, "Emerging Measures and Models," identifies the defining features of the personality disorder diagnosis as "moderate or greater impairment" in self and interpersonal functioning (Criterion A), coupled with the presence of pathological personality traits (Criterion B). On the basis of relative severity of impairments in self and interpersonal functioning, the AMPD classifies personality disorders across a spectrum of severity using the Level of Personality Functioning Scale.

Because of the close correspondence between the TFP-E model of personality functioning and disorder and the atheoretical AMPD, we are able to provide the reader with an *explanatory framework* for the AMPD as well as a *specific treatment approach* linked to the AMPD—both emerging from within the theory of psychodynamic object relations theory.

Psychodynamic Diagnostic Manual, 2nd Edition

The *Psychodynamic Diagnostic Manual*, 2nd Edition (PDM-2; Lingiardi and McWilliams 2017), represents another approach to diagnosis and classification of personality functioning, intended to serve as an alternative, or complement, to the DSM and ICD systems. The PDM-2 was developed by a group of psychodynamically informed researchers and clinicians, with the stated intent of providing a model of classification that can be used to *guide clinical treatment*. The model of personality and personality functioning adopted in the PDM-2 is highly consistent with our own. In particular, the PDM-2 does the following: adopts a dimensional model of personality functioning spanning from healthy functioning to the greatest level of impairment; emphasizes the centrality of the dimension of severity in personality pathology; embraces an approach to classification that combines the level of personality organization with personality style or type; emphasizes the need for comprehensive assessment of personality and psychological functioning; and highlights the clinical reality that symptoms are expressed within the context of the individual's personality. Because of the compatibility between the TFP-E model and the model underlying the PDM-2, TFP-E can offer clinicians a systematic approach to treatment of personality pathology that is a natural extension of the PDM-2 model.

For Whom Did We Write This Book?

We wrote this book for both students and experienced clinicians, and we hope that it will be of interest to researchers as well. Depending on the needs of the reader, this volume can serve a wide variety of functions. For the most general audience, we provide a coherent model of personality functioning and pathology, classification, and assessment. This diagnostic assessment provides information about prognosis and anticipates clinical difficulties likely to emerge not only in longer-term treatment but also in the setting of acute management and short-term intervention. Given the ubiquity of personality disorders in the general population and in clinical settings (Torgersen 2014), the early sections of the book, which focus on the TFP-E model of pathology and assessment, should be of benefit to general clinicians in virtually any clinical setting. Clinicians have made use of the TFP-E model not only in outpatient therapy but also in psychopharmacology practice, on inpatient units, in emergency rooms, and on consultation-liaison and substance abuse services (Hersh 2015; Zerbo et al. 2013).

For our more specialized readers interested in psychotherapy of personality disorders, we provide an in-depth, principle-driven description of the treatment. For students of psychotherapy, we emphasize the principles guiding intervention and provide extensive clinical illustrations. For experienced psychotherapists, we provide an integrated and innovative synthesis of contemporary psychodynamic approaches to psychotherapy embedded in a contemporary model of psychopathology. For clinicians not engaged in longer-term treatments, we offer discrete clinical principles, strategies, and techniques, described here in the context of an integrated, longer-term treatment model, which can be pragmatically utilized in supportive and shorter-term treatments, as well as in the acute management of patients with personality disorders. For clinicians interested in learning more about such applications, we also recommend *Fundamentals of Transference-Focused Psychotherapy* (Hersh et al. 2016), which elaborates application of various elements of our treatment approach in general psychiatric and medical settings. For researchers and other experts in psychopathology research and the range of empirically supported therapeutic interventions, we provide relevant discussion, supporting footnotes, and useful references that link our treatment approach to current research.

Comments on Longer-Term Dynamic Therapy

In the course of psychotherapy, the success and long-term outcome of the treatment depend on much more than the particular techniques used. Patient pathology, therapist qualities, and the match between patient and therapist are all potent factors in treatment outcome (Crits-Christoph et al. 2013). This book describes treatment principles that are used judiciously by therapists who create a particular structure and atmosphere with each individual patient. We emphasize the structure of the treatment, established collaboratively through the process of assessment, setting of treatment goals, and formation of a treatment contract that provides the setting within which specific techniques are utilized.

This book does not prescribe techniques in a step-by-step way for every patient, such as that described in a cognitive-behavioral therapy treatment manual. Rather, each TFP-E treatment is tailored to the individual patient who has specific areas of dysfunction and a specific level of personality organization; this principle-driven treatment provides direction but also flexibility for the moment-to-moment judgment of the empathic clinician. Throughout the treatment, the TFP-E therapist maintains ongoing attention to the relationship between patient and therapist as a source of live, immediate information on how the patient perceives, conceptualizes, and relates to others—information that is especially important in a treatment that targets self and interpersonal functioning. TFP-E also involves an active attitude toward the patient: a positive and supportive interest in all that the patient reports, and respectful neutrality among the various forces that guide the patient's behavior.

Organization of the Book

The reader will find that the chapters of this book are not organized in chronological order, beginning, for example, with assessment and the opening phase and moving through to the ending of treatment. Instead, we have organized the book and chosen the sequence of chapters to help the reader develop the best possible understanding of the model and the treatment—both the specific techniques and the rationale for selecting those techniques. Our primary emphasis is not on answering specific questions such as "What do I do when…?" Rather, our aim is to enable readers to answer for themselves questions such as these: "How do I systematically go about deciding what to do now?" "What are my objectives in this moment?" and "What is my conceptualization of how this intervention might promote change?"

We have divided the book into six sections, anticipating that different sections are likely to be of particular interest to different readers. Section I covers the **object relations theory model of personality**, personality pathology, and classification of personality disorders. These chapters are an essential foundation for the clinical chapters that follow and provide an accessible synthesis for the reader wishing to become familiar with this approach to personality and personality disorders. Section II provides an **overview of TFP-E at the level of clinical theory**, including an introduction to core constructs, discussion of the therapeutic relationship, and description of the strategies organizing the treatment. Section II will be of particular interest to the reader who wants a general understanding of the TFP-E model and its objectives, and who is perhaps less interested in implementation.

Section III covers **patient assessment and treatment planning,** under the umbrella of the therapeutic consultation. This section builds on material introduced in Section I, as we further describe the TFP-E model of classification in the context of discussion of assessment. (Readers most interested in classification and assessment may wish to read Section III immediately following Section I, and then circle back to clinical considerations in Section II.) The model of assessment we present can be useful to clinicians in a variety of clinical settings; the model is reflected in a semistructured interview, the Structured Interview of Personality Organization—Revised (STIPO-R; Clarkin et al. 2016). The second half of Section III tackles sharing the diagnostic impression, describing how, as consultants, we help our patients gain an understanding of their difficulties within the framework of TFP-E.

Section IV describes the **treatment frame,** its functions, and how it is established and maintained within our treatment model; we provide clinical recommendations that should be of interest to the reader encountering patients with personality pathology in any of a variety of clinical settings. We next move on in Section V to discussion of **clinical work,** elaborating general principles of psychotherapy for personality pathology as we describe the specific tactics and techniques employed in each session; we provide in-depth discussion of the interpretive process, working with countertransference, and the role of supportive and structuring interventions, including contracting and limit setting. The sixth and final section of the book covers **phases of treatment,** taking the reader through expected developments that characterize the early, middle, and late phases of treatment. We end with a brief conclusion.

At the end of each chapter, we provide a summary of key clinical concepts discussed in that chapter. We also provide illustrative video clips, as described in the Video Guide that follows this Preface.

Clinical Material

At the outset, we want to comment on the nature of the clinical material that we present in this book. When writing about the clinical situation, the writer is always torn between the wish to provide actual and true-to-life clinical material and the need to protect patient confidentiality. We have found that even when patients' identities are disguised, it is impossible to accurately present clinical material while respecting patient confidentiality; at the very least, the patients whose therapy sessions are cited recognize themselves in the clinical material. As a result, we have chosen not to present actual patients or actual clinical material in this book. Instead, each clinical vignette is a composite of several patients we have treated and/or whose treatment we have supervised over the years.

Pronouns

Finally, the reader will notice that we often use *he* or, alternatively, *she* when we might more accurately have used or *he or she*. While we are not entirely satisfied with this choice, we do so in order to write as clearly as possible, with the aim of making relatively difficult material easier to read.

Acknowledgments

We gratefully acknowledge Ms. Gina Atkinson for her editorial assistance.

References

American Psychiatric Association: Diagnostic and Statistical Manual of Mental Disorders, 5th Edition. Arlington, VA, American Psychiatric Association, 2013

Bender DS, Skodol AE: Borderline personality as a self-other representational disturbance. J Pers Disord 21(5):500–517, 2007 17953503

Caligor E, Kernberg OF, Clarkin JF: Handbook of Dynamic Psychotherapy for Higher Level Personality Pathology. Washington, DC, American Psychiatric Publishing, 2007

Clarkin JF, Yeomans FE, Kernberg OF: Psychotherapy for Borderline Personality. New York, Wiley, 1999

Clarkin JF, Levy KN, Lenzenweger MF, Kernberg OF: Evaluating three treatments for borderline personality disorder: a multiwave study. Am J Psychiatry 164(6):922–928, 2007 17541052

Clarkin JF, Caligor E, Stern BL, Kernberg OF: Structured Interview of Personality Organization—Revised (STIPO-R), 2016. Available at: www.borderlinedisorders.com. Accessed September 20, 2017.

Crits-Christoph P, Gibbons MBC, Mukherjee D: Psychotherapy process-outcome research, in Bergin and Garfield's Handbook of Psychotherapy and Behavior Change, 6th Edition. Edited by Lambert MJ. Hoboken, NJ, Wiley, 2013, pp 298–340

Doering S, Hörz S, Rentrop M, et al: Transference-focused psychotherapy v. treatment by community psychotherapists for borderline personality disorder: randomised controlled trial. Br J Psychiatry 196(5):389–395, 2010 20435966

Fischer-Kern M, Doering S, Taubner S, et al: Transference-focused psychotherapy for borderline personality disorder: change in reflective function. Br J Psychiatry 207(2):173–174, 2015 25999334

Gunderson JG, Lyons-Ruth K: BPD's interpersonal hypersensitivity phenotype: a gene-environment-developmental model. J Pers Disord 22(1):22–41, 2008 18312121

Hersh RG: Using transference-focused psychotherapy principles in the pharmacotherapy of patients with severe personality disorders. Psychodyn Psychiatry 43(2):181–199, 2015 26039227

Hersh RG, Caligor E, Yeomans FE: Fundamentals of Transference-Focused Psychotherapy: Applications in Psychiatric and Medical Settings. Cham, Switzerland, Springer, 2016

Horowitz LM: Interpersonal Foundations of Psychopathology. Washington, DC, American Psychological Association, 2004

Kernberg OF: Structural diagnosis, in Severe Personality Disorders: Psychotherapeutic Strategies. New Haven, CT, Yale University Press, 1984, pp 3–26

Kernberg OF: Contemporary Controversies in Psychoanalytic Theory, Techniques, and Their Applications. New Haven, CT, Yale University Press, 2004

Kernberg OF, Caligor E: A psychoanalytic theory of personality disorders, in Major Theories of Personality Disorder, 2nd Edition. Edited by Lenzenweger MF, Clarkin JF. New York, Guilford, 2005, pp 114–156

Levy KN, Meehan KB, Kelly KM, et al: Change in attachment patterns and reflective function in a randomized control trial of transference-focused psychotherapy for borderline personality disorder. J Consult Clin Psychol 74(6):1027–1040, 2006 17154733

Lingiardi V, McWilliams N (eds): Psychodynamic Diagnostic Manual, 2nd Edition. New York, Guilford, 2017

Livesley WJ: Conceptual and taxonomic issues, in Handbook of Personality Disorders: Theory, Research, and Treatment. Edited by Livesley WJ. New York, Guilford, 2001, pp 3–38

Meyer B, Pilkonis PA: An attachment model of personality disorders, in Major Theories of Personality Disorder, 2nd Edition. Edited by Lenzenweger MF, Clarkin JF. New York, Guilford, 2005, pp 231–281

Pincus AL: A contemporary integrative interpersonal theory of personality disorders, in Major Theories of Personality Disorder, 2nd Edition. Edited by Lenzenweger MF, Clarkin JF. New York, Guilford, 2005, pp 282–331

Torgersen S: Prevalence, sociodemographics, and functional impairment, in The American Psychiatric Publishing Textbook of Personality Disorders, 2nd Edition. Edited by Oldham J, Skodol A, Bender D. Washington, DC, American Psychiatric Publishing, 2014, pp 109–129

Yeomans F, Clarkin JF, Kernberg OF: Transference-Focused Psychotherapy for Borderline Personality Disorder: A Clinical Guide. Washington, DC, American Psychiatric Publishing, 2015

Zerbo E, Cohen S, Bielska W, Caligor E: Transference-focused psychotherapy in the general psychiatry residency: a useful and applicable model for residents in acute clinical settings. Psychodyn Psychiatry 41(1):163–181, 2013 23480166

Video Guide

WE HAVE CREATED A SERIES OF SEVEN BRIEF video clips that illustrate some of the basic principles and techniques of TFP-E. Although the videos are based on real therapy cases, the clips we provide are fictitious composites created to protect the confidentiality of our patients. All the patients who appear in the videos are actors, not actual patients, and any resemblance to real persons is purely coincidental. Each video is linked to material described in the text and is accompanied by written commentary (see also the later section in this guide, "Videos Discussed by Chapter" for additional text discussion):

- In Video 1, "Assessment of Identity Integration: Borderline Level of Personality Organization," Dr. Caligor evaluates identity formation in a male patient presenting with thoughts of self-harm. This video illustrates how difficult it can be for BPO patients to provide a realistic or coherent self description.
- In contrast to Video 1, in Video 2, "Assessment of Identity Integration: Self-Description; Normal Identity Formation," Dr. Caligor invites a female patient presenting with anxiety and problems with self-esteem to provide a self-description. In this clip the patient is able to provide a rich and reflective view of herself.
- In Video 3, "Contracting," Dr. Yeomans discusses the TFP-E treatment contract with a patient with borderline personality disorder, focusing on contracting around self-harm and structured activity.
- Video 4, "Identifying the Dominant Object Relations," illustrates Dr. Yeomans maintaining a neutral stance while elaborating the object relations organizing his patient's experience.
- In Video 5, "The Interpretive Process: Borderline Level of Personality Organization" and Video 6 "The Interpretive Process: Neurotic Level of Personality Organization," respectively, Dr. Caligor illustrates the interpretive process with two different patients, first a patient with a personality disorder and second a patient with subsyndromal personality pathology.

- Finally, in Video 7, "Therapeutic Neutrality," Dr. Yeomans illustrates maintaining a neutral stance while helping his patient appreciate that it is not Dr. Yeomans's demands that are creating pressure within him, but rather the patient's own internal conflicts.

Video Access

Video cues provided in the text identify the videos by title and approximate run time, as shown in the following example:

 Video Illustration 1:
Assessment of Identity Integration:
Borderline Level of Personality Organization (8:33)

The video illustrations are streamed via the Internet and can be viewed online by navigating to www.appi.org/caligor and using the embedded video player. The videos are optimized for most current operating systems, including mobile operating systems.

Videos Discussed by Chapter

Chapter 7

Video 1. Assessment of Identity Integration: Borderline Level of Personality Organization (8:33)
Description: Dr. Caligor and a 35-year-old man after his self-harm attempt

Video 2. Assessment of Identity Integration: Self-Description; Normal Identity Formation (3:36)
Description: Dr. Caligor and a 32-year-old married female classical musician

Chapter 8

Video 3. Contracting (4:52)
Description: Dr. Yeomans and a 26-year-old woman with a history of chronic depression, who is unemployed and supported by the family for many years

Chapter 9

Video 4. Identifying the Dominant Object Relations (4:35)
Description: Dr. Yeomans and a 34-year-old single woman diagnosed with histrionic personality disorder

Chapter 10

Video 5. Interpretive Process: Borderline Level of Personality Organization (8:56)
Description: Dr. Caligor and a 28-year-old woman who presents with problems with interpersonal and intimate relationships

Video 6. Interpretive Process: Neurotic Level of Personality Organization (6:30)
Description: Dr. Caligor and a 40-year-old man who presents with marital problems; he is organized at a neurotic level

Chapter 12

Video 7. Therapeutic Neutrality (3:20)
Description: Dr. Yeomans and a 28-year-old single male college dropout working in a clerical position.

Acknowledgments

The authors wish to thank the following for their creation and production of the videos:
Executive Producer: Cara Blumstein
Producer: Jacob Snyder
Directed by Ian Rice and Jacob Sussman

Introduction

A Model of Treatment Targeting Self and Interpersonal Functioning

IN THIS BOOK, WE PRESENT A PARTICULAR model of treatment for personality disorders that we call *transference-focused psychotherapy—extended* (TFP-E). Rather than focusing on a particular type of personality disorder or constellation of symptoms or behaviors, our approach is organized in relation to modification of self and interpersonal functioning. We present general clinical principles applicable to the treatment of all personality pathology, coupled with an organized approach to their adaptation and modification for patients who represent different levels of severity of pathology and who have different clinical presentations.

Our understanding of self and interpersonal functioning is embedded in contemporary psychodynamic object relations theory and is organized in relation to the construct of identity (Kernberg 2006). This model is intimately linked with a coherent approach to classification of personality disorders, in which severity of self and interpersonal pathology is described based on characterization of identity, object relations, defenses, moral functioning, and aggression. Classification, in turn, dovetails with our approach to assessment, which incorporates both a clinical interview, the Structural Interview (Kernberg 1984), and a more formal, semistructured interview, the Structured Interview of Personality Organization— Revised (STIPO-R; Clarkin et al. 2016).

It has been our long-term goal to expand the accessibility of psychodynamic models of pathology and treatment to the wider community of psychotherapists. Clinicians are routinely faced with a wide array of patients presenting with various difficulties in self and interpersonal functioning, yet many clinicians may lack a coherent model for conceptualizing and treating these disorders. Without a coherent model of personality pathology and treatment, there is a risk of treatments devolving into repetitive cycles of chasing symptoms, or unfocused pursuit of psychological exploration. It is our aim to provide clinicians of all orientations with a clinically near framework within which to conceptualize problems in self and interpersonal functioning, as well as an understanding of how this framework can be used to organize a systematic approach to assessment, treatment formulation, and clinical work.

This effort is timely; there have been major developments in the conceptualization and treatment of personality pathology that are consistent with our orientation. The conceptualization of personality pathology has advanced from a list of criteria (DSM-III; American Psychiatric Association 1980) to focus on self and other functioning (DSM-5 Section III; American Psychiatric Association 2013); the field is shifting its focus from identifying and studying discrete categories of pathology to dimensional assessment and investigation of domains of personality functioning (Clarkin et al. 2015c). Dissatisfaction with the typology of personality pathology in the DSM system has led to alternative typologies based on dimensional traits (Kotov et al. 2017) and psychodynamic conceptualizations of functioning (Lingiardi and McWilliams 2017). Different treatment approaches have much in common, especially those that focus on the patient's self and interpersonal functioning. Psychodynamic treatments of personality disorders, including our own approach, have been found to be as effective as alternative approaches (Fonagy 2015; Leichsenring et al. 2015).

Current Status of Personality Disorders

The decades since 1980, when the current DSM classification of personality disorders was introduced in DSM-III (American Psychiatric Association 1980), have seen rapid advancement of our knowledge of personality disorders and evolution of our systems of classification. The DSM system adopted a categorical, polythetic approach to diagnosis, emphasizing symptoms and maladaptive behaviors to define discrete disorders. In this system, personality disorders are conceptualized as stable across time and situations. The limitations of this system have been extensively documented (Kotov et al. 2017; Livesley and Clarkin 2015), and in some sense, out of these ashes has emerged consensus on a new, more ecologically valid and clinically useful approach to understanding personality disorders.

Relevant limitations of the traditional approach include extensive comorbidity among disorders, failure to account for the dimensional nature of pathology, discontinuity with normal personality functioning, and poor coverage of the spectrum of presentations of personality disorders. Perhaps most central is the failure of the DSM system to define what is essential to and shared by all personality disorders, and the resulting failure to provide a framework that could organize coherent approaches to treatment.

While much remains controversial, there is convergence across the field on a number of central issues, reflecting developing knowledge and study of personality disorders. There is now general acceptance of the following:

- Personality disorders are best described dimensionally rather than categorically.
- The dimension of severity (however it may be defined) is perhaps the most powerful predictor of prognosis and clinical outcome (Crawford et al. 2011; Hopwood et al. 2011).
- The natural course of personality disorders is more variable than initially assumed (Lenzenweger 2010), involving both stability and change across time (Morey and Hopwood 2013) and variability across individuals (Hallquist and Lenzenweger 2013).
- Personality disorder symptoms—and to a lesser degree, functional impairment—fluctuate over a lifetime, presumably in relation to positive and challenging life events, as well as to biology.
- Personality disorders are far more responsive to treatment than initially assumed (e.g., Cristea et al. 2017).

Self and Interpersonal Functioning

At this point in time, there is an emerging consensus that core and defining features of personality and personality disorders lie in the domains of self and interpersonal functioning—that is, that different forms of personality disorder can be described in terms of varying pathology of self and interpersonal functioning (Bender and Skodol 2007; Gunderson and Lyons-Ruth 2008; Horowitz 2004; Kernberg and Caligor 2005; Livesley 2001; Meyer and Pilkonis 2005; Pincus 2005; Sharp et al. 2015). This convergence of expert opinion is formally recognized in the Alternative Model for Personality Disorders presented in DSM-5 Section III, "Emerging Measures and Models." According to this alternative model, personality disorders are conceptualized first in terms of **shared features**—impairments in self and interpersonal functioning characterized across a continuum of severity; and second in the nature of **personality traits**—their extremity and rigidity.

Agreement on the centrality of self and interpersonal functioning in personality pathology provides a new framework for developing and refining treatment models; rather than directing treatment simply toward individual symptoms or behaviors (e.g., self-destructiveness, affective dysregulation, lack of goal-directedness), clinicians can now also target underlying processes that organize *all* personality disorders. General principles emerge applicable to the treatment of the range of personality disorders (i.e., across the various manifestations of pathology of self and interpersonal functioning), whereas specific tactics and techniques of treatment can be modified according to the severity and nature of personality pathology.

Internal Representations

A parallel development in the knowledge of personality disorders has been a general recognition of the centrality of internal representations of self in relation to other, organized as cognitive-affective units, in organizing self and interpersonal functioning (Clarkin and Livesley 2016). Overlapping formulations can be identified in the constructs of *internal object relations* (object relations theory) (Kernberg and Caligor 2005), *working models of attachment* (attachment theory) (Bowlby 1980), *cognitive schemas* (cognitive-behavioral theory) (Pretzer and Beck 2005), and *maladaptive interpersonal signatures* (interpersonal theory) (Benjamin 2005; Cain and Pincus 2016). These approaches have contributed to our understanding of the development of normal and disordered self and interpersonal functioning and of their organization and expression in the here and now. These models can inform the development of clinical strategies for modifying self and interpersonal functioning, depending on the organization of psychological structures and attachment style.[1]

Assessment

Recent advances in the knowledge of personality disorders, coupled with advances in contemporary object relations and attachment theories, have profound implications not only for the understanding of personality disorders and their treatment, but also for the TFP-E approach to clinical assessment. These developments imply that assessment should target not only current symptoms and dysfunction, but also underlying domains of functioning central to personality and personality disorder, focusing on self and interpersonal functioning, representations of self and others, and the nature of attachment. In addition to sophisticated clinical approaches to the evaluation of personality pathology, there are now validated interviews and self-report assessments focusing on self and interpersonal functioning and attachment style (Clarkin et al. 2018).

Implications for Treatment

All these advances together are leading to meaningful changes in the psychotherapeutic treatment of personality disorders. We are seeing the emergence of a consensually agreed-upon model of pathology that transcends individual theoretical frameworks and identifies specific targets for intervention. This model can inform the development of clinical interventions; principle-driven treatments can be organized in relation to modifying central aspects of self and interpersonal functioning characteristic of personality disorders across the range of severity. General principles organizing treatment can be developed and then tailored to the individual patient on the basis of severity and nature of pathology, accounting for shifts across time. The TFP-E approach to the treatment of personality disorders embraces this strategy.

---

[1]All these contributions, including our own, are compatible with the overarching Cognitive-Affective Processing System framework developed by Mischel and Shoda (2008) for conceptualizing personality functioning. In this model, a cognitive-affective unit is an organized pattern of psychological processes—including conceptions of self and others, expectancies and beliefs, affects, goals and values, and self-regulatory strategies—that are rooted in genetic and epigenetic predispositions. Cognitive-affective units are expressed behaviorally in specific contexts, generating responses from the environment and, in the process, modifying it. Responses from the environment feed back to the individual's expectancies over time, leading to construction of the individual's typical environment.

Object Relations Theory and TFP-E

Object Relations Theory

Object relations theory comprises a cluster of somewhat loosely related psychodynamic and psychoanalytic models of psychological motivation and functioning that view the internalization of early patterns of relating as a central feature of psychological development and psychological functioning. In this frame of reference, the term *object* is used to refer to a person (for historical reasons, and rather unfortunately) with whom the subject has a relationship. Similarly, the term *object relations* refers to the quality of the subject's relationships with others. Turning from the external, interpersonal world to the internal world of the subject, we use the term *internal object* to refer to the representation or presence of another within the mind of the subject, and the term *internal object relation* to refer to the representation of a relationship pattern within the mind of the subject (Caligor and Clarkin 2010).

TFP-E is embedded in a particular model of object relations theory developed by Otto Kernberg and colleagues at the Personality Disorders Institute of Weill Cornell Medical College (Kernberg and Caligor 2005). This model provides an overarching conceptualization of normal and disordered personality functioning within a psychodynamic frame of reference. The theoretical framework and understanding of psychopathology provided by contemporary object relations theory is compatible with recent developments in the understanding of personality disorders outlined above, and has been refined in response to ongoing developments in the fields of personality disorder research, attachment theory, developmental psychology, and neuroscience, in conjunction with our clinical experience.

The framework of object relations theory organizes the TFP-E approach to the classification and treatment of personality disorders and informs the understanding of each clinical moment as therapists work with their patients. The model identifies specific treatment goals and targets for clinical intervention, with the longer-term objective of modifying self and interpersonal functioning. Finally, the model is embedded in a clinically near model of personality change and growth.

Psychological Structures

Central to the object relations theory model of personality pathology is the construct of a *psychological structure*. In a psychodynamic frame of reference, *structures* are stable patterns of psychological functioning that are repeatedly and predictably activated in particular contexts. This is to say that psychological structures are not structures in the concrete sense, but rather are psychological *processes* that can be conceptualized as dispositions to organize subjective experience and behavior in certain predictable ways.

At the level of clinical observation, the nature of psychological structures can be inferred, and also systematically assessed, on the basis of their impact on descriptive aspects of personality functioning—in particular, an individual's behavior, interpersonal relations, and subjective experience. For example, *conscience* is a familiar psychological structure comprising the psychological processes involved in moral functioning. Ethical (and unethical) behavior, feelings of guilt, and commitment to moral values and ideals are descriptive features of personality functioning that are organized by the various processes that together form the structure *conscience*. Similarly, the defensive operation *denial* is a psychological process manifested descriptively in the predictable tendency to minimize the emotional impact of painful experiences.

The cornerstone of all psychodynamic models of personality disorders is that descriptive features of personality pathology that characterize a particular personality disorder can be seen to reflect the nature and organization of underlying psychological structures. Treatments that lead to changes in psychological structures will at the same time lead to changes in descriptive features of personality pathology and to improvement in psychological functioning.

The Centrality of Internal Object Relations

Within the object relations theory model of personality, the most basic psychological structures are cognitive-affective units referred to as *internal object relations*. An internal object relation is a mental representation of a relationship pattern consisting of a representation of the self, referred to as a *self representation*, interacting with a representation of another, referred to as an *object representation*, linked to a particular affect state (Kernberg 1980). The object relations theory of personality disorders places these internalized representations of self and other at the center of the understanding of psychological experience, psychopathology, and psychotherapeutic treatment; internal object relations are seen to be both the organizers of subjective experience and the building blocks of higher-order structures.

Internal Object Relations and Subjective Experience

Different object relations will be activated in different contexts and will organize the individual's expectations and experience of that setting. From this perspective, internal object relations function as latent *schemas*, ways in which the individual can potentially organize her experience, which will be activated in particular contexts (Kernberg and Caligor 2005). Once activated, internal object relations will color the individual's subjective experience—in particular, the individual's conception of self as defined in relation to others—and will lead him to feel and act in ways that correspond to the internal object relation currently activated. We think of this process in terms of the individual's enacting, or *living out*, his internal object relations in his daily life. When internal object relations are enacted, psychological structures are actualized.

The following examples illustrate how internal object relations are conceptualized in their role as organizers of subjective experience: Consider an object relation of a small, childlike self interacting with a powerful authority figure in which the interaction is linked to feelings of fear, or, alternatively, the image of a small, childlike self and a caring protective figure associated with feelings of gratification and safety. In these illustrations, these internal object relations will become manifest in the adult to the degree that they function to organize the individual's expectations and experience as he enters a dependent relationship—coloring the experience of the self and of the person depended on, while activating anxiety and fear as affective experience in the first case, and an experience of gratification and safety in the second case.

Origins of Internal Object Relations: The Past in the Present and the Role of Conflict

Internal object relations are derived from affectively charged experiences with significant others. Specifically, Kernberg (1980; see also Kernberg and Caligor 2005) suggests that internal object relations emerge from the interaction of inborn affect dispositions and attachment relationships; from the earliest days of life, constitutionally determined affect states are activated in relation to, regulated by, and cognitively linked to interactions with caretakers. Over time, these interactions are internalized as relationship patterns, which are gradually organized to form the enduring, affectively charged psychological structures that we refer to as internal object relations. Thus, internal object relations can be seen to represent the impact of early relational experience on current psychological functioning.

In its emphasis on the centrality of internal representations in personality functioning, the object relations theory model overlaps with other major models, including cognitive-behavioral, interpersonal, and attachment theories (Clarkin et al. 2016). However, what distinguishes object relations theory from other overlapping models is that object relations theory invokes a relatively complex, "dynamic" relationship between early attachment relationships and the psychological structures that come to organize adult experience; because object relations theory is a *psychodynamic* model (in contrast to a purely developmental one), internal object relations are not conceptualized simply as historically valid representations of early experience with others. Rather, internal object relations are viewed as constructions, not only deriving from early experience—colored by the cognitive developmental level at the time—but also reflecting psychodynamic factors, including the individual's psychological conflicts, defenses, and fantasies.

This is to say that internal object relations—the affectively charged representations of self and other that organize self and interpersonal functioning—are motivational structures viewed as reflecting early experience as organized in relation to the individual's defenses and conflicts, needs and wishes, all of which become a focus of clinical exploration. Thus, in their role as organizers of psychological experience, internal object relations form a bridge not only between the developmental past and the lived present, but also between psychological defenses and conflicts and subjective experience. In sum, the nature and quality of internal object relations are seen to reflect a condensation of temperamental factors (e.g., inborn affect dispositions), developmental experience, conflict, and defense.[2]

Internal Object Relations, Identity Formation, and Treatment Goals

Within the object relations theory model, clusters or networks of internal object relations are seen to work in concert to constitute higher-order structures. In particular, the object relations theory model focuses on the object relations organizing the individual's sense of self and sense of others, and how these object relations are organized in relation to one another to constitute identity formation (Kernberg and Caligor 2005).

Normal identity formation is understood as an expression of an adaptive, flexible, and stable organization of component object relations, a process referred to as *identity consolidation*, whereas pathology of identity formation is understood in terms of inadequate or rigid organization of component internal object relations. Identity formation is a central organizer of normal and disordered self and interpersonal functioning; a fully consolidated identity characterizes the normal personality, whereas the personality disorders are characterized by pathology of identity formation.

Clinical intervention in the treatment of personality disorders is directed toward promoting, at the level of psychological structures, the coalescence of individual internal object relations to attain progressive degrees of identity consolidation (*structural change*). To the extent that clinical intervention promotes identity consolidation, the therapist will see corresponding improvement in self and interpersonal functioning, along with amelioration of the complaints, symptoms, and subjective distress that bring patients with personality disorders to clinical attention.

Object Relations Theory in Context

Personality, both normal and disordered, reflects the dynamic integration of behavior patterns that have their roots in the interaction of temperamental factors, cognitive capacities, character, and internalized value systems (Kernberg 2016); personality is best understood as an emergent property, a complex end product unique to each individual, which cannot

---

[2]To illustrate the potential role of defense and conflict in determining the nature of internal object relations, we return to our earlier example of an internal object relation composed of a small, childlike self and a powerful, threatening authority figure linked to feelings of fear. We suggest that for a particular individual, the self experience of powerlessness and fear in the setting of dependent relationships may reflect not only actual early experiences with a frightening caregiver, but also defensive needs or fantasy. For example, this object relation might be a defensive construction in relation to conflictual wishes to hurt a parental figure. Here we would speak of *projection*, as if to say: "She is the aggressive and sadistic one, not me; I am weak and frightened. Therefore, I need not feel guilty for having sadistic feelings." Alternatively, for someone with more severe personality pathology, a more extreme and highly affectively charged version of this same object relation might function as part of a defensive effort to protect the fantasy of a wished-for, perfectly gratifying parental figure. This is an example of *splitting*: "This feels terrible, but nevertheless it means that I can still hope to find a perfect caretaker." Similarly, the more positive representation of the dependent relationship we described, colored by feelings of safety and gratification, might reflect early positive interactions with a caregiver, or an idealized version of an imperfect caregiving relationship, or a wished-for relationship, perhaps in the setting of a history of parental neglect or hostility.

be reduced to its component parts (Lenzenweger 2010). Normal personality development is characterized by the accomplishment of a number of age- and stage-relevant tasks from infancy through adulthood (Cicchetti 2016). These tasks include the development of the capacity for regulation of emotions, the formation of cooperative and satisfying relationships with others, the development and integration of a cohesive and positive sense of self, and successful adjustment to school and work.

This complex conceptual framework has provided the background for advances in the object relations theory model of personality disorders, advances that reflect the mutual influence of growing empirical knowledge and evolving theoretical formulations. Our current understanding of both normal personality functioning and personality dysfunction or disorder reflects emerging convergence among leading theoretical articulations of personality functioning, findings of experimental studies that challenge various aspects of personality functioning (see Clarkin et al. 2015c), electronic diary studies known as *ecological momentary assessment* (Trull et al. 2008), assessment of neurocognitive functioning with instruments such as functional magnetic resonance imaging, and prospective developmental studies (Clarkin et al. 2015b). This larger context enables us to more clearly identify the enduring insights of object relations theory, its consistency with empirical advances, its similarity to near-neighbor theories, and its limitations.

Development of the Object Relations Theory Model of Personality and Treatment

Object relations theory emerged initially from clinical observation of patients studied in detail and treated in psychoanalysis and psychoanalytic psychotherapy; intensive treatment of patients with various forms of psychopathology provided a rich ground for insight into patients' internal representations of themselves in relation to others (Kernberg 1975). In addition to clinical observations, Kernberg's early theoretical formulations drew on contributions of a generation of twentieth-century psychoanalytic pioneers, notably Melanie Klein, Ronald Fairbairn, Edith Jacobson, Margaret Mahler, and Erik Erikson (for a review, see Kernberg 2004).

However, whereas classical psychoanalytic approaches to mental functioning and intrapsychic conflict had been conceptualized in terms of conflicts between drives and defenses, Kernberg (1992, 2004) suggested that psychological conflicts may be better conceptualized in terms of conflicts among different needed, desired, or feared internalized object relations.

Thus, Kernberg placed affectively charged, internalized representations of relationships at the center of psychological motivation and conflict.

Internal Conflicts and External Functioning

In another break with established psychoanalytic tradition, Kernberg's model placed equal emphasis on psychological conflict and current, external functioning, especially the nature of the individual's interactions with others. In this conceptualization and approach to personality pathology, attention is directed simultaneously to internal structures and to related symptoms and observable behaviors in classifying personality disorders (Kernberg 1984). Clinically, a patient's relative strengths and weaknesses in both domains—mental structures and observable behaviors—contribute to understanding psychopathology and to tailoring intervention, moment to moment, to the individual patient. This focus on real-time functioning is consistent with advances in social neurocognitive science (Clarkin and De Panfilis 2013) and ecological momentary assessment (Trull et al. 2008), and contributes to the understanding of interpersonal dynamics between patient and therapist in the treatment setting.

Systematic Assessment

In the 1980s, Kernberg further advanced an object relations theory–based approach to personality functioning and personality disorders by articulating an organized clinical interview, the *Structural Interview* (SI; Kernberg 1984). The SI is designed to assess a patient's representations of self and others, and to yield a diagnosis focused on severity of personality disorder, conceptualized in terms of *level of personality organization* (see Chapter 2 for definitions of levels of personality organization and related discussion). Our clinical research group subsequently devised both a self-report questionnaire that yields a rating of identity, level of defenses, and reality testing—the Inventory of Personality Organization (Lenzenweger et al. 2012)—and a semistructured interview version of Kernberg's SI—the STIPO-R (Clarkin et al. 2016). The complete STIPO-R interview and score sheet, which includes subscales as well as overall ratings, can be found at www.borderlinedisorders.com.

Transference-Focused Psychotherapy

The project of developing and studying a systematic approach to classification and treatment of personality disorders based in object relations theory was further advanced by the development of *transference-focused psychotherapy* (TFP; Yeomans et al. 2015), a specific, empirically supported treatment for severe personality disorders based on object relations theory. TFP targets failure of identity formation in patients with personality disorders. Clinical intervention focuses on internal representations of self and other as they are enacted in the patient's relationships, both with the therapist and in the patient's interpersonal life.

We have demonstrated that attachment coherence and reflective functioning change significantly in a positive direction in patients with borderline personality disorder in response to TFP, but this is not the case with either dialectical behavior therapy or supportive treatment (Levy et al. 2006). This result suggests that the focus on internal representations in TFP may lead to important modifications of these internal structures. There is preliminary evidence that such changes in TFP are also reflected in brain functioning, with increases in prefrontal control over emotional centers (Perez et al. 2016).

The Influence of Attachment Theory

As mentioned earlier, the object relations theory model of personality pathology and treatment has been influenced by and refined in relation to a variety of theoretical, empirical, and clinical developments introduced within near-neighbor disciplines. Contributions from attachment theory have been especially influential—in particular, in relation to the role of *internal working models*, *mentalization*, and *reflective functioning* in psychopathology and treatment.

Attachment theory was introduced by John Bowlby (1973, 1977), a British psychiatrist and psychoanalyst who studied children reared in adoption agencies. The main focus of attachment theory is on the nature and quality of the affective bond between infant and caregiver early in development, and how this affects attachment style later in life. A smooth, coordinated, empathic, and caring interaction between infant and caregiver results in the infant's felt security, whereas disruptions in this attachment bond result in various forms of insecure (anxious and avoidant) attachment, leaving the developing individual prone to psychopathology. An important link to object relations theory is reflected in Bowlby's belief that as a result of repeated interactions with the caregiver, the infant develops mental representations of self and others with expectations about these relationships. These internal representations are referred to as *internal working models* to indicate that they guide and direct future relationships but are open to new information and modification (Bretherton and Munholland 2016).

Attachment theory has benefited from the development of procedures and instruments to identify attachment status. Ainsworth's Strange Situation (Ainsworth et al. 1978) provided a laboratory assessment of the child's attachment style toward the maternal caregiver. A further advance was the introduction of the Adult Attachment Interview by Mary Main and colleagues (Main et al. 2003), which provided the first assessment of the mental representations of attachment status. There is at present a robust and rapidly developing research base for attachment theory, focusing on measures of attachment, the impact of caregiving behavior and of trauma on attachment style, neural and physiological correlates of attachment, and the relationship between attachment status and psychopathology (Cassidy and Shaver 2016).

Attachment theory has found clinical expression in mentalization-based treatment (MBT) for patients with borderline personality disorder (Bateman and Fonagy 2006). MBT is based not only on the trait-like status of attachment style but more centrally on the functional incapacity to *mentalize*—that is, to understand self and others in terms of emotions and intentions in daily interactions. MBT has significantly influenced our own treatment approach by focusing our attention more specifically on the therapeutic potential of promoting reflection and the capacity to entertain alternative perspectives in our patients, especially those with more severe personality pathology.

Key Clinical Concepts

- Psychological structures are central to an object relations theory model of personality functioning.

- Internal object relations are psychological structures composed of mental representations of self and other in interaction, linked with an affect state.

- Kernberg's theoretical articulation of object relations theory focuses on self and interpersonal functioning and the role of affectively invested representations of self and others in personality disorders.

- The object relations theory model of personality functioning and disorder overlaps with many contemporary theories of personality and personality disorders.

References

Ainsworth MDS, Blehar M, Waters E, Wall S: Patterns of Attachment: A Psychological Study of the Strange Situation. Hillsdale, NJ, Erlbaum, 1978

American Psychiatric Association: Diagnostic and Statistical Manual of Mental Disorders, 3rd Edition. Washington, DC, American Psychiatric Association, 1980

American Psychiatric Association: Diagnostic and Statistical Manual of Mental Disorders, 5th Edition. Arlington, VA, American Psychiatric Association, 2013

Bateman A, Fonagy P: Mentalization-Based Treatment for Borderline Personality Disorder. New York, Oxford University Press, 2006

Bender DS, Skodol AE: Borderline personality as a self-other representational disturbance. J Pers Disord 21(5):500–517, 2007 17953503

Benjamin L: Interpersonal theory of personality disorders: the structural analysis of social behavior and interpersonal reconstructive therapy, in Major Theories of Personality Disorder, 2nd Edition. Edited by Lenzenweger MF, Clarkin JF. New York, Guilford, 2005, pp 157–230

Bowlby J: Attachment and Loss, Vol 2: Separation: Anxiety and Anger. London, Hogarth Press and Institute of Psycho-Analysis, 1973

Bowlby J: The making and breaking of affectional bonds. I: Aetiology and psychopathology in the light of attachment theory, II: Some principles of psychotherapy. Br J Psychiatry 130:201–210; 421–431, 1977

Bowlby J: Attachment and Loss, Vol 3: Loss: Sadness and Depression. London, Hogarth Press and Institute of Psycho-Analysis, 1980

Bretherton I, Munholland KA: The internal working model construct in light of contemporary neuroimaging research, in Handbook of Attachment: Theory, Research, and Clinical Applications, 3rd Edition. Edited by Cassidy J, Shaver PR. New York, Guilford, 2016, pp 102–127

Cain NM, Pincus AL: Treating maladaptive interpersonal signatures, in Integrated Treatment for Personality Disorder: A Modular Approach. Edited by Livesley WJ, Dimaggio G, Clarkin JF. New York, Guilford, 2016, pp 305–324

Caligor E, Clarkin J: An object relations model of personality and personality pathology, in Psychodynamic Psychotherapy for Personality Disorders: A Clinical Handbook. Edited by Clarkin J, Fonagy P, Gabbard G. Washington, DC, American Psychiatric Publishing, 2010, pp 3–36

Cassidy J, Shaver PR (eds): Handbook of Attachment: Theory, Research, and Clinical Applications, 3rd Edition. New York, Guilford, 2016

Cicchetti D: Socioemotional, personality, and biological development: illustrations from a multilevel developmental psychopathology perspective on child maltreatment. Annu Rev Psychol 67:187–211, 2016 26726964

Clarkin JF, De Panfilis C: Developing conceptualization of borderline personality disorder. J Nerv Ment Dis 201(2):88–93, 2013 23364115

Clarkin JF, Livesley WJ: Formulation and treatment planning, in Integrated Treatment for Personality Disorder: A Modular Approach. Edited by Livesley WJ, Dimaggio G, Clarkin JF. New York, Guilford, 2016, pp 80–100

Clarkin JF, Cain N, Livesley WJ: The link between personality theory and psychological treatment: a shifting terrain, in Personality Disorders: Toward Theoretical and Empirical Integration in Diagnosis and Assessment. Edited by Huprich SK. Washington, DC, American Psychological Association, 2015a, pp 413–433

Clarkin JF, Fonagy P, Levy KN, Bateman A: Borderline personality disorder, in Handbook of Psychodynamic Approaches to Psychopathology. Edited by Luyten P, Mayes LC, Fonagy P, et al. New York, Guilford, 2015b, pp 353–380

Clarkin JF, Meehan KB, Lenzenweger MF: Emerging approaches to the conceptualization and treatment of personality disorder. Can Psychol 56:155–167, 2015c

Clarkin JF, Caligor E, Stern BL, Kernberg OF: Structured Interview of Personality Organization—Revised (STIPO-R), 2016. Available at: www.borderlinedisorders.com. Accessed September 20, 2017.

Clarkin JF, Livesley WJ, Meehan KB: Clinical assessment, in Handbook of Personality Disorders: Theory, Research, and Treatment, 2nd Edition. Edited by Livesley WJ, Larstone R. New York, Guilford, 2018, pp. 367–393

Crawford MJ, Koldobsky N, Mulder R, Tyrer P: Classifying personality disorder according to severity. J Pers Disord 25(3):321–330, 2011 21699394

Cristea IA, Gentili C, Cotet CD, et al: Efficacy of psychotherapies for borderline personality disorder: a systematic review and meta-analysis. JAMA Psychiatry 74(4):319–328, 2017 28249086

Fonagy P: The effectiveness of psychodynamic psychotherapies: an update. World Psychiatry 14(2):137–150, 2015 26043322

Gunderson JG, Lyons-Ruth K: BPD's interpersonal hypersensitivity phenotype: a gene-environment-developmental model. J Pers Disord 22(1):22–41, 2008 18312121

Hallquist MN, Lenzenweger MF: Identifying latent trajectories of personality disorder symptom change: growth mixture modeling in the longitudinal study of personality disorders. J Abnorm Psychol 122(1):138–155, 2013 23231459

Hopwood CJ, Malone JC, Ansell EB, et al: Personality assessment in DSM-5: empirical support for rating severity, style, and traits. J Pers Disord 25(3):305–320, 2011 21699393

Horowitz LM: Interpersonal Foundations of Psychopathology. Washington, DC, American Psychological Association, 2004

Kernberg OF: Object Relations Theory and Clinical Psychoanalysis. New York, Jason Aronson, 1975

Kernberg OF: The conceptualization of psychic structure: an overview, in Internal World and External Reality: Object Relations Theory Applied. New York, Jason Aronson, 1980, pp 3–18

Kernberg OF: Structural diagnosis, in Severe Personality Disorders: Psychotherapeutic Strategies. New Haven, CT, Yale University Press, 1984, pp 3–26

Kernberg OF: Aggression in Personality Disorders and Perversions. New Haven, CT, Yale University Press, 1992

Kernberg OF: Contemporary Controversies in Psychoanalytic Theory, Techniques, and Their Applications. New Haven, CT, Yale University Press, 2004

Kernberg OF: Identity: recent findings and clinical implications. Psychoanal Q 75(4):969–1004, 2006 17094369

Kernberg OF: What is personality? J Pers Disord 30(2):145–156, 2016 27027422

Kernberg OF, Caligor E: A psychoanalytic theory of personality disorders, in Major Theories of Personality Disorder, 2nd Edition. Edited by Lenzenweger MF, Clarkin JF. New York, Guilford, 2005, pp 114–156

Kotov R, Krueger RF, Watson D, et al: The Hierarchical Taxonomy of Psychopathology (HiTOP): a dimensional alternative to traditional nosologies. J Abnorm Psychol 126(4):454–477, 2017 28333488

Leichsenring F, Luyten P, Hilsenroth MJ, et al: Psychodynamic therapy meets evidence-based medicine: a systematic review using updated criteria. Lancet Psychiatry 2(7):648–660, 2015 26303562

Lenzenweger MF: Current status of the scientific study of the personality disorders: an overview of epidemiological, longitudinal, experimental psychopathology, and neurobehavioral perspectives. J Am Psychoanal Assoc 58(4):741–778, 2010 21115756

Lenzenweger MF, McClough JF, Clarkin JF, Kernberg OF: Exploring the interface of neurobehaviorally linked personality dimensions and personality organization in borderline personality disorder: the Multidimensional Personality Questionnaire and Inventory of Personality Organization. J Pers Disord 26(6):902–918, 2012 23281675

Levy KN, Meehan KB, Kelly KM, et al: Change in attachment patterns and reflective function in a randomized control trial of transference-focused psychotherapy for borderline personality disorder. J Consult Clin Psychol 74(6):1027–1040, 2006 17154733

Lingiardi V, McWilliams N (eds): The Psychodynamic Diagnostic Manual, 2nd Edition. New York, Guilford, 2017

Livesley WJ: Conceptual and taxonomic issues, in Handbook of Personality Disorders: Theory, Research, and Treatment. Edited by Livesley WJ. New York, Guilford, 2001, pp 3–38

Livesley WJ, Clarkin JF: Diagnosis and assessment, in Integrated Treatment for Personality Disorder: A Modular Approach. Edited by Livesley WJ, Dimaggio G, Clarkin JF. New York, Guilford, 2015, pp 51–79

Main M, Goldwyn R, Hesse E: Adult attachment scoring and classification system. Unpublished manuscript, University of California at Berkeley, 2003

Meyer B, Pilkonis PA: An attachment model of personality disorders, in Major Theories of Personality Disorder, 2nd Edition. Edited by Lenzenweger MF, Clarkin JF. New York, Guilford, 2005, pp 231–281

Mischel W, Shoda Y: Toward a unified theory of personality: integrating dispositions and processing dynamics within the cognitive-affective processing system, in Handbook of Personality: Theory and Research, 3rd Edition. Edited by John OP, Robins RW, Pervin LA. New York, Guilford, 2008, pp 208–241

Morey LC, Hopwood CJ: Stability and change in personality disorders. Annu Rev Clin Psychol 9:499–528, 2013 23245342

Perez DL, Vago DR, Pan H, et al: Frontolimbic neural circuit changes in emotional processing and inhibitory control associated with clinical improvement following transference-focused psychotherapy in borderline personality disorder. Psychiatry Clin Neurosci 70(1):51–61, 2016 26289141

Pincus AL: A contemporary integrative interpersonal theory of personality disorders, in Major Theories of Personality Disorder, 2nd Edition. Edited by Lenzenweger MF, Clarkin JF. New York, Guilford, 2005, pp 282–331

Pretzer J, Beck AT: A cognitive theory of personality disorders, in Major Theories of Personality Disorder, 2nd Edition. Edited by Lenzenweger MF, Clarkin JF. New York, Guilford, 2005, pp 43–113

Sharp C, Wright AG, Fowler JC, et al: The structure of personality pathology: both general ('g') and specific ('s') factors? J Abnorm Psychol 124(2):387–398, 2015 25730515

Trull TJ, Solhan MB, Tragesser SL, et al: Affective instability: measuring a core feature of borderline personality disorder with ecological momentary assessment. J Abnorm Psychol 117(3):647–661, 2008 18729616

Yeomans F, Clarkin JF, Kernberg OF: Transference-Focused Psychotherapy for Borderline Personality Disorder: A Clinical Guide. Washington, DC, American Psychiatric Publishing, 2015

Section I

Personality and Personality Disorders Through the Lens of Object Relations Theory

A COMPREHENSIVE DESCRIPTION OF ANY form of psychotherapy will begin with the following:

- A description of the frame of reference within which the treatment is embedded (e.g., psychodynamic, cognitive-behavioral, interpersonal)
- Elaboration of a clearly specified model of the pathology being treated (i.e., identifying what is "wrong" with the patient?)
- Designation of which aspects of psychopathology are the targets of the treatment (i.e., clarifying what will be changed in the patient if treatment is successful?)
- A theory of how the treatment can lead to the targeted changes (i.e., a model for mechanisms of change)

Object relations theory provides an integrated theoretical foundation for conceptualizing, classifying, and assessing personality disorders, and has led to the development of transference-focused psychotherapy—extended (TFP-E). Object relations theory places pathology of identity formation at center stage, as the organizer of the various disruptions of self and interpersonal functioning that are defining features of personality disorders. The goal of TFP-E is to promote progressive degrees of identity consolidation, corresponding with the development of a coherent and increasingly complex experience of self in relation to others.

In Section I of this volume (Chapters 2 and 3), we present an overview of the object relations theory–based model of personality and personality disorders. In Chapter 2, we discuss descriptive and structural features of normal and disordered personality functioning and the approach to classification of personality disorders that emerges from this framework. We focus in particular on identity as the organizer of self and other functioning, as well as the related dimensions of object relations, defenses, moral functioning, and quality of aggression.

In Chapter 3, we cover dynamic features of personality within an object relations theory frame of reference—the model of conflicts, anxieties, and defenses that attempts to explain the psychological motivations underlying maladaptive personality functioning and to account for their resistance to change. Together, these chapters provide the conceptual foundation for the clinical chapters to follow. As we review the object relations theory model of personality disorder, we emphasize the relationship between theory and clinical work.

Personality and Personality Disorders Within the Framework of Object Relations Theory

THE TERM AND CONCEPT OF PERSONALITY refer to the dynamic organization of enduring patterns of behavior, cognition, emotion, motivation, and ways of experiencing and relating to others that are characteristic of an individual (Kernberg 2016). The individual's personality is an integral part of his experience of himself and of the world—so much so that it may be difficult for him to imagine being any different. Personality develops out of the interaction of inborn temperamental and genetic factors, developmental experience, and psychological conflict and defense.

When DSM-III introduced personality disorder into the diagnostic system in 1980 (American Psychiatric Association 1980), it was with the assumption that personality disorder characteristics are stable over time. Many clinicians have retained this assumption and remain pessimistic about the possibility of truly modifying personality dysfunction. However, empirical research on personality and personality disorders has progressed, and data now support a more complex and less static view, a view more optimistic about the long-term prognosis of individuals with personality disorders. Current data suggest that personality involves both stability and change (see Clarkin et al. 2015), and longitudinal data support the position that disordered personality functioning can be modified as a result of maturation, the passage of time, and life experience (Lenzenweger 2010), as well as by successful treatment (Bateman and Fonagy 2008).[1]

Part 1

Psychodynamic Description of Personality and Personality Disorder

A *PSYCHODYNAMIC* DESCRIPTION OF PERsonality and personality pathology within the framework of object relations theory is characterized by 1) descriptive, 2) structural, and 3) dynamic features of personality functioning. In this chapter, we discuss normal personality and personality disorders from *descriptive* and *structural* perspectives. In Chapter 3, we elaborate the *dynamic* features of personality disorders, focusing on the relationship between dynamics and structure.

Together, descriptive and structural assessments offer the clinician a clear appreciation of the patient's objective and subjective difficulties and provide the information needed to make a diagnosis and to guide treatment planning. The descriptive features of personality disorder are rela-

---

[1]Longitudinal studies have revealed that personality disorder, as defined and identified by DSM criteria and traits, tends to decline categorically and dimensionally over time, both in community (Lenzenweger 2010; Lenzenweger et al. 2004) and clinical (Grilo et al. 2004; Zanarini et al. 2005) samples. In general, symptoms classified as diagnostic criteria often decline, but functioning remains suboptimal (Zanarini et al. 2012).

tively variable and may be more malleable in treatment, whereas the structural aspects of personality pathology are more enduring and require special focus if they are to change. Transference-focused psychotherapy—extended (TFP-E) is a treatment approach that attempts to change both the descriptive and structural features of personality disorder through an understanding and examination of the dynamic features.

From a *descriptive* perspective, an individual's personality, normal or disordered, can be described in terms of clusters of *personality traits*. Personality traits are the relatively stable and enduring patterns of behavior, cognition, emotion, and interpersonal relatedness that are organized to form the directly observable components of personality functioning. For example, conscientiousness, altruism, optimism, rebelliousness, selfishness, entitlement, self-destructiveness, and impulsivity are all personality traits, some more adaptive and more desirable than others. Clinically, assessment of descriptive features of personality pathology provides information about presenting complaints and problems, maladaptive personality traits, and relationships with significant others. Such assessment can be used to formulate a *descriptive diagnosis*. This is the approach taken with the personality disorders in DSM-5 Section II, "Diagnostic Criteria and Codes" (American Psychiatric Association 2013); assessment of descriptive features of personality pathology enables the clinician to make a categorical DSM-5 diagnosis.

From a *structural* perspective, an individual's personality can be described in terms of the relatively stable and enduring patterns of psychological *functions* or *processes* that underlie and organize the individual's behavior, perceptions, and subjective experience in predictable ways.[2] A stable pattern of psychological functions that in concert organize a particular aspect of psychological life is referred to as a psychological *structure*; psychological structures are stable patterns of psychological functioning that are repeatedly and predictably activated in particular contexts. At the level of cognitive neuroscience, the neural correlates of what we think of as psychological structures can be conceptualized as associations among neuronal circuits, or *associational networks*, that tend to be activated in

---

[2]There is growing consensus that the optimal way to conceptualize personality pathology is by domains of dysfunction rather than solely by categories and diagnoses. However, a lack of consensus remains as to which domains are essential to capture personality pathology (for a review of this topic, see Clarkin 2013). We opt for the domains specified by object relations theory and captured by the Structured Interview of Personality Organization—Revised (STIPO-R; Clarkin et al. 2016) to focus assessment and treatment.

concert (Westen and Gabbard 2002). Motivational systems, coping mechanisms, patterns of relating, and processes that function to regulate mood and impulses are all examples of psychological structures. The nature and organization of psychological structures are characteristic of the individual and tend to be relatively stable over time.

Within the framework of psychodynamic object relations theory, a *structural diagnosis* provides information about the *severity* of personality pathology (Kernberg 1984). While there is growing agreement among personality disorder researchers that *severity* of personality dysfunction is central to assessment and treatment planning (see Livesley et al. 2015),[3] there is little unanimity about how to measure it in actual practice.[4] Within the framework of object relations theory, severity of personality pathology is defined through the lens of the individual's experience of herself and her significant others; the quality of her relationships, or object relations; the nature of her defensive operations; and the stability of her reality testing (Kernberg 1984). A similar approach to describing personality functioning and pathology has been adopted in the Level of Personality Functioning Scale, presented in the Alternative Model for Personality Disorders in DSM-5 Section III (American Psychiatric Association 2013, pp. 775–778), an alternative approach to describing personality disorders that characterizes them according to the severity of impairment in self and interpersonal functioning. Likewise, proposals for ICD-11 focus on the presence or absence of personality disorder and ratings of severity (i.e., mild, moderate, or severe; Tyrer et al. 2011).

When it comes to *classification* of personality disorders, the model

---

[3]Severity of personality dysfunction has been found to predict outcome better than diagnostic category. Hopwood et al. (2011) found that generalized severity was the most predictive of current and future dysfunction, but that personality style indicated specific areas of difficulty.

[4]There is a diversity of opinion on how to measure severity of personality dysfunction. Suggested approaches include the following: examining failures in cooperating and coping with the interpersonal world (Parker et al. 2004), Global Assessment of Functioning Scale scores (Widiger et al. 2013), the sum of all criteria observed across all personality disorders (Tyrer and Johnson 1996), and ratings of areas of interpersonal dysfunction (Bornstein 1998). While researchers are looking for the optimal way in which to arrive at a summary score for severity, it may be more clinically useful to identify areas of deficit indicative of severity that are likely to be modifiers of treatment response. For example, the multidimensional space defined by object relations theory includes both prototypical categories of disorder and dimensional ratings of key domains of dysfunction.

based on object relations theory combines a dimensional classification of personality disorders according to the severity of structural pathology, focusing on identity formation, with a second-order classification based on descriptive features or personality traits. Thus, both clinically and conceptually, the object relations theory approach relies on first characterizing the severity of personality pathology by assessing the nature, organization, and degree of integration of psychological structures, and then characterizing descriptive features of personality pathology to make a diagnosis of personality "type" or "style."[5] Our two-axial approach reflects the clinical reality that similar personality styles or maladaptive traits may be seen across a broad spectrum of pathology, with markedly different prognostic implications (Hopwood et al. 2011). From a clinical perspective, the degree of severity of personality pathology/dysfunction is of far greater importance with regard to prognosis and differential treatment planning than is personality "type" (Crawford et al. 2011).

The Alternative Model for Personality Disorders in DSM-5 Section III reflects a two-pronged approach to classification, very similar to our own. The DSM-5 Section III model combines 1) dimensional assessment of impairment of self and interpersonal functioning with 2) descriptions of pathological personality traits to characterize the various personality disorders. The DSM-5 Section III model of diagnosis and related assessment is described as a "hybrid" approach, combining dimensional ratings of self and interpersonal (i.e., other) functioning and dimensional assessment of traits. These dimensional ratings are combined with a categorical diagnosis of one of six personality disorder categories.

Trait-Based Diagnosis of Personality Disorders and DSM-5 Section II

Trait-based approaches to personality disorders characterize both normal personality and the personality disorders in terms of personality *traits—*

---

[5]The categorical organization of personality disorders as defined from DSM-III to DSM-5 does not hold up to empirical scrutiny (see Wright and Zimmerman 2015). Data gathered on a large inpatient sample and subjected to a bifactor statistical analysis revealed a large general factor of personality pathology that extends across the 10 categories of personality disorder recognized in DSM-5 (Sharp et al. 2015). The authors suggested that this factor structure is consistent with Kernberg's articulation of borderline personality organization.

habitual patterns of behavior, cognition, emotion, and interpersonal relatedness that are characteristic of the individual. Within this framework,
individual personality disorders are defined on the basis of clusters of
more or less maladaptive traits that tend to hang together, and in concert
constitute a particular personality "type" or "style." This is the approach
traditionally taken in the DSM system, in which traits associated with a
particular personality disorder are listed as diagnostic criteria used to
make a categorical diagnosis. (In a categorical diagnostic system, one either does or does not have a particular personality disorder, based on
meeting or failing to meet a particular diagnostic threshold.)

Everyone has personality traits. It is the flexibility versus rigidity with
which traits are activated, and the degree to which traits are normative
and adaptive rather than extreme and maladaptive, that distinguishes
normal personality from pathology at the level of traits.[6] In the normal
personality, personality traits are not extreme and are flexibly and adaptively activated in different settings; the traits fall within the range of what
is culturally accepted as normal, and the individual is able to flexibly limit
their expression to settings in which they are appropriate and adaptive.
For example, an individual can be attentive to detail in a flexible and
adaptive fashion—able to make a quick decision in a pinch or capable of
overlooking details to complete a task when it is deemed necessary to do
so. Similarly, an individual can be in general reserved but still able to con-
verse in a socially appropriate fashion when called on to do so. When
traits are not extreme and are flexibly and adaptively activated, an individual may be said to have a particular personality "style"—for example,
obsessive-compulsive or introverted—in the absence of psychopathology.

Moving across the range of normal personality functioning toward
pathology, personality traits become progressively more rigid and extreme, interfering with the individual's functioning more profoundly and
more globally as personality pathology becomes more severe. When traits
are rigid, the individual is unable to change his behavior, even when it is
highly maladaptive not to do so and even if he purposefully attempts to
do so. Rather than learning from experience and modifying maladaptive
patterns, in the setting of personality rigidity, the individual will activate

---

[6]Traits provide a general view of personality functioning but have limitations for
the clinician insofar as they fail to capture intra-individual variation across environmental situations. For example, an individual may have a strong aggressive
trait, but that fact does not provide information about when, with whom, or in
what circumstances the individual is aggressive (Meehan and Clarkin 2015).

the same behaviors, emotional responses, and ways of relating time and time again, in a broad array of circumstances, regardless of whether these behaviors are appropriate to the setting.

For example, the individual who is rigidly attentive to detail will be unable to temporarily loosen his standards, even when his boss calls on him to do so or when failing to do so means missing an important deadline. Similarly, the introverted individual will not be able to come out of her shell to behave appropriately in a job interview or on a date. When personality traits are extreme, they demonstrate an increasingly wide deviation from commonly encountered and culturally normative behaviors and ways of functioning. Thus, the first individual is not merely attentive to detail but must reread a document five times and then have three others read it before he approves it. And the second individual, as she becomes increasingly introverted, may move from being reserved to being reclusive, unable to interact comfortably with others, and shying away from social contact.

At the most severe end of the spectrum are individuals whose traits are not only extreme and maladaptive, but also mutually contradictory. For example, an individual who is typically excessively detail oriented might periodically submit a document riddled with glaring omissions and errors, or someone who is habitually avoidant, to the point of social isolation, may play the role of the life of the party at a large social gathering.

From a descriptive perspective, an individual whose personality rigidity reaches the point that it significantly, consistently, and chronically interferes with daily functioning, and/or causes significant distress to the individual or those around him, is said to have a *personality disorder*.

Structural Diagnosis of Personality Disorders and DSM-5 Section III

The structural approach to personality pathology characterizes personality disorders in terms of pathology of key psychological structures; both normal and disordered personality functioning are understood in terms of the level of integration of psychological structures organizing subjective experience and behavior, with lower levels of integration corresponding with more severe pathology. Within the framework of object relations theory, the structural approach to personality pathology focuses in particular on the core construct of identity in understanding and classifying the personality disorders.

Identity is the psychological structure that organizes the individual's experience of self and the experience of others in interaction (Kernberg 2006; Kernberg and Caligor 2005). Identity consolidation distinguishes between normal personality and higher-level personality disorders on the one hand and more severe personality disorders on the other (Kernberg 1984; Kernberg and Caligor 2005). The central position assigned to identity in the object relations theory model of personality pathology is mirrored in the DSM-5 alternative model's general criteria for personality disorder, in which moderate or greater impairment in self and interpersonal functioning (Criterion A) is identified as a defining feature of any personality disorder diagnosis.

Along with its focus on identity, the object relations theory model focuses on the closely related constructs of quality of object relations (internal working models of relationships and interpersonal relations), defensive operations (customary ways of coping with external stress and internal conflict), reality testing (appreciation of conventional notions of reality), and moral functioning (ethical behavior, ideals, and values) (Kernberg and Caligor 2005).

The structural approach to personality disorders describes a continuous spectrum of personality functioning and pathology across the dimension of severity, spanning the normal to the most severe personality disorders. In the normal personality, 1) identity is fully consolidated, corresponding with a well-integrated, stable, and realistic sense of self and a corresponding sense of significant others, along with the capacity to identify and pursue long-term goals; 2) relations with others are marked by a capacity for concern, mutual dependency, and intimacy; 3) mature defenses predominate and allow for adaptation to life and flexible management of psychological conflict; 4) moral functioning is internalized, stable, and linked to personally and consistently held values and ideals; and 5) reality testing is stable even in areas of conflict or in the setting of affect activation (Horz et al. 2012).

In contrast, with the introduction of personality pathology, deterioration—though sometimes uneven deterioration—is evident in functioning in all these domains, progressively worsening as pathology becomes more severe. Thus, in the setting of the more severe personality disorders, 1) identity is poorly consolidated, reflected in an experience of self and others that is distorted, superficial, unstable, and highly affectively charged, and the capacity to identify and pursue long-term goals is impaired; 2) relations with others are superficial, based on need fulfillment, and are increasingly exploitative as pathology becomes more severe; 3) lower-level, splitting-based defenses predominate and maintain a dissociated, black-

and-white quality of experience while introducing severe rigidity and poor adaptation; 4) moral functioning is inconsistent, and at the most severe end of the spectrum is characterized by antisocial features and an absence of internalized values or ideals; and 5) reality testing is vulnerable in the setting of affect activation, psychological conflict, or interpersonal stressors (Horz et al. 2012).

Part 2

Classification of Personality Pathology Within the Model of Object Relations Theory

Level of Personality Organization and STIPO-R Dimensional Profiles

Careful characterization of identity, object relations, defenses, moral functioning, and reality testing enables the clinician to describe a patient's *personality organization*, a dimensional assessment of personality pathology reflecting severity and clinical prognosis, which will guide treatment planning (Kernberg 1984; Kernberg and Caligor 2005). Within the model of object relations theory, there are two complementary approaches to classification of personality organization: 1) level of personality organization (or structural diagnosis) and 2) dimensional profiles based on the Structured Interview of Personality Organization—Revised (STIPO-R; Clarkin et al. 2016).

The first approach, more familiar and most often based on clinical assessment (see Chapter 7), describes a patient's *level of personality organization*, or *structural diagnosis* (Figure 2–1). Within this framework, patients can be described as having normal personality organization, a neurotic level of personality organization (NPO), a high borderline level of personality organization (high BPO), a middle borderline level of personality organization (middle BPO), or a low borderline level of personality organization (low BPO); these terms describe the trajectory from the healthiest to the most severe pathology. There are two important considerations regarding this approach:

1. We anticipate the possibility that some readers may by confused as to why high BPO designates the least severe group and low BPO the most severe. Within the object relations theory framework, "high" and "low" refer *not* to severity, but to level of organization, with higher levels of organization and integration corresponding with higher levels of psychological health.
2. We also want to make clear the distinction between the DSM-5 borderline personality disorder (BPD) and the borderline level of personality organization (BPO). BPD is a specific personality disorder, diagnosed on the basis of a constellation of descriptive features. BPO is a much broader category based on structural features, in particular, pathology of identity formation. The BPO diagnosis (Kernberg 1984) subsumes the DSM-5 BPD diagnosis as well as all of the severe personality disorders. See Figure 2–2 for further clarification of the relationship between the DSM-5 Section II diagnostic categories and levels of personality organization.

In Figure 2–1, we define the different levels of personality organization. In Figure 2–2, we illustrate the relationship between the structural approach to personality disorders and the more familiar DSM-5 Section II personality disorders, emphasizing the dimension of severity.

The Level of Personality Functioning Scale (LPFS)[7] in DSM-5 Section III provides five levels of personality health and pathology (0=little or no impairment; 4=extreme impairment), focusing on the dimensions of self and interpersonal functioning. The five levels described in LPFS correspond quite closely with the five levels of personality organization (see Figure 2–1) described in the object relations theory model.[8]

An alternative and less familiar approach to the classification of personality organization is based on a semistructured interview, the Structured Interview of Personality Organization—Revised (STIPO-R; Clarkin

---

[7]The LPFS can be found in the appendix of helpful resources at the back of this book and is also located in the Alternative Model for Personality Disorders in DSM-5 Section III.

[8]A major difference between the two classification systems is that the LPFS focuses solely on self and interpersonal functioning, with minimal attention given to the role of moral functioning and aggression in the classification of severity of personality disorder.

Lowest severity ————————————————————————▶ Highest severity

	Normal personality organization	Neurotic personality organization	Borderline level of personality organization[a]		
			High	Middle	Low
Personality rigidity	None	Mild-moderate	Moderately extreme	Extreme	Very extreme
Identity	Consolidated	Consolidated	Mild–moderate pathology	Moderate–severe pathology	Severe pathology
Object relations	Deep, mutual	Deep, mutual	Some mutual	Need-fulfilling	Exploitative
Predominant defensive style	Mature	Repression-based	Splitting-based and repression-based	Splitting-based	Splitting-based
Moral functioning	Internalized Flexible	Internalized Rigid	Uneven/inconsistent Mild pathology	Mild–moderate pathology	Severe pathology
Reality testing	Intact Stable Social reality testing intact	Intact Stable Social reality testing intact	Intact Some social deficits	Vulnerable to stress Transient psychotic states Social deficits	Vulnerable to stress Transient psychotic states Social deficits

FIGURE 2–1. **Structural approach to classification of personality pathology.**

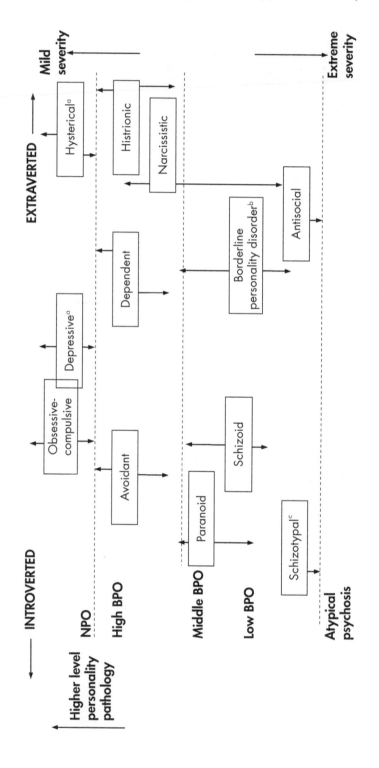

FIGURE 2–2. **Relationship between levels of personality organization and DSM-5 Section II diagnoses.**

Severity ranges from mildest, at the top of the figure, to extremely severe at the bottom. Arrows indicate range of severity. BPO=borderline level of personality organization; NPO=neurotic level of personality organization.

[a]Neither depressive personality nor hysterical personality is included in DSM-5 (although the former was included in DSM-IV-TR Axis II as a criteria set for further research). Because neither personality meets the severity criteria for a personality disorder, these personalities are best characterized as common forms of subsyndromal personality pathology (also referred to as higher level personality pathology [Caligor et al. 2007]). They are included here because they are widely recognized and described in the clinical literature and frequently encountered in outpatient clinical practice.

[b]Note the distinction between the DSM-5 borderline personality disorder (BPD) and the borderline level of personality organization (BPO). BPD is a specific personality disorder, diagnosed on the basis of a constellation of descriptive features. BPO is a much broader category based on structural features, in particular, pathology of identity formation. The BPO diagnosis (Kernberg 1984) subsumes the DSM-5 BPD diagnosis as well as all of the severe personality disorders.

[c]We include schizotypal personality disorder here because it was retained in DSM-5 Section II. However, based on family and genetic studies, it appears that schizotypal personality disorder is best described not as a personality disorder but rather as a schizophrenia spectrum disorder.

Source. Adapted from Caligor et al. 2007, p. 20.

et al. 2016). The STIPO-R evaluates the domains of identity, object relations, defenses, aggression, and moral values. The patient's functioning in each domain is rated on a 5-point scale of severity (1 = normal; 5 = most severe). The ratings for each of the five STIPO-R domains are combined to provide an individualized profile of the level of personality functioning and pathology (e.g., see Figure 2–3, a profile for the patient described in Clinical Illustration 1 later in this chapter).

The anchors for STIPO-R ratings provide descriptions of identity, object relations, defenses, aggression, and moral values as they manifest in the normal personality and in different levels of severity of personality pathology. Review of these anchors provides a clinically and conceptually useful overview of the dimensional framework of structural classification of personality pathology. In the appendix of helpful resources at the back of this book, we provide a clinician-friendly version of the STIPO-R anchors for overall ratings of identity, object relations, defenses, aggression, and moral values. We encourage the reader to review them as a way to become conversant with the structural approach to classification. The complete STIPO-R interview and score sheet, which includes subscales as well as overall ratings, can be found at www.borderlinedisorders.com.

In the illustrative vignettes later in this chapter, we provide for each patient *both* the level of personality organization (in the heading) and the STIPO-R dimensional profile (in a figure) to facilitate the reader's developing familiarity with these approaches to classification.

Prototypes and Dimensional Profiles

Before moving ahead to discuss clinical perspectives on personality organization, we want to comment on the conceptual relationship between 1) the levels of personality organization and the LPFS levels of personality functioning presented in DSM-5 Section III, both of which are typically diagnosed on the basis of a clinical interview; and 2) the dimensional profiles provided by the STIPO-R semistructured interview. The different levels of personality organization—normal personality organization, NPO, high BPO, middle BPO, and low BPO—as well as the corresponding LPFS levels 0 through 4, represent diagnostic *prototypes* (e.g., see Table 2-1 for the relationship between level of personality organization prototypes and STIPO-R dimensional ratings). These prototypes have proved extremely useful clinically; they convey critical information about severity and prognosis of pathology, guide treatment planning, and facilitate communication among clinicians (Caligor and Clarkin 2010).

In contrast, the STIPO-R does not provide a structural diagnosis, level of personality organization, or diagnostic prototypes; rather, the STIPO-R provides a dimensional description of personality functioning across each of the core domains (e.g., see Figure 2–3 in Clinical Illustration 1 later in this chapter). The dimensional approach to classification adopted in the STIPO-R is more cumbersome than a prototype but leaves more room to account for variability within a given level of personality organization (i.e., not all high-BPO patients are the same). The more nuanced classification provided by the STIPO-R profile can be helpful not only in research settings but in the clinical arena as well, especially when working with patients who do not fit neatly into a particular level of personality organization prototype (e.g., a patient who appears to best fit into the high-BPO range, but who demonstrates significant moral pathology) and those best described as on the border between two levels of personality organization (e.g., a patient who seems to fall into the area of transition between high BPO and NPO).

In sum, there are advantages to both prototypic and dimensional approaches to classification; the prototypic approach, aimed at determining a level of personality organization, is more familiar and corresponds more closely with how clinicians tend to organize clinical data—that is, by making use of implicit or explicit prototypes developed through clinical experience (Westen 1997; Westen and Shedler 2000). The dimensional profiles provided by the STIPO-R are more specific and leave more room for individual variability, providing greater opportunity to consider potential moderators of severity and of change in personality disorders. Table 2–1 describes the relationship between the five levels of personality organization and the STIPO-R five-point ratings.

Higher Level Personality Pathology

We have used the term *higher level personality pathology* (see Caligor et al. 2007) to describe a relatively healthy group of patients composed of those organized at a neurotic level, along with those with hybrid structures falling on the border between high BPO and NPO. In addition to the traditional neurotic personality types, the higher level personality pathology cohort includes a relatively healthy subset of patients with avoidant, narcissistic, or histrionic personality disorder who resemble high-BPO patients insofar as they present with a combination of dissociative and repression-based defenses, but resemble NPO patients insofar as they benefit from a reasonably stable sense of self. The designation of *higher*

TABLE 2–1. Relationship between levels of personality organization and STIPO-R dimensional scores[a]

STIPO-R dimension	STIPO-R score	Level of PO×STIPO-R dimensional rating by domain				
		Normal PO	NPO	High BPO	Middle BPO	Low BPO
Identity	Prototype score	1	2	3	4	4 or 5
	Range of scores	1	2	3	3–5	4–5
Object relations	Prototype score	1	2	3	4	5
	Range of scores	1	1–2	2–3	3–5	4–5
Defenses	Prototype score	1	2	3	4	4 or 5
	Range of scores	1	2–3	3	4–5	4–5
Aggression	Prototype score	1	2	3	4	4 or 5
	Range of scores	1	1–2	2–3	3–4	4–5
Moral values	Prototype score	1	2	3	4	5
	Range of scores	1	1–2	2–3	3–4	4–5

Note. BPO=borderline level of personality organization; NPO=neurotic level of personality organization; PO=personality organization; STIPO-R= Structured Interview of Personality Organization—Revised (Clarkin et al. 2016).

[a]As an example, for the STIPO-R domain Identity, the normal personality organization is associated with a STIPO-R Identity rating of 1; NPO with a STIPO-R Identity rating of 2; high BPO with a STIPO-R Identity rating of 3; and middle and low BPO with STIPO-R Identity ratings of 4 and 5, respectively, with some variability.

level personality pathology is clinically meaningful; as a group, these individuals do well in the less structured form of TFP-E that we outline in this book for the treatment of NPO patients; this form of TFP-E is also described in depth by Caligor et al. (2007).

Clinical Perspectives

As described thus far in this book, the object relations theory approach to classification of personality disorders is organized first and foremost in relation to the construct of identity. The structural approach to classification of personality disorders begins by distinguishing between two groups: 1) those with milder pathology, in whom identity consolidation and a predominance of repression-based defenses are seen, constituting higher level personality pathology and referred to as *neurotic level of personality organization* (NPO); and 2) those with more severe pathology, in whom clinically significant identity pathology and a predominance of splitting-based or dissociative defenses are seen, referred to as *borderline level of personality organization* (BPO) (Kernberg 1984; Kernberg and Caligor 2005).

To illustrate application of the STIPO-R to clinical assessment and classification, we present and discuss four cases (using representative patients Ms. N, Ms. B, Mr. H, and Mr. L) across different levels of personality organization. Each case presentation includes discussion of the specific STIPO-R ratings for the representative patient (for each 1–5 rating, a series of descriptors is provided for each anchor, in which 1 = normal and 5 = most severe pathology). The STIPO-R anchors are intended to serve as general guidelines. It is expected that some, but not all, descriptors will apply to a particular patient. Because much of the assessment of personality pathology comes down to pattern recognition, we hope that these vignettes and related discussion can provide the reader with ready prototypes to draw upon when assessing patients with personality disorders. For complete list of all descriptors for each anchor, see "STIPO-R Clinical Anchors for Personality Organization: Identity, Object Relations, Defenses, Aggression, and Moral Values Across the Range of Severity" in the appendix at the back of this book.

Neurotic Level of Personality Organization

In individuals with the less severe, neurotic level of personality organization, we see maladaptive personality rigidity (Shapiro 1965) in the setting of 1) consolidated identity; 2) a predominance of higher-level, repression-based, defensive operations; and 3) intact and stable reality testing. This group includes individuals with obsessive-compulsive and depressive personality disorders (the latter omitted from DSM-5), individuals with the higher-level hysterical personality disorder (omitted from DSM-5), a relatively healthy subset of patients with avoidant personality disorder, and the large group of patients seen in clinical practice who present with personality pathology not of sufficient severity to meet criteria for a DSM personality disorder (Westen and Arkowitz-Westen 1998).[9] Individuals organized at a neurotic level generally function well in many domains, and their maladaptive personality traits typically interfere predominantly in focal areas of functioning and/or cause subjective distress.

Clinical Illustration 1: Neurotic Level of Personality Organization

Ms. N, a 28-year-old single woman who teaches in an elementary school, was seen in consultation with the complaint of "problems with men." Ms. N was attractive, charming, and quietly seductive. She described feeling inadequate and unattractive relative to her friends and coworkers, shy with men, and sexually inhibited, yet she acknowledged that she was often surprised to find herself the center of attention in social settings. She felt that her insecurities explained why she had not yet found a life partner, whereas many of her friends were married or engaged, and she explained that lately her inability to move ahead had left her feeling "down."

Ms. N also described a tendency to shy away from conflict, leaving her at times excessively accommodating to the needs or wishes of others. Although she did not have a boyfriend, she had a group of female friends, some of whom she had known as far back as elementary school; she de-

---

[9]We choose to use the term *personality pathology* in contrast to *personality disorder* when describing the neurotic level of personality organization. This reflects the relatively mild severity of these disorders and the high level of functioning typical of individuals with these disorders. Our choice of terminology is consistent with the DSM-5 Section III general criteria for personality disorders, which identify "moderate or greater impairment" in personality functioning as Criterion A. As noted in Figure 2–2, neither depressive personality nor hysterical personality is included in DSM-5. Because neither personality meets the severity criteria for a personality disorder, these personalities are best characterized as common forms of subsyndromal personality pathology (also referred to as higher level personality pathology [Caligor et al. 2007]). These disorders are widely recognized and described in the clinical literature and are frequently encountered in outpatient clinical practice.

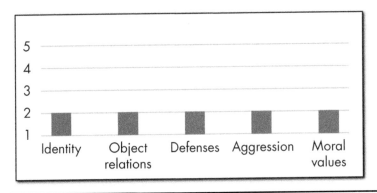

FIGURE 2–3. STIPO-R profile for Ms. N (NPO).

STIPO-R ratings: Identity—Level 2; Object relations—Level 2; Defenses—Level 2;
Aggression—Level 2; Moral values—Level 2.

NPO=neurotic level of personality organization; STIPO-R=Structured Interview of
Personality Organization—Revised (Clarkin et al. 2016).

scribed the group as "close-knit and supportive." When asked, she was
able to provide a three-dimensional and nuanced description of her best
friend: "She is strong, independently minded, sometimes stubborn, but always thoughtful, caring, and considerate of others. I greatly admire her,
in addition to loving her."

Ms. N characterized her work as an elementary school teacher as both
challenging and fulfilling, noting that the warmth she felt toward her students helped her cope with her as yet unfulfilled wishes to have her own
children. She explained that "giving back" was important to her and had
been part of her decision to pursue a career in education. She described
herself as an overall level-headed person, but she was aware that at times
she placed extremely high demands on herself and could become excessively self-critical when she did not meet her own expectations.

By the end of a 90-minute interview, the consultant felt that he had a
vivid impression of Ms. N, of her difficulties, and of the important people
in her life.

Figure 2–3 shows the STIPO-R profile for Ms. N, followed by discussion of the STIPO-R ratings for this patient.

Guide to STIPO-R Ratings for Ms. N (NPO)

Identity. Ms. N presents with an overall experience of self and others
that is complex, stable, and continuous across time. She is highly invested
in her career, which she finds deeply satisfying. The clinician can detect
some distortion in her sense of self and her experience of others' assessment of her, limited to the appraisal of her sexual attractiveness. This sta-

ble, focal distortion in Ms. N's sense of self and others distinguishes her identity formation from what would be seen as normal, and reflects the impact of repression-based defenses on the sense of self in a young woman with a consolidated identity in the setting of conflicts in relation to sexuality and competitive aggression.

> **STIPO-R Identity Rating: Level 2   Consolidated identity, but with some areas of slight deficit**—Sense of self and others is well integrated for the most part, but with mild superficiality, instability, or distortion, and/or with some difficulty in investment in work/school or recreation.

Object Relations.   Ms. N presents with a fully developed capacity for object relations in depth. She has established stable, long-lasting friendships that are mutually supportive and relatively free of conflict. However, in contrast to the normal personality, there is evidence of a focal but significant problem with romantic/sexual relationships, characterized by severe inhibition expressed in limited dating experience and her failure to have found a long-term intimate partner, as would be normative for her social group.

> **STIPO-R Object Relations Rating: Level 2   Attachments are generally strong,** durable, realistic, nuanced, and sustained over time, with some conflict or incomplete satisfaction; relationships are not seen in terms of need fulfillment; capacity for interdependence and empathy is fully developed; there is some degree of impairment or conflict in intimate/sexual relationships.

Defenses.   The clinician sees little to no evidence of lower-level defenses; defenses are characterized by a combination of flexible, adaptive coping (mature/healthy defenses)—in particular, sublimation of her wish to have children and her altruism in relation to her students. The clinician also sees the impact of repression-based defenses in focal areas of conflict—in particular, sexuality and aggression, leading to rigidity in the form of inhibitions interfering with the formation of romantic relationships and maladaptive coping strategies involving avoidance of confrontation and competition.

> **STIPO-R Defenses Rating: Level 2   Adaptive coping strategies are used with less consistency or efficacy,** or in some areas but not others, with general resilience to stress. Some lower-level defenses are endorsed (may be limited to idealization and/or devaluation), but

these are clearly not the predominant defensive style of the respondent; limited or no impairment in functioning is seen from use of lower-level defenses.

Aggression.   Ms. N demonstrates good control of aggression. Her functioning in this domain is distinguished from the normal personality by some inhibition in the adaptive expression of aggression, leaving her with difficulty asserting herself and a tendency to avoid confrontation.

> **STIPO-R Aggression Rating: Level 2   Relatively good control of aggression**—maladaptive expressions of aggression are limited to inhibitions (failure to express aggression), minor self-destructive behaviors or neglect, a controlling interpersonal style, or occasional verbal outbursts.

Moral Values.   Ms. N demonstrates fully internalized moral values and ideals. She takes pleasure in "giving back." Her functioning in this domain is distinguished from the normal personality on the basis of mild rigidity, expressed in self-criticism when she fails to meet the high standards that she sets for herself.

> **STIPO-R Moral Values Rating: Level 2   Internal moral compass is autonomous and consistent, with rigidity and/or ambiguity involving questionable opportunities for personal gain;** no evidence is seen of frankly amoral or immoral behavior; the individual demonstrates some rigidity (either excessive or some laxity) in sense of concern and responsibility for potentially hurtful or unethical behavior; the individual experiences guilt, but in such a way that ruminative self-recrimination is more prevalent than proactive efforts to make amends.

Summary.   Ms. N can be classified dimensionally using the STIPO-R ratings as follows: Identity—Level 2; Object Relations—Level 2; Defenses—Level 2; Aggression—Level 2, and Moral Values—Level 2. Referring to Table 2–1, in addition to this dimensional assessment, the clinician can describe Ms. N as organized at a neurotic level of personality organization. Her prognosis is excellent, and the clinician can anticipate a relatively smooth treatment course.

Borderline Level of Personality Organization

In the personality disorders organized at a borderline level, patients present with severely maladaptive personality rigidity in the setting of 1) clinically significant identity pathology; 2) a predominance of lower-level, splitting-based, defensive operations; and 3) variable reality testing (in which ordinary reality testing is grossly intact but can be vulnerable in the setting of affect activation) and impairment of the more subtle capacities to appreciate social conventions and to accurately perceive the inner states of others. Most of the personality disorders described in DSM-5 are found in this more severe group of personality disorders, including dependent, histrionic, narcissistic, borderline, paranoid, schizoid, and antisocial personality disorders. Individuals organized at a borderline level have pervasive difficulties that adversely compromise functioning in many if not all domains, and maladaptive traits are more extreme and more rigid than those of individuals in the NPO group.

Clinical Illustration 2: Borderline Level of Personality Organization

Ms. B, a 28-year-old, single, employed woman was seen in consultation. Like Ms. N (in Clinical Illustration 1), Ms. B presented with a chief complaint of "problems with men." Physically attractive, Ms. B wore a short skirt and low-cut blouse to the interview. Though she was cooperative, her manner was sexually provocative in a way that left the male consultant uncomfortable. When the consultant asked her about her style of dress, Ms. B explained that she "needed a lot of attention" and that she had a history of throwing temper tantrums when she did not get it. This latter comment had the air of a veiled threat.

Ms. B described a series of brief relationships with men that according to her report always ended badly. She began each relationship with the feeling that "this is the one who will solve all my problems," only to find herself disappointed and frustrated down the road. Ms. B told the consultant that when her feelings toward her boyfriends changed, she found it difficult to control her anger with them; on one occasion, she had verbally assaulted and threatened a man whom she had been dating, to such an extent that he called the police.

When asked about her relationship with her parents, Ms. B shrugged as she explained that she had been estranged from them since they discovered she had on one occasion taken "just 20 dollars" from her mother's purse ("I was desperate"); when the interviewer asked if Ms. B could sympathize with her parents' feelings, Ms. B responded that she had hoped they would "give me a break." She otherwise denied a history of stealing or of any other illegal activity.

She had a scattered group of friends—"more acquaintances, actually"—who came and went. Her sister was the only person whom she trusted or felt attached to. Since dropping out of community college after one semester, she had held a series of jobs; she was currently working as a receptionist. She found her work dreary, boring, and pointless, although she could not think of anything else that she would rather be doing for

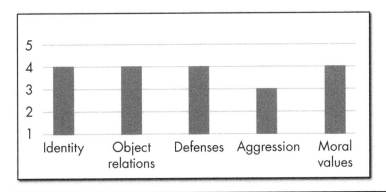

FIGURE 2–4.   STIPO-R profile for Ms. B (BPO).

STIPO-R ratings: Identity—Level 4; Object relations—Level 4; Defenses—Level 4; Aggression—Level 3; Moral values—Level 4.

BPO = borderline level of personality organization; STIPO-R = Structured Interview of Personality Organization—Revised (Clarkin et al. 2016).

work or a career. She routinely spent time on the job doing online shopping and making social calls on her phone, and she frequently called in sick; she justified these behaviors on the basis of the boring and routine nature of her work.

Ms. B described feeling unhappy and resentful much of the time; she enjoyed shopping but otherwise had few interests. She felt her life was "going nowhere," and she was plagued by chronic feelings of emptiness. When asked to describe herself, her initial retort was hostile: "I suck and I always get the short end of the stick—is that what you want to hear?!" During the interview, the consultant found himself feeling increasingly burdened by the profound and pervasive emptiness that characterized Ms. B's narrative and experience, along with the chaotic level of her functioning in multiple domains.

Figure 2–4 shows the STIPO-R profile for Ms. B, followed by discussion of the STIPO-R ratings for this patient.

Guide to STIPO-R Ratings for Ms. B (BPO)

Identity.   In the case of Ms. B, the clinician sees extensive evidence of relatively severe identity pathology. Her sense of both herself and others was superficial, polarized, and unstable; her views of her boyfriends alternated between dissociated, idealized, and paranoid attitudes. She had no personal interests or investments and was unable to identify goals for herself in any domain of functioning. She suffered from painful feelings of chronic emptiness, a hallmark of severe identity pathology.

> STIPO-R Identity Rating: Level 4   Moderate identity pathology—
> Sense of self and others is poorly integrated (significant superficiality or incoherence; markedly unstable, contradictory, and distorted), with little capacity to invest in work/school or recreation.

Object Relations.   The clinician sees extreme poverty of interpersonal relations; she describes only one stable attachment, with her sister, and otherwise her relationships are extremely superficial, with others described as "acquaintances." Interpersonal interactions are based on need fulfillment and in particular, her need for attention and sexual admiration from others. She demonstrates no capacity for empathy, either with her boyfriends or with her parents, and her attempts to seek intimacy are chaotic and invariably fail.

> STIPO-R Object Relations Rating: Level 4   Attachments are few and highly superficial; relationships are consistently viewed in terms of need fulfillment; there is little capacity for empathy; despite any demonstrated efforts to seek intimacy, few to no intimate relationships have developed.

Defenses.   Ms. B demonstrates extensive use of splitting-based defenses, leading to gross impairment in functioning. In this brief vignette, there is idealization and devaluation in her relationships with boyfriends, externalization ("I always get the short end of the stick"), and a suggestion of projective identification in the uneasiness she stimulated in the interviewer. The clinician can infer that Ms. B's social isolation reflects a level of paranoia compatible with lower-level projection.

> STIPO-R Defenses Rating: Level 4   Lower-level defenses are consistently endorsed; shifts in perception of self and others are relatively severe and pervasive. Clear evidence of impairment in respondent's life is seen from use of lower-level defenses.

Aggression.   Ms. B shows evidence of moderately extreme forms of externally directed aggression in her history of frequent verbally abusive outbursts, manipulative tantrums, and threats to her boyfriends, on one occasion leading to police involvement. The absence of physical assault or acts of violence distinguishes Ms. B's functioning in this domain from that of persons at Level 4.

> STIPO-R Aggression Rating: Level 3   Moderately poor control of aggression—maladaptive expressions of aggression include significant self-destructive or higher-risk behaviors, self-neglect or non-

compliance, and/or frequent tantrums or outbursts of hateful verbal aggression, chronic hostile control of others, and/or deriving sadistic pleasure from others' discomfort or misfortune.

Moral Values. The clinician sees significant laxity of moral functioning; Ms. B acknowledged having stolen money from her mother, rationalizing that because she was in need and the sum was small, her behavior was not problematic. Ms. B's exploitation of her employers by frequently calling in sick when she was not ill and spending work time on personal matters is further evidence of failure of moral functioning; her behavior is ego-syntonic, and even though she knows the difference between right and wrong, she relies on rationalization when her actions are questioned, demonstrating a lack of appropriate guilt or concern. The absence of more extensive antisocial behavior or exploitation distinguishes Ms. B's functioning in this domain from that of persons at STIPO-R Level 5.

> **STIPO-R Moral Values Rating: Level 4** **Moral values and internal standards are weak, inconsistent, and/or corrupt;** moral orientation is toward not getting caught and may include presence of aggressive antisocial behavior (e.g., robbery, forgery, blackmail); such behavior may involve confrontation of victims, but without assault, and any violence that occurs is generally not premeditated; exploitation of others is ego-syntonic and the individual freely pursues opportunities for personal gain at the expense of others; guilt or remorse is lacking.

Summary. Ms. B can be classified dimensionally using the STIPO-R ratings as follows: Identity—Level 4; Object Relations—Level 4; Defenses—Level 4; Aggression—Level 3; and Moral Values—Level 4. Referring to Table 2–1, in addition to this dimensional assessment, the clinician can describe Ms. B as organized at a middle borderline level of personality organization. Ms. B's pathology of moral functioning presents potential treatment challenges.

Dimensional Nature of Classification and High, Middle, and Low Borderline Personality Organization

Despite the apparently categorical nature of our framework, as it is described in this chapter and represented in Figure 2–1 and Figure 2–2, the structural approach in fact assumes a dimensional perspective on personality pathology (Kernberg and Caligor 2005). As a result, the demarcation between neurotic and borderline levels of personality organization is dimensional, and there are patients with mild identity pathology who present with mixed features. Similarly, patients with neurotic personality organization, characterized by essentially normal identity formation, nevertheless may present with subtle, largely focal pathology in the sense of self and others. Most important, there is a broad spectrum of pathology within the BPO spectrum.

The group of personality disorders falling into the borderline level of personality organization is large and heterogeneous and can be further characterized according to severity on the basis of 1) quality of object relations and 2) moral functioning, along with increasing severity of identity pathology. Within the BPO group, evaluation of these additional dimensions leads to identification of *high-level borderline organization* (i.e., healthier individuals with less pathology of object relations, more intact moral functioning, and a better prognosis) and *low-level borderline organization* (i.e., those with more severe personality pathology, grossly impaired object relations, severe pathology of moral functioning, and a poor prognosis). Between these two categories is *middle-level borderline organization* (i.e., individuals falling between the previous two groups in relation to severity and having an intermediate prognosis) (see Figure 2–1 and Figure 2–2). Middle-level and low-level BPO represent *severe personality disorders* (Kernberg 1984).

An essential distinction between the high-BPO group and the middle- and low-BPO groups is the role played by aggression in psychological functioning and pathology. Psychopathology in the low-BPO group, and to a lesser but nonetheless significant degree in the middle-BPO group, is characterized by the expression of poorly integrated forms of aggression, which may be inwardly and/or outwardly directed and are a central cause of anxiety. Aggression is less central in individuals with high-level borderline pathology, who struggle primarily with anxieties related to dependency and self-esteem maintenance, and only secondarily with aggression. The high-BPO group includes dependent, histrionic, and more disturbed avoidant personalities, as well as the healthier end of the narcissistic spectrum. The low-BPO group includes antisocial personality disorder and more severe forms of narcissistic personality disorder presenting with prominent antisocial features, including malignant narcissism.

The remaining personality disorders—borderline, schizoid, paranoid, and schizotypal—typically fall into the middle borderline range; these personality disorders may also fall into the low borderline range, depending on the presence of comorbid antisocial and narcissistic features. Ms. B, introduced in Clinical Illustration 2 in the foregoing section, is illustrative of personality disorders falling in the middle borderline range.

Clinical Illustration 3: High Borderline Level of Personality Organization

Mr. H, a 38-year-old married lawyer without children, was seen in consultation for complaints of anxiety. Dressed in a suit and tie, Mr. H was overweight, slightly disheveled, and visibly sweating, and made limited eye contact. He described his work at a small law firm as challenging and potentially beyond his abilities. He told the consultant he spent significant amounts of time while in the office in an anxious state, feeling that his colleagues were looking down on him and wondering whether they were speaking about him behind his back. He described at times becoming so uncomfortable that he felt compelled to flee the office, ultimately bingeing on ice cream.

Mr. H also described procrastination; he routinely put off tasks until the very last minute, which had compromised the quality of his work and on occasion led to his missing deadlines. In response to questions about his overall performance at work, Mr. H explained that his formal reviews had indicated problems and a need for improvement, but there had been no talk of letting him go, and despite his anxiety, he felt relatively secure in his position.

Mr. H described himself as shy, socially awkward, and passive, always comparing himself to others and feeling inferior. He admiringly described his wife as more powerful and effective than he, adding that she routinely bossed him around; she also criticized him for being overweight and for neglecting his health, "but rightfully so." When asked how he felt about his marital relationship, Mr. H said that he had "a great marriage." When asked to describe his wife, he responded, "Strong, wonderful—without her I'd be lost."

Mr. H had no close friends. He described hanging out once a week with a group of "drinking buddies" dating back to high school, and he stayed in touch with a college roommate who lived in another city. Mr. H enjoyed online poker and participated in several ongoing games, but otherwise had no outside interests. After hearing Mr. H's story, the consultant found himself concerned about the impact of Mr. H's personality pathology on his ability to retain a job, and wondered whether Mr. H had the necessary motivation to commit to longer-term treatment.

Figure 2–5 shows the STIPO-R profile for Mr. H, followed by discussion of the STIPO-R ratings for this patient.

Guide to STIPO-R Ratings for Mr. H (High BPO)

Identity.   The clinician sees evidence of identity pathology, most clearly in Mr. H's consistently idealized, superficial experience of his wife and his

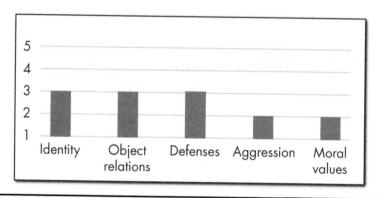

FIGURE 2–5. STIPO-R profile for Mr. H (high BPO).

STIPO-R ratings: Identity—Level 3; Object relations—Level 3; Defenses—Level 3; Aggression—Level 2; Moral values—Level 2.

BPO=borderline level of personality organization; STIPO-R=Structured Interview of Personality Organization—Revised (Clarkin et al. 2016).

correspondingly devalued self representation. Identity pathology is not extremely severe, although it is clinically significant; the clinician does not see the profoundly unstable and incoherent experience of self and others that characterizes more severe pathology. Mr. H demonstrated goal-directed behavior in having graduated from law school and in working in the legal profession. His investment in his career, however, seems somewhat superficial, and his personal interests are limited to online poker.

> **STIPO-R Identity Rating: Level 3   Mild identity pathology—**
> Sense of self and/or others is somewhat poorly integrated (evident superficiality or incoherence and instability, at times contradictory and distorted), with clear impairment in capacity to invest in work/ school and/or recreation; or individual invests largely to meet narcissistic needs.

Object Relations.   Mr. H demonstrates moderately severe pathology of object relations. His most significant relationship is with his wife. Although this relationship is stable and long-lasting, it is based on brittle idealization and fulfillment of Mr. H's dependency needs. Other relationships, although sustained over time, are distant and superficial.

> **STIPO-R Object Relations Rating: Level 3   Attachments are present but are superficial,** brittle, and marked by conflict and lack of satisfaction; relationships tend to be viewed in terms of need ful-

fillment; there is some capacity for concern for the other or some degree of empathy; sexual relationships have limited intimacy.

Defenses.   The clinician sees some evidence of repression-based defenses (inhibitions in relation to aggression in the form of submitting to his wife; procrastination at work), with predominant and consistent use of lower-level defenses in the form of stable idealization of his wife and denial of problems in both his marriage and work, with occasional acting out by bingeing on ice cream.

> **STIPO-R Defenses Rating: Level 3   Lower-level defenses have a mixed pattern of endorsement;** shifts in perception of self and others are present. Some impairment in functioning is seen from use of lower-level defenses.

Aggression.   Mr. H shows relatively mild pathology of aggression, which is limited predominantly to self-defeating behavior, self-neglect (he is overweight and generally neglects his health), and inhibited expression of aggression. No evidence of other-directed aggression is present.

> **STIPO-R Aggression Rating: Level 2   Relatively good control of aggression**—maladaptive expressions of aggression are limited to inhibitions (failure to express aggression), minor self-destructive behaviors or neglect, a controlling interpersonal style, or occasional verbal outbursts.

Moral Values.   Mr. H demonstrates no evidence of frankly amoral or immoral behavior, although the clinician notes an absence of appropriate feelings of responsibility or concern in relation to his performance at work.

> **STIPO-R Moral Values Rating: Level 2   Internal moral compass is autonomous and consistent, with rigidity and/or ambiguity involving questionable opportunities for personal gain;** no evidence is seen of frankly amoral or immoral behavior; the individual demonstrates some rigidity (either excessive or some laxity) in sense of concern and responsibility for potentially hurtful or unethical behavior; the individual experiences guilt, but in such a way that ruminative self-recrimination is more prevalent than proactive efforts to make amends.

Summary.   Mr. H can be classified dimensionally using the STIPO-R ratings as follows: Identity—Level 3; Object Relations—Level 3; Defenses—

Level 3; Aggression—Level 2; and Moral Values—Level 2. Referring to Table 2–1, in addition to this dimensional assessment, the clinician can describe Mr. H as organized at a high borderline level of personality organization, with a relatively positive prognosis for treatment.

Clinical Illustration 4: Low Borderline Level of Personality Organization

Mr. L, a 38-year-old, married, unemployed lawyer without children, was seen in consultation with complaints of "depression" and "problems with work." Mr. L initially told the consultant that his greatest problem was that he procrastinated, explaining that this was a reflection of his being "too conscientious." However, as the interview proceeded, it emerged that since graduating from law school 10 years earlier, Mr. L had been fired from a series of jobs because he had failed to complete projects and often missed deadlines; he also had a history of falsifying time sheets, frequently calling in sick, and getting into power struggles with his bosses. His experience of the jobs and of being let go was of having been treated unfairly, with no sense of personal responsibility for negative consequences. He had most recently worked as a paralegal, a job he found demeaning, and he had been fired 6 months before the consultation after physically threatening a coworker and then pushing him against a copy machine, an act he described as "fully justified under the circumstances."

Mr. L was emotionally distant and subtly hostile and devaluing in the interview. He described himself as alternating between feeling smarter than everyone else and feeling like a "dumb loser," and he reported that his wife complained that he provided neither financial nor emotional support. Mr. L explained that he had lost sexual interest in his wife early in the marriage and that he routinely visited prostitutes. He stayed in the marriage because his wife owned the apartment they lived in, and he enjoyed living off her income. When asked to describe his wife, to provide a lifelike, three-dimensional picture of her, Mr. L responded: "She's boring, complains all the time, and I'm sick of her." When the interviewer prompted him for additional information, perhaps something positive about his wife, Mr. L responded, "She earns good money and lets me stay in her apartment."

Mr. L complained of feeling empty and restless. He wanted the consultant to tell him how to feel less dysphoric and anxious, and how to have a more stable sense of himself as exceptional. At the end of a 90-minute interview, the consultant found himself with only a superficial, caricature-like sense of Mr. L and an even more shadowy image of his wife. The consultant noted feeling put off by Mr. L's dishonesty, exploitiveness, and devaluation.

Figure 2–6 shows the STIPO-R profile for Mr. L, followed by discussion of the STIPO-R ratings for this patient.

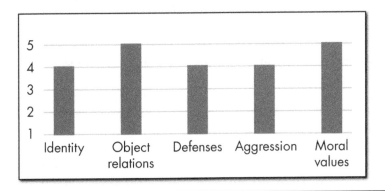

FIGURE 2–6. STIPO-R profile for Mr. L (low BPO).
STIPO-R ratings: Identity—Level 4; Object relations—Level 5; Defenses—Level 4;
Aggression—Level 4; Moral values—Level 5.
BPO = borderline level of personality organization; STIPO-R = Structured Interview of
Personality Organization—Revised (Clarkin et al. 2016).

Guide to STIPO-R Ratings for Mr. L (Low BPO)

Identity. In Mr. L, the clinician sees moderately severe identity pathology
expressed in poorly integrated, superficial, polarized, and contradictory experiences of self, colored by idealization and devaluation, as well as by a
markedly superficial, vague, devalued, and caricature-like experience of his
wife. Although Mr. L managed to graduate from law school, at present, he
is unemployed and demonstrates no longer-term goals or investments.

> **STIPO-R Identity Rating: Level 4   Moderate identity pathology—**
> Sense of self and others is poorly integrated (significant superficiality
> or incoherence; markedly unstable, contradictory, and distorted),
> with little capacity to invest in work/school or recreation.

Object Relations. The clinician sees a man with no social connections
other than with his wife. Mr. L's relationship with her is expressly need-
fulfilling and overtly exploitive; beyond gratification of these needs, he
demonstrates no interest in relationships, with no capacity for empathy
or attempts at intimacy.

> **STIPO-R Object Relations Rating: Level 5   No true relationships**
> **exist** (may have acquaintances); the individual may be severely iso-
> lated, lacking even acquaintances; any relations that exist are based
> exclusively on need fulfillment; there is no demonstrated capacity

for empathy; no capacity for intimacy and/or no attempts at intimacy are evident.

Defenses.   Mr. L's pervasive reliance on splitting, idealization, and devaluation leads to extreme shifts and distortions in his experience of himself that interfere with functioning and are the cause of constant distress. His experiences of others, such as his wife, are either similarly shifting or consistently devalued and distorted.

> **STIPO-R Defenses Rating: Level 5   Lower-level defenses are used pervasively across situations.** Severe, radical shifts in perception of self and others are to a degree that grossly interferes with functioning, with multiple examples of instability and distortion.

Aggression.   Mr. L demonstrates poor control of poorly integrated aggression, outwardly directed. Aggression is expressed in frequently hateful and abusive verbal outbursts, power struggles with bosses, verbal threats, and the physical assault of a coworker.

> **STIPO-R Aggression Rating: Level 4   Poor control of aggression—** If self-directed, aggression is severe to lethal, but somewhat less pervasive, less chronic (i.e., more episodic), and/or less life-threatening than aggression in item 5. If other-directed, aggression is episodic but frequent, with hateful verbal abuse of others, frequent verbal and physical threats to hurt self or other, and/or physical intimidation that may involve physically threatening or assaulting the other, with pleasure in hurting and/or hostile control of others.

Moral Values.   Although he has not found himself in trouble with the law, Mr. L appears to have no comprehension of moral values. He demonstrates no sense of guilt or remorse in relation to his violent behavior in the workplace, financial exploitation of his wife, or use of prostitutes, nor any regret in relation to his behavior in the workplace; all are fully ego-syntonic and in his mind justified.

> **STIPO-R Moral Values Rating: Level 5   No comprehension of the notion of moral values** is evident; the presence of violent, aggressive antisocial behavior (assault, battery, premeditation) or frank psychopathy (no comprehension or notion of moral values) with or without violent behavior is evident; there is no sense of guilt or remorse.

Summary. Mr. L can be classified dimensionally using the STIPO-R ratings as follows: Identity—Level 4; Object Relations—Level 5; Defenses—Level 4; Aggression—Level 4; and Moral Values—Level 5. Referring to Table 2–1, in addition to this dimensional assessment, the clinician can describe Mr. L as organized at a low borderline level of personality organization. His severe pathology of both object relations and moral values leave him with an extremely guarded prognosis, and his motivation for treatment is extremely superficial and unrealistic.

Part 3

Psychological Structures and Levels of Personality Disorder

Identity

As described in the text, the construct of identity anchors the object relations theory model of personality disorders—and identity consolidation distinguishes the normal personality and neurotic-level personality disorders on the one hand, from the personality disorders organized at a borderline level on the other (see Figure 2–1). In the TFP-E approach, normal identity and identity pathology are described from the perspective of the impact of identity formation on the individual's internal and external functioning, and also from the perspective of the organization and level of integration of the internal object relations that function as the building blocks of identity and that organize subjective experience.

Normal Identity Formation

Identity Consolidation

Normal identity formation, or *identity consolidation*, corresponds with an integrated sense of self, which is manifested subjectively in experiences both of the self and of significant others that are complex, realistic, and continuous across time and situations. Normal identity formation is manifested in the ability to invest, over time, in professional, intellectual, and recreational interests, and to "know one's own mind" with regard to one's values, opinions, tastes, and beliefs. The coherent sense of self conferred by normal identity formation is basic to healthy self-esteem, the capacity to make and derive pleasure from commitments to relationships and to work, and the ability to pursue long-term goals. A coherent and integrated conception of others, in addition, is associated with the ability to accurately appreciate the internal experience of others, contributing to the capacity for empathy and social tact, and thus confers the ability to interact and relate successfully with others (Kernberg 2006).

Identity formation also has bearing on the nature of *affective experience*; identity consolidation is associated with the capacity to experience a range of complex and well-modulated affects in the setting of a predominantly positive affective experience. Identity consolidation also confers the capacity to experience even states of high affective arousal without the risk of loss of impulse control or compromise of *reality testing*, reflecting the role of a consistent and stable self in contextualizing and making sense of intense affect states (Kernberg 2016).

Internal Object Relations and the Contextualization of Experience

Within the object relations theory model of personality disorders developed in this manual, the focus on internal object relations centers on their function both as the building blocks of higher-order structures and as the organizers of subjective experience. In the normal personality, the internal object relations organizing the individual's experience of self and others are *well integrated*. These well-integrated object relations coalesce to form a stable and flexible overarching structure that corresponds with normal identity consolidation, conferring the experience of a stable, continuous, and realistic sense of self and others. When internal object relations are well integrated, they are associated with affects that are complex and well modulated, and representations are well differentiated, characterized by subtlety and depth, and include shades of gray.

In normal identity, these well-integrated internal object relations naturally *coalesce*: they come to be stably organized in relation to one another, forming an overarching structure, such that the internal object relations activated and organizing moment-to-moment experience remain at the same time embedded in an ongoing sense of self and significant others. As a result, in the setting of identity consolidation, different, relatively well-integrated and realistic internal object relations are fluidly activated across different situations and emotional states, while the individual's experience remains anchored by and embedded in a stable structure that provides a continuous and consistent sense of self and others.

It is this structural configuration that confers the capacity to pull together different aspects of another person to make up a coherent "whole" image of the other, as well as to maintain a continuous sense of self across time and situations. *Normal personality functioning* implies not only integration but also flexibility; normal identity consolidation confers the capacity to flexibly contain within the overall structure of identity even those experiences of self and other that are *conflictual* (i.e., potentially threatening to the individual's sense of himself and his world). This capacity to flexibly manage conflictual object relations corresponds with the impact of mature defensive operations on psychological functioning.

Identity in the Neurotic Level of Personality Organization

In the setting of the neurotic level of personality organization, identity formation closely resembles the organization that characterizes the normal personality. In individuals at this level, consolidation of well-integrated internal object relations helps to form a stable, continuous, and largely realistic experience of self and others. However, in contrast to what is seen in the normal personality, in which conflictual object relations are fluidly contained and managed within an overarching sense of self, in the setting of NPO, the more extreme and highly affectively charged experiences of self and others associated with psychological conflict are excluded from, rather than contained within, a stable and relatively well-integrated sense of self, and remain stably out of conscious awareness. This configuration reflects the impact of repression-based defenses, which operate to exclude conflictual object relations from an otherwise consolidated identity; the conflictual experiences of self and other associated with these object relations are not part of conscious self experience and instead are repressed. This structural situation results in minor distortions in the experience of self and others in the setting of consolidated identity; in focal areas of conflict, the experience of self and others is rigid, somewhat distorted, and to some degree superficial or "washed out" (see Clinical Illustration 1, earlier in chapter).

Pathology of Identity Formation: Syndrome of Identity Diffusion

Normal identity contrasts with pathological identity formation, which in its more extreme version is sometimes referred to as the syndrome of *iden-*

tity diffusion (Kernberg 1980; Kernberg and Caligor 2005), the structural hallmark of the severe personality disorders (those organized at low and middle borderline levels). In the setting of poorly consolidated identity, the individual lacks an overarching, coherent sense of self and of significant others. Instead, the subjective experience of self and others is unstable, fragmented across time, and distorted—polarized ("all good" or "all bad," idealized or paranoid), poorly differentiated, and superficial. Individuals with identity diffusion lack the capacity to accurately "read" others (Donegan et al. 2003; Wagner and Linehan 1999) and may be unable to respond tactfully to subtle social cues. They demonstrate a paucity of meaningful investments in professional, intellectual, and recreational pursuits. Tastes, opinions, and values are inconsistent, typically adopted from others in the environment, and may shift easily and dramatically with changes in milieu. In the setting of poorly consolidated identity, affective experience is superficial and poorly integrated, and in the setting of conflict, affective experience is often extreme and poorly modulated. Identity diffusion is characterized by the predominance of negative affective experience, often in the form of chronic dysphoria, free-floating anxiety, or feelings of emptiness, with limited capacity for enjoyment, pleasure, or contentment. In addition, in the setting of identity diffusion, states of high affective arousal may be associated with loss of impulse control and may transiently compromise reality testing.

The structural correlate of identity diffusion is the failure of internal object relations to coalesce to form a stable, realistic, and flexible experience of self and others. In the setting of identity diffusion, individual internal object relations are *poorly integrated*. When internal object relations are identified as poorly integrated, they are associated with affects that are highly charged, lacking in complexity, and typically highly positive or highly negative; these affect states are linked to representations that are extreme, poorly differentiated, superficial, or caricature-like, and polarized into either all good or all bad. The poorly integrated quality of internal object relations in the setting of the failure of identity consolidation reflects the impact of splitting-based defenses on psychological organization and functioning (see next section, "Defenses," for a discussion of splitting).

These poorly integrated and highly affectively charged object relations do not coalesce to form a stable core sense of self, but instead are only loosely organized in relation to one another. In this setting, different internal object relations will be activated in different situations and emotional states, without being anchored in or contextualized in relation to a continuous and consistent sense of self. The outcome is a relatively fragmented and affectively charged series of superficial and contradictory experiences of self and other, each organized by a particular internal object relation, with one experience poorly related to the next.

Clinical Illustration 5: Identity Diffusion in High Borderline Level of Personality Organization

A young woman with the diagnosis of histrionic personality disorder with dependent features organized at a high borderline level was seen in consultation. She had graduated from college and then worked at a series of jobs in a variety of fields, including publishing, home decorating, landscaping, and data analysis; none had been particularly interesting or meaningful to her, and she had been unable to identify longer-term career goals. She enjoyed reading novels and spending time on social media, but otherwise denied personal interests or hobbies.

When the consultant asked her to describe herself, she could come up with little to say but did comment that most of the time she felt depressed, empty, and aimless. She added that it was difficult to describe herself because her view of herself and her mood state frequently shifted, depending on where she was or whom she was with (friends, family, coworkers); she would change her style of dress, taste in music, and patterns of speech to suit her latest group of friends. When asked about the important people in her life, she explained that boyfriends came and went; typically, they seemed great at first but quickly became controlling and abusive. Her descriptions of others in her life were vague, general, and polarized—for example, she characterized individuals as "nice," "pretty," and "funny," or "selfish" and "heartless."

Clinical Illustration 4 *(continued)*: Identity Diffusion in Low Borderline Level of Personality Organization

Mr. L, the unemployed lawyer introduced earlier in this chapter, was diagnosed with narcissistic personality disorder organized at a low borderline level. He had been out of work for many months, spending his days watching television or wandering about the city. When asked about goals and interests, he said that he had no goals, enjoyed watching football on television, and otherwise did not have personal interests or hobbies. When with his wife, Mr. L was withdrawn and hostile. When socializing at his gym, however, he behaved entirely differently: he was outgoing, charming, and flirtatious. Mr. L's references to his wife were superficial, vague, and one-dimensional, adding up to more of a caricature than a complex and realistic description of another person. When asked specifically to describe his wife, Mr. L could only provide a string of negative adjectives: "boring," "nagging," and "no fun," and he explained that he had never derived any pleasure from their relationship. Even when prompted, he could think of nothing positive to say about her, though he acknowledged that she "provides income" and "takes care of the house." When asked to describe himself, he acknowledged that most of the time he felt "better and smarter" than others, but said that this view of himself would at times collapse, leaving him feeling "like a worm."

Although most clearly evident in DSM-5 borderline personality disorder, some degree of identity pathology characterizes all personality disorders (see Figure 2–2). There are different degrees of identity pathology and different ways in which it may become manifest. Borderline personality disorder is in many ways the prototype of the personality disorders characterized by identity disturbance; both the sense of self and the sense of others are polarized, vague, unrealistic, and unstable. Temporal discontinuity tends to be an especially prominent subjective manifestation of identity pathology in individuals with borderline personality disorder.

In contrast, in narcissistic personality disorder, a more stable sense of self, albeit distorted and often fragile, coexists with what is often a dramatically superficial, shadowy, or caricature-like experience of others, even in individuals who are highly intelligent and accomplished. Feelings of inauthenticity tend to be an especially prominent subjective manifestation of identity pathology in the narcissistic group. In contrast, in the schizoid personality, the clinician sees a capacity to appraise others in the absence of any integrated or stable sense of self, in conjunction with prominent feelings of emptiness. In personality disorders falling in the high BPO range, identity disturbance can be relatively mild, characterized by a sense of self that is more complex and less unstable than that characteristic of individuals organized at a low borderline level, along with a better developed capacity to sustain relationships with significant others.

Defenses

Defenses are an individual's automatic psychological response to external stressors or psychological conflict.[10] Different levels of personality pathology are associated with different dominant defensive operations, and defenses operate differently in individuals with consolidated identity than they do in those without. At the healthiest end of the spectrum, defenses

---

[10]Both object relations theory and attachment theory recognize the role of defensive operations, but in somewhat different ways (Levy et al. 2015).

TABLE 2–2.   Classification of defenses

Mature defenses: healthy adaptation and coping

  Suppression

  Anticipation

  Altruism

  Humor

  Sublimation

Repression-based defenses: conflictual aspects of internal experience are banished from consciousness

  Repression

  Isolation of affect

  Intellectualization

  Reaction formation

  Neurotic projection

  Displacement

Splitting-based defenses[a]: aspects of conscious experience are dissociated to avoid conflict

  Splitting

  Projective identification

  Lower-level idealization

  Devaluation

  Omnipotent control

  Lower-level denial

---

[a]Splitting-based defenses are often referred to as "primitive" defenses in the psychodynamic literature. Lower-level idealization and lower-level denial are sometimes referred to as "primitive idealization" and "primitive denial," respectively.

are flexible and adaptive and involve little or no distortion of internal or external reality. At the most pathological end of the spectrum, defenses are highly inflexible and maladaptive, involving gross distortion of reality (Vaillant 1992). Across the spectrum of personality pathology, defensive operations protect the individual from anxiety and pain associated with the expression of conflictual experiences of self and other, but at the cost of introducing maladaptive rigidity and structural pathology into personality functioning.

As shown in Table 2–2, Kernberg (1975) presents an approach to the classification of defenses that divides them into three groups: 1) mature defenses, 2) repression-based or "neurotic" defenses, and 3) splitting-based or lower-level (sometimes referred to as "primitive") defenses. This classification is in many ways consistent with the general consensus within the research community (Perry and Bond 2005), while placing greater emphasis on the psychological mechanisms underlying defensive operations. Mature, or healthy, defenses involve minimal distortion of internal and external reality and are associated with the flexible and adaptive functioning of the normal personality. Neurotic-level defenses avoid distress by repressing, or banishing from consciousness, aspects of the subject's psychological experience that are conflictual or a potential source of emotional discomfort. Splitting-based defenses do not banish mental contents from consciousness per se, but instead compartmentalize, or maintain distance between, conscious mental contents that are in conflict with each other or whose approximation would generate psychological conflict (Kernberg 1975).

Mature Defenses

Mature, or healthy, defenses are best described as adaptive and flexible coping mechanisms that enable the individual to deal with anxiety-provoking situations with a minimum of emotional distress (Vaillant 1992). Mature defenses correspond with the capacity to flexibly contain conflictual internal object relations within an overall positive sense of self and others. They are the predominant defensive style in the normal personality and are associated with flexible and adaptive functioning. Mature defenses do not bar any aspect of a conflict from consciousness, nor do they maintain a distance between aspects of emotional life that are in conflict. Rather, mature defenses allow all aspects of an anxiety-provoking situation into subjective awareness, with little or no distortion, but in a fashion that minimizes psychological distress while optimizing coping (Vaillant 1992).

Suppression, anticipation, altruism, humor, and sublimation are examples of mature defenses. *Suppression* involves intentionally and adaptively putting aside a particular thought or feeling until a time when constructive action can be taken. *Anticipation* involves planning ahead as a way to deal with potentially stressful situations. *Altruism* involves deriving satisfaction vicariously through helping others. *Humor* involves the capacity to see the comic aspects of a stressful situation as a way to reduce discomfort and to create useful distance from immediate events. *Sublimation* involves the constructive and creative redirection of conflictual motivations into nonconflictual areas of functioning, and is a central feature of normal adaptation.

Repression-Based Defenses

Repression-based, or neurotic, defenses serve to avoid distress by repressing, or banishing from consciousness, aspects of the individual's psychological experience that are conflictual or a potential source of emotional discomfort. At a structural level, repression-based defenses correspond with the capacity to stably split off conflictual internal object relations from an otherwise consolidated identity.

Individuals organized at a neurotic level rely predominantly on a combination of repression-based and mature defenses, and the rigidity that characterizes the neurotic level of personality organization reflects the impact of repression-based defenses on psychological functioning (Caligor et al. 2007; Shapiro 1981); conflictual aspects of experience are split off from the dominant sense of self and remain more or less permanently out of conscious awareness, protecting against recognition of conflictual experiences of self and other, but at the cost of introducing rigidity into personality functioning. Within the object relations theory model, enactment of defensive object relations supports repression, as seen in the following vignette.

Clinical Illustration 1 *(continued)*: Repression-Based Defense

Ms. N, the patient introduced earlier to illustrate neurotic level of personality organization, could be seen to make use of repression-based defenses to manage conflicts in relation to sexual competition and aggression. For example, when at a party, Ms. N was unaware of her conflictual wishes to command sexual attention; these wishes, perhaps represented by internal object relations of a powerful, sexually attractive woman-self in relation to 1) an admiring and responsive man and 2) an inferior, defeated woman, with both dyads associated with feelings of triumph and sexual pleasure, were excluded from Ms. N's dominant, conscious sense of self, and were repressed. Instead, enactment of nonconflictual, defensive object relations—for example, of a pleasant but sexually unattractive, girlish self in relation to an approving, friendly other, associated with feelings of security—dominated Ms. N's conscious self experience while supporting repression of conflictual wishes for sexual power and attention. Thus, repression-based defenses managed Ms. N's conflict by protecting her from awareness of conflictual motivations, but at the expense of introducing rigidity into her functioning; Ms. N was unable to behave in an openly sexually provocative manner or to freely enjoy sex, even at times when it would be both adaptive and appropriate to do so.

Repression-based defenses primarily alter the subject's *internal* reality, to some degree washing out affective experience in areas of conflict (Ms. N did not have access to the pleasures of commanding sexual attention and enjoying her sexuality) and causing subtle distortions in the view of self and other (Ms. N was not able to appreciate the extent to which she was a sexually attractive woman). However, repression-based defenses typically do so without grossly distorting the subject's sense of external reality (Ms. N was not unaware that she received sexual attention; she was simply perpetually surprised that she did). Thus, although repression-based defenses are responsible for personality rigidity and may interfere in focal areas of functioning or cause discomfort or distress, in contrast to splitting-based defenses, they typically do not lead to grossly abnormal or disruptive behaviors.

Although there are a variety of neurotic defenses that work in different ways, they all involve repression in the setting of a relatively well-integrated sense of self; some aspect of the subject's experience is split off and barred access to consciousness (Kernberg 1975). In classical *repression*, it is the idea that is repressed, whereas in *isolation of affect*, it is the affect that is repressed. *Intellectualization* is similar to isolation; here affect is repressed while the individual consciously focuses on abstract ideas. In *reaction formation*, both affect and the associated idea vanish and are replaced by their opposites. In *neurotic projection*, it is the connection between the subject and his motives and feelings that is repressed, and in *displacement*, the connection between a motive or feeling and a particular object is repressed.

Although not considered a neurotic defense (i.e., the process is not unconscious), *rationalization* supports repression by providing seemingly rational explanations for behaviors that have unconscious roots. Furthermore, rationalization and denial are often used to support both repression and splitting in the following ways:

- In the case of repression, rationalization provides seemingly rational explanations for behaviors that have unconscious roots, while denial causes the individual to neglect or deny the significance of these behaviors.
- In the more extreme case of splitting, rationalization may provide argument for the reasonableness of manifestly contradictory behaviors and experiences, while lower-level denial allows the individual to entirely shrug off of the significance of evident contradictions.

Splitting-Based Defenses

Whereas the neurotic defenses make use of repression, the lower-level, or splitting-based, defenses make use of dissociation,[11] or splitting, to avoid psychological conflict and emotional distress. In TFP-E, the terms *dissociation* and *splitting*[12] refer to a psychological process in which two aspects of experience that are in conflict are both allowed to emerge fully into consciousness, but either not at the same time or not in conjunction with the same object relation (Kernberg 1975). Instead, they are compartmentalized or split apart. Thus, while nothing is repressed when dissociative defenses are employed, conflicting aspects of psychological experience are not simultaneously experienced in relation to the self, and in this process, conflict is avoided.

Splitting-based defenses are the prototypical defenses seen in patients with severe personality disorders. Splitting is intimately tied to identity pathology in patients organized at a borderline level; splitting can be seen as responsible for maintaining the polarized, superficial, idealized, and paranoid experiences of self and others that characterize identity pathology across the BPO spectrum. In individuals organized at middle and low borderline levels, splitting-based defenses cause severe personality rigidity and are responsible for flagrant distortion of interpersonal reality, causing problems in the interpersonal lives of individuals with these personality

---

[11]We distinguish between dissociation as a defensive operation and dissociative states. *Dissociative states* involve the defensive operation of dissociation, but they also involve an altered state of consciousness; *dissociation* as a defensive operation does not involve an altered state of consciousness.

[12]In the psychodynamic literature, the terms *dissociative defenses* and *splitting* are often used more or less interchangeably. *Splitting* is used most frequently when referring to the dissociation of *idealized* (strongly positive) and *persecutory* (strongly negative), or loving and hateful, aspects of experience, whereas *dissociation* is more frequently used when referring to the separation of other aspects of self experience (e.g., sexual and dependent motivations) that are in conflict. The splitting-based defenses were first systematically described by Melanie Klein (1946/1975, 1952/1975) and include, in addition to splitting proper, lower-level idealization, devaluation, projective identification, omnipotent control, and lower-level denial. Klein suggested that the predominance of this constellation of defensive operations is a central feature of what she referred to as the *paranoid schizoid position*, a level of psychological development and mental organization that she viewed as quite primitive and characteristic of patients with severe psychopathology. As a result, she referred to the group of splitting-based defenses as *primitive defenses*, and she contrasted them with the classical neurotic defenses that are based on repression.

disorders. In this setting, splitting-based defenses typically have behavioral manifestations and frequently result in disruptive behaviors.

Individuals falling in the high BPO range rely on a combination of splitting-based defenses, which tend to be less extreme than those seen in more severe pathology, and repression-based defenses. This defensive organization is typically characterized by moderately stable but rigid functioning in many domains. However, in the setting of stress or in areas of psychological conflict, the individual is subject to intrusion into consciousness of more highly affectively charged, split experiences of self and others, leading to interpersonal distortions and often resulting in maladaptive behaviors.

In the setting of the failure of identity consolidation, splitting manages psychological conflict by segregating internal object relations associated with positive affect from those associated with negative affect. This splitting results in two dissociated, affectively charged, and equally distorted sectors of experience: one highly positive (referred to as *idealized*) and the other highly negative (referred to as *persecutory*, *paranoid*, or *devalued*). At the level of subjectivity, this leads to experiences of self and other that are polarized, superficial, and unrealistic—for example, *perfectly* gratifying caretaker or a source of *unbearable* frustration; a *perfect* protector or an object who *threatens to obliterate* the self; an *omnipotent* self or a feeble self devoid of *any* power.

Because splitting militates against integrative processes, these highly affectively charged and polarized internal object relations do not coalesce to form an overarching structure; as a result, when activated, they are not experienced as embedded in an ongoing experience of self and others. The outcome of this structural configuration is a fragmented and discontinuous, sometimes abruptly shifting and contradictory series of experiences that are poorly contextualized in relation to other experiences; whichever polarized and affectively charged object relation is the organizing experience in the moment comes to take over the entirety of the individual's subjectivity. In this setting, the distinction between internal experience and external reality can become blurred, lending a *concrete* quality to experience in the moment; it is as if the person could say, "How I experience it now is all there is, and there is no room to think about alternative perspectives; it is not that you are frustrating me now, but rather that you are a frustrating person."

Clinical Illustration 2 *(continued)*: Splitting-Based Defense

Ms. B, the patient introduced earlier in this chapter, was referred for individual dynamic therapy. During the first weeks of the therapy, she repeatedly told the therapist what a good listener he was, how well he understood her, and how helpful she found him to be, contrasting him with her "cold," "dull," and "uninsightful" previous treaters. Several weeks into the treatment, the therapist for the first time handed Ms. B a bill. Ms. B came to her next session in a rage and began to viciously attack the therapist; she called him "a charlatan," untrustworthy and incompetent, and said that she had been a fool to be in treatment with someone who clearly cared nothing about her as a person and was just using her to make money. The therapist commented that he was struck by the contradiction between Ms. B's current experience of him on the one hand, and, on the other hand, the positive attitude that had characterized their interactions up until this point and her previous experience of him as a good listener and as helpful. Ms. B responded that she remembered having had those thoughts, but they were irrelevant in the present; she now saw the therapist for who he truly was, and that was the only thing that mattered.

This brief vignette illustrates the unstable, widely polarized, superficial, and unrealistic views of others (and associated views of self) that are typical manifestations of splitting. In this setting, "all-good," idealized views of significant others temporarily ward off awareness of "all-bad," paranoid, and hateful object relations, with both views equally distorted. Initially, Ms. B enacts an idealized relationship with the therapist. When the therapist hands her a bill, her view of the therapist, and of herself in relation to the therapist, makes a dramatic shift, and highly negatively charged, paranoid object relations flood Ms. B's experience, while the idealized ones are lost to her; though remembered, they hold no emotional significance in that moment. Thus, both idealized and paranoid images of the therapeutic relationship are consciously experienced, but only at different times. When the therapist calls Ms. B's attention to the rapid shift in her view of him, Ms. B denies the emotional significance of her earlier idealized view of their relationship. This enables Ms. B to continue to separate the idealized aspect from the paranoid side of her experience.

The group of splitting-based defenses includes, in addition to splitting proper, projective identification, lower-level ("primitive") idealization, devaluation, omnipotence, and lower-level ("primitive") denial. In the setting of BPO, *splitting* most commonly involves separating sectors of experience associated with positive affects, along with idealized representations of self and others, on the one hand, from those sectors associated with negative affects and devalued or paranoid (also referred to as *persecutory*) object relations on the other. *Projective identification* involves splitting off aspects of one's internal experience and projecting them into another person so that the projected aspects of the self are experienced as part of the other person. At the same time, the individual using projective identification will interact with the other person to elicit responses consistent with what has been projected. (This is to say that in projective identification, projections tend to be actualized.)

Lower-level ("primitive") idealization is a form of splitting that involves seeing others as all good so as to avoid anxieties associated with negative feelings. Idealization is often followed by its opposite, *devaluation*. In *omnipotent control*, a grandiose self magically controls a depreciated, emotionally degraded other. *Lower-level ("primitive") denial* supports splitting by maintaining a disregard for aspects of the internal or external world that are either contradictory or potentially threatening. As illustrated in the vignette of Ms. B, when lower-level denial is employed, the individual is cognitively aware of a threatening experience, but this awareness fails to evince the corresponding emotional reaction.

Individuals organized at a neurotic level also make use of defenses based on dissociation and splitting.[13] However, in contrast to severe personality disorders, here the impact of splitting and dissociation is on the psychological experience of an individual who has a consolidated identity and a relatively well-integrated sense of self and experience of significant others. In this setting, splitting and dissociation are less extreme and more stable than in more severe personality pathology, and they do not lead to the highly polarized, rapidly shifting, and affectively charged experiences of internal and external reality that are characteristic of the severe personality disorders.

Rather than the highly distorted and affectively charged experiences seen in conjunction with splitting in BPO, in individuals organized at a neurotic level, splitting and dissociation are associated with the segregation of aspects of psychological experience that are relatively well integrated but in conflict, and with the more or less subtle dissociation of conflictual motivations from dominant self experience (Caligor et al. 2007). For example, a young man was sexually timid and at times impotent with his girlfriends, but when unattached would have one-night stands in which he was sexually adventurous, free of his usual inhibitions, and "not at all like myself." This young man demonstrated an inability to integrate tender and passionate feelings within the same relationship. In contrast to Ms. N, who used repression to manage her sexual conflicts,

---

[13]For a discussion of splitting proper in the NPO patient, see the Chapter 3 clinical illustration "Dynamic Relationship Between Paranoid and Depressive Orientations in a Patient Organized at a Neurotic Level" for an example and discussion of "splitting of the depressive position."

this young man relied on dissociation. He acted on his sexual motivations, but only in a manner dissociated from his dominant self experience; both tender and sexual motivations were consciously experienced and enacted, but not at the same time or in relation to the same person.

Another example is a female patient who, despite being generally quite critical and devaluing of the men in her life, quietly idealized her husband; she rarely found fault with him, avidly defending him when others criticized him, and felt herself extremely fortunate to have found "such an unusual and wonderful man." This woman demonstrated an inability to integrate tenderness and hostility; she relied on idealization and dissociation to protect her relationship with her husband from hostile feelings. Like the young man mentioned just previously in relation to sexual motivations, this woman fully experienced both tender and hostile feelings toward men, but only by dissociating them; she dissociated all hostility from her relationship with her husband, while criticizing and devaluing the other men in her life.

Quality of Object Relations

Quality of object relations refers to the internal beliefs, expectations, and capacities that organize an individual's interpersonal relations, as well as to the capacity to establish and sustain mutual and intimate attachments. In the normal personality, the ability to maintain mutually dependent relationships is based on an understanding of give and take, the ability to appreciate and care about the needs of the other independent of the needs of the self, and a capacity for concern. The normal personality is also associated with the capacity to integrate intimacy and sexuality in romantic love. The neurotic level of personality organization, too, is associated with the capacity for mutual dependency and concern, but often in the context of a failure to fully integrate intimate and mutually dependent relations with sexuality. Thus, an individual who is able to establish mutually dependent intimate relationships may repeatedly find himself unable to sustain an enjoyable sexual life with an intimate partner.

In contrast, the borderline level of personality organization is characterized by pathology of object relations. In low and middle borderline levels of personality organization, pathology of object relations is relatively severe, and a need-fulfilling orientation toward interpersonal relations predominates. Relations are viewed and evaluated in terms of the extent to which they meet the needs of the self; this orientation is often tied to the assumption that relations are organized on a quid pro quo basis (i.e., "If I do something for you, I expect to receive something in return"). Pathology of quality of object relations is most extreme in the antisocial personality, for which all human interactions are based on usage and exploitation of others.

Individuals organized at a high borderline level are most clearly distinguished from those with more severe pathology by virtue of their capacity for at least some—and, outside areas of conflict, often quite highly developed—capacity for mutual dependency and for maintaining relationships that transcend a self-serving orientation. In contrast, narcissistic pathology is characterized by pathology of object relations that is severe relative to the overall level of functioning. For example, Mr. L, the unemployed lawyer described in Clinical Illustration 4 earlier in this chapter, explained to the consultant that even though he no longer had any positive or sexual feelings for his wife, he stayed with her because she had the means to support him financially; he avoided close friendships because he did not want anyone to feel he "owed" them anything.

Moral Values

The normal personality is associated with a commitment to values and ideals and a "moral compass" that is consistent, flexible, and fully integrated into the sense of self. In the neurotic level of personality organization, there is a commitment to values and ideals and an absence of antisocial behavior, reflecting a fully integrated and internalized sense of values and ideals. However, moral rigidity, a tendency to hold the self to unreasonably high standards (i.e., to be excessively self-critical or to anguish over the temptation to stray), is a common feature of personality disorders organized at a neurotic level.

In contrast, the borderline level of personality organization is characterized by a variable degree of pathology in moral functioning. At one end of the spectrum, the clinician finds a relatively well-developed but rigid and excessively severe level of moral functioning characterized by severe anxiety and subjective distress, in the form either of self-criticism or of anticipated criticism from others in relation to not adhering to internal standards. At the other end of the spectrum, the clinician sees the absence of any internal moral compass and a lack of capacity for guilt or remorse, characteristic of patients organized at a low borderline level, and in particular those with antisocial personality disorder or severe narcissistic pathology.

Returning to Mr. L (introduced in Clinical Illustration 4), during the consultation, it emerged that he was perfectly comfortable exploiting his wife financially, and he routinely lied to her about using prostitutes. He experienced no discomfort in relation to these behaviors, never giving them a second thought. When his therapist called the patient's attention to his lying, the patient denied the significance of his behavior and rationalized that he did it "to smooth things out."

It is common for individuals organized at a high borderline level to demonstrate excessively harsh moral standards that may comfortably co-exist with glaring lacunae in moral functioning. Splitting and denial underlie the capacity to maintain frankly contradictory attitudes toward moral functioning.

Reality Testing and Reflective Capacities

Sustained loss of perceptual reality testing is not a feature of personality disorders. When a patient presents with frank and persistent loss of reality testing, evaluating and treating psychosis becomes the highest priority, and the issue of personality pathology is deferred until psychotic symptoms resolve. However, *transient* loss of reality testing can be seen in some of the more severe personality disorders, especially in highly stressful or affectively charged settings (as well as in the context of alcohol or drug abuse). This process is understood not in terms of psychosis, but rather in terms of the highly concrete quality of experience that can accompany splitting in the setting of conflict and affect activation. In these cases, the individual's experience in the moment, often paranoid or at times idealized, is "all there is," and takes on the quality in the moment of absolute truth; from the patient's perspective, there is no distinction between her internal reality and external reality, and what she thinks and feels is how it is, leaving no room for entertaining alternative perspectives. The patient's subjectivity is entirely dominated by the impact of a single object relation, with no sense of an observing self to consider alternative perspectives or to reflect on what might be happening.

For example, Ms. B, the young woman described in Clinical Illustration 2 who presented with unstable relationships with men, noted that many of her breakups were precipitated by her feeling convinced that her boyfriend was lying to her. Nothing he or anyone else could say or do would change her view; she had no doubt that the boyfriend was an untrustworthy, exploitative liar. These episodes, though very dramatic, were time-limited; after cutting him off, she would realize she had misjudged him and would then desperately attempt to reestablish the relationship.

In personality disorders as a rule, thinking tends to be more concrete in areas of conflict; as pathology becomes more severe, so too does the vulnerability to concrete thinking, with a parallel decline in the capacity to reflect on internal states in self and other (i.e., the capacity to *mentalize*[14]). These observations have important clinical implications, and our treatment approach takes into account the need to address the concrete nature of the patient's experience in the moment before initiating exploratory work (see the description of therapeutic tact and timing in Chapter 11).

Turning from reality testing proper to what we refer to as *social reality testing*, we see that individuals organized at a borderline level frequently present with deficits in this area. Social reality testing is responsible for the ability to read social cues, understand social conventions, and respond tactfully in interpersonal settings, all of which are characteristic of the normal personality and are also seen in NPO. Deficits in social reality testing can lead individuals who are organized at a borderline level to behave inappropriately in social settings, typically without being aware of doing so, and misinterpretation of social cues may lead to transient feelings of paranoia or fears of being abandoned.

For example, Ms. B not only frequently misjudged her boyfriends, but also often misread social cues in a variety of settings and failed to understand conventions; she could be excessively seductive with both women and men, including at her workplace, in a way that made others uncomfortable, and she had no awareness of doing so. She was routinely late for work and she often arrived inappropriately dressed, in a fashion that was either excessively casual or excessively revealing—again, with no appreciation that her behavior was off-putting.

---

[14]The concept of *mentalization* is broad, overlapping with other concepts such as mindfulness, empathy, and affect consciousness (Choi-Kain and Gunderson 2008). A more circumscribed view of mentalization has been articulated by Kernberg (2012) as it relates to therapeutic intervention with patients manifesting severe personality dysfunction. The complex process of interpretation in transference-focused psychotherapy (i.e., steps of clarification, confrontation, and interpretation in the here and now, as described throughout this volume) contributes to the patient's ability to mentalize—that is, to the ability to act on a relatively accurate, balanced, and complex conception of self and others, even under conditions of extreme affect arousal.

Part 4

Clinical Implications of the Structural Model of Personality Disorders

THE DISTINCTIONS BETWEEN NPO AND BPO, on the one hand, and among high, middle, and low borderline levels of personality organization, on the other, have important implications for a patient's prognosis, differential treatment planning, and clinical process. Patients in each of these groups have different clinical needs and benefit from treatments specifically targeting their psychopathology.

Transference-focused psychotherapy—extended (TFP-E) is conceptualized as helping patients at all levels of personality pathology to attain progressively higher levels of personality organization, reflected in improved self and interpersonal functioning (Table 2–3). For patients organized at a borderline level who present with clinically significant identity pathology, treatment is organized around promoting the integration and coalescence of dissociated, idealized, and paranoid internal object relations, with the goal of establishing a more coherent, stable, better-differentiated, and complex experience of self and others—that is, identity consolidation (Yeomans et al. 2015). For patients organized at a neurotic level who present with personality rigidity in the setting of normal identity formation, treatment is organized around promoting the integration of repressed or dissociated internal object relations into an already consolidated, stable, and relatively complex sense of self, with the goal of reducing personality rigidity and enriching affective experience in an area of conflict (Caligor et al. 2007).

Across all levels of severity of personality pathology, psychotherapy is organized around exploration of the patient's internal object relations as they are played out in current interpersonal relationships, including the relationship with the therapist. Therapeutic inquiry focuses on the here and now, attending closely to the patient's current life situation and to his immediate and affectively dominant experience in the treatment hour. Through exploration of the internal object relations enacted in each session, the therapist gains access to the patient's internal world. Throughout

---

TABLE 2–3. Goals of transference-focused psychotherapy—extended

---

Across the range of personality organization

  Higher level of personality organization

  Improved self and interpersonal functioning

Borderline level of personality organization

  Identity consolidation

  Integration of dissociated, idealized, and paranoid internal object relations

  Coherent, differentiated experience of self and others

Neurotic level of personality organization

  Decreased personality rigidity and enriched affective experience in area of conflict

  Integration of repressed or dissociated internal object relations into self experience

  Flexible and adaptive functioning in area of conflict

---

the treatment process, the TFP-E therapist remains mindful that the internal object relations enacted in a particular moment or setting may serve defensive functions, protecting the patient in the moment from awareness of more threatening or painful, conflictual experiences of self and other.

As treatment progresses, the therapist can anticipate relatively predictable developments and shifts in the object relations organizing the patient's communications and experience in the clinical setting, as defenses and conflicts are explored and worked through. The clinical chapters of this book outline how to apply general psychotherapeutic principles, strategies, and tactics to best meet the needs of patients with personality disorders across the range of severity, tailoring them to each patient's moment-to-moment psychological functioning and phase of treatment (Table 2–4).

Structural Goals of Treatment: Targeting Identity Consolidation

The object relations theory model of personality disorders identifies identity pathology and associated defensive operations as the *targets* of clinical intervention. The *structural goal* of treatment is to promote progressive levels of personality organization, beginning with identity consolidation and then, at a higher level of integration, progressing to containment and contextualization of conflictual object relations within an overall, stable, and integrated sense of self. At the level of the patient's subjectivity, the structural goals of treatment correspond with helping the patient develop a re-

---

TABLE 2–4. Clinical approach of transference-focused psychotherapy—extended

---

Explore internal object relations played out in interpersonal relationships, including relationship with therapist.

Work in the here and now.

Focus on patient's immediate, affectively dominant experience in session.

Focus on patient's life situation.

Employ overarching clinical principles and techniques across the range of severity and different phases of treatment.

Tailor techniques to individual patient and phase of treatment.

---

alistic, complete, and continuous experience of herself and a corresponding experience of significant others, both characterized by depth and complexity, while flexibly containing aspects of self and others that are conflictual. These changes at the level of the patient's subjective experience correspond with, at the level of the patient's *functioning*, the development of improved self and interpersonal functioning. In sum, to the extent that the structural goal of promoting progressive levels of personality organization is attained, presenting problems and areas of difficulty will improve.

Key Clinical Concepts

- Personality disorders can be classified according to severity of structural pathology, or level of personality organization, combined with a description of dominant personality traits.

- The level of structural pathology is determined by identity formation, quality of object relations, defenses, moral functioning, and reality testing.

- The overarching goal of TFP-E is to help the patient attain higher levels of personality organization and integration.

- Within the object relations theory model, personality integration is conceptualized in terms of progressive coalescence of the internal object relations that organize the individual's sense of self and others.

- Integrative changes will be manifested in improved self and interpersonal functioning, symptomatic improvement, deepening affective experience, and flexible adaptation to life's challenges.

References

American Psychiatric Association: Diagnostic and Statistical Manual of Mental Disorders, 3rd Edition. Washington, DC, American Psychiatric Association, 1980

American Psychiatric Association: Diagnostic and Statistical Manual of Mental Disorders, 5th Edition. Arlington, VA, American Psychiatric Association, 2013

Bateman A, Fonagy P: 8-year follow-up of patients treated for borderline personality disorder: mentalization-based treatment versus treatment as usual. Am J Psychiatry 165(5):631–638, 2008 18347003

Bornstein RF: Dependency in the personality disorders: intensity, insight, expression, and defense. J Clin Psychol 54(2):175–189, 1998 9467762

Caligor E, Clarkin J: An object relations model of personality and personality pathology, in Psychodynamic Psychotherapy for Personality Disorders: A Clinical Handbook. Edited by Clarkin J, Fonagy P, Gabbard G. Washington, DC, American Psychiatric Publishing, 2010, pp 3–36

Caligor E, Kernberg OF, Clarkin JF: Handbook of Dynamic Psychotherapy for Higher Level Personality Pathology. Washington, DC, American Psychiatric Publishing, 2007

Choi-Kain LW, Gunderson JG: Mentalization: ontogeny, assessment, and application in the treatment of borderline personality disorder. Am J Psychiatry 165(9):1127–1135, 2008 18676591

Clarkin JF: The search for critical dimensions of personality pathology to inform diagnostic assessment and treatment planning: a commentary on Hopwood et al. J Pers Disord 27(3):303–310, 2013 23735039

Clarkin JF, Fonagy P, Levy KN, Bateman A: Borderline personality disorder, in Handbook of Psychodynamic Approaches to Psychopathology. Edited by Luyten P, Mayes LC, Fonagy P, et al. New York, Guilford, 2015, pp 353–380

Clarkin JF, Caligor E, Stern BL, Kernberg OF: Structured Interview of Personality Organization—Revised (STIPO-R), 2016. Available at: www.borderlinedisorders.com. Accessed September 20, 2017.

Crawford MJ, Koldobsky N, Mulder R, Tyrer P: Classifying personality disorder according to severity. J Pers Disord 25(3):321–330, 2011 21699394

Donegan NH, Sanislow CA, Blumberg HP, et al: Amygdala hyperreactivity in borderline personality disorder: implications for emotional dysregulation. Biol Psychiatry 54(11):1284–1293, 2003 14643096

Grilo CM, Sanislow CA, Gunderson JG, et al: Two-year stability and change of schizotypal, borderline, avoidant, and obsessive-compulsive personality disorders. J Consult Clin Psychol 72(5):767–775, 2004 15482035

Hopwood CJ, Malone JC, Ansell EB, et al: Personality assessment in DSM-5: empirical support for rating severity, style, and traits. J Pers Disord 25(3):305–320, 2011 21699393

Horz S, Clarkin JF, Stern B, Caligor E: The Structured Interview of Personality Organization (STIPO): an instrument to assess severity and change of personality pathology, in Psychodynamic Psychotherapy Research: Evidence-Based Practice and Practice-Based Evidence. Edited by Levy RA, Ablon JS, Kachele H. New York, Humana, 2012, pp 571–592

Kernberg OF: Object Relations Theory and Clinical Psychoanalysis. New York, Jason Aronson, 1975

Kernberg OF: Internal World and External Reality: Object Relations Theory Applied. New York, Jason Aronson, 1980

Kernberg OF: Severe Personality Disorders: Psychotherapeutic Strategies. New Haven, CT, Yale University Press, 1984

Kernberg OF: Identity: recent findings and clinical implications. Psychoanal Q 75(4):969–1004, 2006 17094369

Kernberg OF: Mentalization, mindfulness, insight, empathy, and interpretation, in The Inseparable Nature of Love and Aggression. Washington, DC, American Psychiatric Publishing, 2012, pp 57–80

Kernberg OF: What is personality? J Pers Disord 30(2):145–156, 2016 27027422

Kernberg OF, Caligor E: A psychoanalytic theory of personality disorders, in Major Theories of Personality Disorder, 2nd Edition. Edited by Lenzenweger MF, Clarkin JF. New York, Guilford, 2005, pp 114–156

Klein M: Notes on some schizoid mechanisms (1946), in Envy and Gratitude and Other Works, 1946–1963. New York, Free Press, 1975, pp 1–24

Klein M: Some theoretical conclusions regarding the emotional life of the infant (1952), in Envy and Gratitude and Other Works, 1946–1963. New York, Free Press, 1975, pp 61–93

Lenzenweger MF: Current status of the scientific study of the personality disorders: an overview of epidemiological, longitudinal, experimental psychopathology, and neurobehavioral perspectives. J Am Psychoanal Assoc 58(4):741–778, 2010 21115756

Lenzenweger MF, Johnson MD, Willett JB: Individual growth curve analysis illuminates stability and change in personality disorder features: the longitudinal study of personality disorders. Arch Gen Psychiatry 61(10):1015–1024, 2004 15466675

Levy KN, Scala JW, Temes CM, Clouthier TL: An integrative attachment theory framework of personality disorders, in Personality Disorders: Toward Theoretical and Empirical Integration in Diagnosis and Assessment. Edited by Huprich SK. Washington, DC, American Psychological Association, 2015, pp 315–343

Livesley WJ, Dimaggio G, Clarkin JF (eds): Integrated Treatment for Personality Disorder: A Modular Approach. New York, Guilford, 2015

Meehan KB, Clarkin JF: A critical evaluation of moving toward a trait system for personality disorder assessment, in Personality Disorders: Toward Theoretical and Empirical Integration in Diagnosis and Assessment. Edited by Huprich SK. Washington, DC, American Psychological Association, 2015, pp 85–106

Parker G, Hadzi-Pavlovic D, Both L, et al: Measuring disordered personality functioning: to love and to work reprised. Acta Scandinavia 110(3):230–239, 2004 15283744

Perry JC, Bond M: Defensive functioning, in The American Psychiatric Publishing Textbook of Personality Disorders. Edited by Oldham JM, Skodol AE, Bender DS. Washington, DC, American Psychiatric Publishing, 2005, pp 523–540

Shapiro D: Neurotic Styles. New York, Basic Books, 1965

Shapiro D: Autonomy and Rigid Character. New York, Basic Books, 1981

Sharp C, Wright AG, Fowler JC, et al: The structure of personality pathology: both general ('g') and specific ('s') factors? J Abnorm Psychol 124(2):387–398, 2015 25730515

Tyrer P, Johnson T: Establishing the severity of personality disorder. Am J Psychiatry 153(12):1593–1597, 1996 8942456

Tyrer P, Crawford M, Mulder R, et al: The rationale for the reclassification of personality disorder in the 11th revision of the International Classification of Diseases (ICD-11). Personality and Mental Health 5:246–259, 2011

Vaillant G: Ego Mechanisms of Defense: A Guide for Clinicians and Researchers. Washington, DC, American Psychiatric Press, 1992

Wagner AW, Linehan MM: Facial expression recognition ability among women with borderline personality disorder: implications for emotion regulation? J Pers Disord 13(4):329–344, 1999 10633314

Westen D: Divergences between clinical and research methods for assessing personality disorders: implications for research and the evolution of Axis II. Am J Psychiatry 154(7):895–903, 1997 9210738

Westen D, Arkowitz-Westen L: Limitations of Axis II in diagnosing personality pathology in clinical practice. Am J Psychiatry 155(12):1767–1771, 1998 9842791

Westen D, Gabbard GO: Developments in cognitive neuroscience, II: implications for theories of transference. J Am Psychoanal Assoc 50(1):99–134, 2002 12018876

Westen D, Shedler J: A prototype matching approach to diagnosing personality disorders: toward DSM-V. J Pers Disord 14(2):109–126, 2000 10897462

Widiger TA, Costa PT, McCrae RR: Diagnosis of personality disorder using the five-factor model and the proposed DSM-5, in Personality Disorders and the Five-Factor Model of Personality, 3rd Edition. Edited by Widiger TA, Costa PT Jr. Washington, DC, American Psychological Association, 2013, pp. 285–310

Wright AGC, Zimmerman J: At the nexus of science and practice: answering basic clinical questions in personality disorder assessment and diagnosis with quantitative modeling techniques, in Personality Disorders: Toward Theoretical and Empirical Integration in Diagnosis and Treatment. Edited by Huprich SK. Washington, DC, American Psychological Association, 2015, pp. 109–144

Yeomans F, Clarkin JF, Kernberg OF: Transference-Focused Psychotherapy for Borderline Personality Disorder: A Clinical Guide. Washington, DC, American Psychiatric Publishing, 2015

Zanarini MC, Frankenburg FR, Hennen J, et al: The McLean Study of Adult Development (MSAD): overview and implications of the first six years of prospective follow-up. J Pers Disord 19(5):505–523, 2005 16274279

Zanarini MC, Frankenburg FR, Reich DB, Fitzmaurice G: Attainment and stability of sustained symptomatic remission and recovery among patients with borderline personality disorder and Axis II comparison subjects: a 16-year prospective follow-up study. Am J Psychiatry 169(5):476–483, 2012 22737693

Clinical Psychodynamics Within the Framework of Object Relations Theory

Conflict, Anxiety, Defense, and Internal Object Relations

UP TO THIS POINT IN THE BOOK, WE HAVE focused diagnostic and structural perspectives on personality disorders within the framework of object relations theory. We turn now to dynamic perspectives, focusing on the nature of the psychological conflicts that characterize personality disorders at different levels of severity and on the relationship among internal object relations, defense, and conflict. In the transference-focused psychotherapy—extended (TFP-E) model of treatment, the therapist links the progressive integration of internal object relations and structural change to the working through of psychodynamic conflicts motivating pathogenic defensive operations, focusing on the role of anxieties that interfere with integrative processes. As anxieties are contained and worked through, the patient relinquishes maladaptive defenses, takes responsibility for conflictual motivations, and comes to tolerate ambivalence. These dynamic shifts correspond with identity consolidation, the attainment of higher levels of personality organization, and decreased personality rigidity.

Psychological Conflict Within the Framework of Object Relations Theory

Psychodynamic models of psychological functioning focus on the dynamic interplay of conscious and unconscious psychological processes in organizing an individual's subjective experience and behavior. In particular, psychodynamic models focus on conscious and unconscious motivations, conflicts that emerge among different motivations, and psychological defenses that mediate among these conflicts. Psychological motivations are inborn dispositions shaped by developmental experience. Psychological motivations are expressed as needs, wishes, or fears. Within the psychodynamic model, conflicts among conscious and unconscious psychological motivations are seen as both painful and inevitable. Psychological conflicts generate painful affects, or "anxieties," which stimulate the activation of defensive operations. Psychological defenses are seen to mediate among the conflicting needs that emerge within the individual and in the process to impact psychological functioning in ways that can be more or less adaptive.

Psychodynamic models of personality disorders view psychological conflicts as playing a central role in personality pathology. These conflicts are seen as organized in relation the following:

1. A conflictual motivation (i.e., a motivation that is in conflict with other motivations), sometimes also referred to as an "impulse" or a "drive"
2. Negative affective experience associated with expression of the conflictual motivation, sometimes described in terms of a "danger" or "anxiety-motivating defense"
3. A defense based on either repression or splitting

Conflictual Motivations

Conflictual motivations are powerful, highly motivated wishes, needs, or fears that are incompatible with the individual's values or sense of self, or whose direct expression the individual anticipates would lead to a situation experienced as painful, frightening, or dangerous. Different motivations will be experienced as more or less conflictual by different individuals. For example, one person may experience dependency needs as highly conflictual, anticipating humiliation if these needs were to be expressed, whereas someone else may freely enjoy expression of dependency needs, anticipating feelings of comfort and security to accompany their expression. Motivations that commonly become involved in conflict include those tied to the expression of the following:

- Aggression (anger, sadism, envy, competition, strivings for power)
- Dependency needs (wishes to be loved or taken care of)
- Sexual desire
- Narcissistic needs (strivings for autonomy, attention, admiration, self-regard)

In general, as personality pathology becomes more severe, conflictual motivations become increasingly poorly integrated, and aggression becomes more central to psychological conflict and personality functioning. In the more severe personality disorders (i.e., those at a low or middle borderline level of personality organization; BPO), the centrality of poorly integrated forms of aggression is expressed with full access to consciousness, for example, in the form of hatred, sadism, or envy. At the other end of the spectrum, at a neurotic level of personality organization (NPO), conflicts are typically organized around somewhat better-integrated forms of aggressive, sexual, dependent, and narcissistic motivations that when conflictual are stably repressed. In high BPO, condensations of conflicts around dependency and narcissistic needs with conflicts in relation to aggression often play a central role.

Psychological Anxieties and Defense

Expression of a conflictual motivation is associated with a particular "anxiety," "danger," or fear (e.g., "If I am aggressively competitive, it would make me a bad person, or people won't like me"; "If I unleash my sadism, I will destroy everything I value, or I will be hated and isolated"; "If I allow myself to be dependent, I will be flooded with painful feelings of envy and inferiority"). The anxieties associated with expression of a conflictual motivation may be fully conscious or fully unconscious; however, anxieties often are "preconscious"—that is, accessible to consciousness but out of awareness.

The specific nature of the danger or anxiety associated with expression of a conflictual motivation will vary depending on the particular motivations involved, the individual's level of personality organization, and the individual's personal history. As pathology becomes more severe, anxieties become more poorly integrated, overwhelming, and ultimately catastrophic, as shown in the following examples:

1. An individual organized at a neurotic level who presents with conflicts in relation to competitive aggression might have the fear that "If I am too competitive, it would make me a bad person, or people won't like me, or I will be punished."
2. Someone organized at a high borderline level with conflicts around dependency and aggression might fear that "Expression of my hostility will leave me in a world where there is no hope of positive attachment."
3. An individual organized at a middle borderline level with conflicts in relation to narcissistic needs and aggression might fear that "If I allow myself to be vulnerable in any way, I will be viciously attacked and humiliated."
4. Anxieties are most extreme at the low borderline level, where extremely poorly integrated expressions of aggression predominate, and the projection of aggression is associated with highly paranoid anxieties, such as "He will annihilate me, and the only protection is for me to destroy him first."

Regardless of the specific nature of the danger or anxiety associated with the expression of a conflictual motivation, it will always be linked to a particular negative affect, most commonly anxiety, fear or terror, paranoia, loss, shame, guilt, or depression. For example, in the numbered list above, in the first item (that of an individual organized at a neurotic level), we see guilt in relation to expression of competitive aggression; in the second item (that of someone organized at a high borderline level), we see despair in relation to expression of aggression; and in the third and fourth items, we see terror and paranoia in relation to poorly integrated, projected aggression in someone organized at a middle or low borderline level.

In the setting of psychological conflict, defensive operations are automatically and involuntarily activated to ward off the negative affects associated with expression of a conflictual motivation. Defenses reduce negative affect by splitting off awareness of conflictual motivations from the dominant, conscious sense of self. Defenses based on repression permanently banish the conflictual motivation from consciousness, while defenses based on dissociation or splitting put conflictual motivations out of mind in the moment.

As we discussed in Chapter 2, in personality disorders, defenses that function to keep potentially threatening motivations out of awareness introduce rigidity into personality functioning. Personality rigidity resulting from psychological conflict can thus be understood in terms of the need to fend off awareness of painful and threatening internalized relationship patterns and associated affect states.

Psychological Conflict and Internal Object Relations

In the object relations theory model, conflictual motivations, anxieties, and defenses are all conceptualized in terms of wished-for, needed, or feared relationships—that is, in terms of internal object relations (Kernberg 1992). Thus, motivations in this frame of reference are conceptualized not simply as "impulses" or "drives," but rather as wishes, needs, and fears directed toward another person, which are represented as highly motivated internal object relations associated with highly charged affect states.

For example, a conflictual sexual motivation, experienced as a physical sexual urge or impulse, might be mentally represented as a hypersexual child self in relation to a sexually stimulating parental object associated with feelings of intense sexual excitement. Or sadistic motivations might be represented in terms of a powerful and cruel self in relation to a depreciated and enraged object associated with hatred. Or the wish to be taken care of might be represented as a happy, dependent self being nurtured by a caring mother.

Similarly, defenses are not conceptualized as "mechanisms" but rather in terms of the defensive enactment of an internal object relation that is relatively nonconflictual and that functions to keep more conflictual object relations out of awareness, via either repression or dissociation (Kernberg and Caligor 2005). For example, defensive enactments of an internal object relation may include the following: defending against the sexual impulse illustrated above, enactment of an internal object relation of a nonsexual child self and a nurturing parental figure, associated with feelings of security; defending against sadistic motivations, a powerful and beneficent self in relation to an adoring object, associated with feelings of gratification; and defending against anxieties associated with dependency, an autonomous, self-sufficient self in relation to distant but admiring others.

Psychological Conflict and TFP-E

In sum, in the setting of psychological conflict, enactment of defensive object relations automatically and involuntarily wards off anxieties associated with the expression of conflictual motivations. However, as described in Chapter 2, in the setting of personality pathology, defenses ward off anxiety at the cost of introducing rigidity into personality functioning and interfering with natural integrative processes. Specifically, in BPO, splitting-based defenses interfere with identity consolidation; in NPO, repression-based defenses interfere with the integration of conflictual internal object relations into an already consolidated identity; and across the spectrum of severity of personality disorders, defenses introduce rigidity into personality functioning and interfere with the individual's attainment of a higher, more flexible, and adaptive level of personality organization.

Described further in this chapter, the specific nature of the conflicts and anxieties motivating defenses is different at different levels of personality organization, but across the spectrum of severity, the clinical objectives are to help patients contain and work through anxieties associated with expression of conflictual motivations, allowing them to adopt more flexible and adaptive defenses. This process corresponds with promoting integrative processes, encouraging identity consolidation, and supporting the attainment of progressively higher levels of personality organization.

Psychological Conflicts, Anxieties, and Level of Personality Organization

Different levels of personality organization are associated with different kinds of conflicts and anxieties (Table 3–1). Thus, accurate diagnosis of a patient's level of personality organization provides information about the nature of the anxieties and conflicts likely to be central to personality functioning, allowing the clinician to anticipate treatment developments as well as problems likely to emerge. In NPO, we tend to see the centrality of better-integrated, depressive anxieties and triadic oedipal conflicts, whereas in BPO, paranoid anxieties and dyadic conflicts are most central.

Neurotic Level of Personality Organization

In NPO, as we have already discussed, the motivational systems that color conscious experience are relatively well integrated, while conflictual mo-

TABLE 3–1.   Conflicts, anxieties, and level of personality organization

Dynamic constellation	NPO	High BPO	Middle and low BPO
Defenses	Predominantly repression-based	Combination of splitting-based and repression-based	Splitting-based
Central conflictual motivations	Sexuality, better-integrated forms of aggression, dependency, narcissistic needs	Dependency and narcissistic needs, with secondary fears in relation to sexuality and aggression	Poorly integrated aggression, need for security in a paranoid world
Anxieties motivating defense	Self-criticism, fear of disapproval, shame, loss of love, loss of loved one	Fear of loss of attachment figure, fear of loss of self-esteem, humiliation	Fear of sadistic attack or exploitation, destruction of the good, loss of all hope of security
Access to consciousness of motivational systems	Motivations accessible to consciousness are relatively well integrated; less well-integrated motivational systems are stably repressed.	Motivations accessible to consciousness are moderately well integrated; poorly integrated motivational systems are partially and unstably repressed.	Poorly integrated motivations are dissociated and fully accessible to consciousness; no capacity for repression.
Nature of dominant conflicts	Conflicts are predominantly depressive; responsibility for conflictual motivations.	Conflicts oscillate between paranoid and depressive; variable sense of responsibility.	Conflicts are predominantly paranoid; conflictual motivations are projected with no sense of responsibility.

Note.   BPO=borderline level of personality organization; NPO=neurotic level of personality organization.

tivations that are more poorly integrated are for the most part repressed and remain inaccessible to consciousness. Psychological conflicts at a neurotic level of personality organization most commonly involve the expression of sexual, competitively aggressive, dependent, narcissistic, and sadistic motivations. Anxieties associated with the expression of conflictual motivations in NPO typically involve self-critical or shameful feelings, fear of disapproval or punishment from others, or anxiety about loss of attachment relationships. Defensive operations are based on repression.

An example of a typical conflict encountered by someone organized at a neurotic level concerns the expression of competitive aggression. If put into words, this person's conflict might sound like this: "If I were to express hostile or competitive feelings toward people I care about, doing so would make me a bad or unlovable person. In the face of this conflict, I automatically defend against awareness of hostile feelings by repressing or projecting them. As a result, I do not consciously experience myself as hostile or competitive; to the extent that my hostility remains repressed, I do not experience anxiety." Subjectively, we see a dominant sense of self here that is relatively complex and realistic, but unable to comfortably accommodate awareness of aggression in the self (or, depending on the individual, awareness of dependency needs, sexual desires, competitive or narcissistic strivings, or sadistic motivations).

Motivational systems that are conflictual and more poorly integrated are repressed, and even when they emerge into consciousness, they lack the overwhelming quality and intensity of conflictual motivations characteristic of the severe personality disorders; similarly, the anxieties associated with expression of conflictual motivations in NPO are typically bad feelings about the self or directed toward the self, or loss of attachments, but do not threaten the safety, integrity, or survival of the self. Anxieties of this type, in which the individual suffers from and ultimately takes responsibility for conflictual motivations, are sometimes referred to as *depressive anxieties* (discussed later in this chapter; see "Anxieties and Conflicts Central to the Treatment of Personality Disorders: Paranoid and Depressive Anxieties and Oedipal Conflicts").

Low and Middle Borderline Levels of Personality Organization

In BPO, conflicts are organized somewhat differently than in NPO; the intensity is much greater, and the stakes are much higher. In low and middle BPO, psychological functioning is dominated by the impact of poorly integrated, aggressive, and destructive motivational systems (sometimes referred to as *primitive aggression*). Further, the predominance of splitting-based defenses means that highly charged object relations associated with poorly integrated aggression are not repressed but are fully accessible to consciousness. The dominant anxieties are that poorly integrated forms of aggression associated with powerful negative affect states and paranoid object relations will swamp and overwhelm idealized sectors of experience. Characteristic expressions of these anxieties are fears of annihilation of the self and destruction of idealized object relations, with attendant loss of all possibility of internal or external security. In this setting, the tendency to project highly aggressive object relations only makes matters worse, often leading to paranoia and even more overwhelming anxiety and fear. This psychological situation is associated with the individual's inability to assume responsibility for his affect states or his actions, which typically feel justified on the basis of perceived (often misperceived) provocation.

If put into words, the typical conflict encountered at a low or middle borderline level of personality organization might sound something like this: "I am filled with overwhelming, often terrifying, poorly integrated, destructive aggression, hatred, sadism, and envy, which threaten to annihilate me and to destroy everything around me. I can try to rid myself of these impulses by projecting them, but now the world feels unbearably dangerous and malevolent. The only hope is to sequester whatever positive aspects of experience I can locate, creating idealized object relations and attempting to protect them via dissociation from aggressively infiltrated, paranoid object relations. I can now try to cling to an idealized sector as an island of safety, but it is all unstable and fragile, a weak defense. The threat of destruction of everything of value, both within me and in the world around me, always looms large."

Anxieties of this "life-and-death" type are sometimes referred to as *paranoid anxieties*; we will discuss this topic further later in this chapter (see "Anxieties and Conflicts Central to the Treatment of Personality Disorders: Paranoid and Depressive Anxieties and Oedipal Conflicts"). We hope to convey the marked contrast between the painful but relatively measured, focused quality of predominantly depressive anxieties that motivate defenses in NPO, on the one hand, and the catastrophic and terrifying quality of the predominantly paranoid anxieties experienced in severe personality disorders, on the other.

High Borderline Level of Personality Organization

Whereas anxieties related to poorly integrated aggression are preeminent in low and middle BPO, in high BPO, anxieties more typically relate to dependency and narcissistic needs, and paranoid concerns and sexual conflicts are often secondary to fears of closeness and vulnerability. In the setting of a combination of repression-based and splitting-based defenses, we often see condensations of conflicts related to dependency, sexuality, and self-esteem maintenance with conflicts around aggression, and with more poorly integrated forms of aggression emerging into consciousness when repressive defenses fail. For example, if put into words, one individual's anxieties might sound like this: "If I allow myself to feel needy or to want something from him, he will disappoint or humiliate me. In the face of this conflict, I can defensively idealize him, or I can attempt to repress or project my dependency needs, or I can pull away and distance myself. However, invariably, in settings that activate my core conflicts or stimulate significant anxiety, I can anticipate being flooded with overwhelming experiences of disappointment, rejection, and humiliation, followed by reactive—and from my perspective, justified—rage and paranoia. These experiences are profoundly unsettling and disruptive, discontinuous with my usual level of psychological functioning."

Internal Object Relations, Defense, and Level of Personality Organization

At all levels of personality organization, the enactment of defensive object relations can be seen to ward off anxiety by protecting against awareness of object relations more closely tied to the expression of conflictual motivations. Because defensive internal object relations are, by definition, less threatening to the individual than are the conflictual motivations they are defending against, at all levels of personality organization, defensive object relations have greater accessibility to consciousness than do the object relations defended against. What this means is that at any moment, in the setting of conflict, the representations of self and other closest to consciousness and organizing the individual's subjective experience can be seen to serve defensive functions, by supporting repression or dissociation of more conflictual object relations. As a result, in treatment, identifying and exploring the defensive object relations that are organizing the patient's conscious experience in session is always the first step in examining the anxieties and conflicts interfering with integrative processes.

In this section, we discuss how internal object relations are organized in the setting of personality pathology to serve defensive functions, pointing to similarities and differences between neurotic and borderline structures. Exploring how internal object relations can be structured to serve defensive functions at different levels of personality organization provides an understanding of the relationships among conflict, defense, and structural pathology in personality disorders. This conceptualization organizes the strategies guiding technique and forms a conceptual link between clinical intervention and structural change.

Internal Object Relations and Defense in the Neurotic Level of Personality Organization

Repression and Layering of Defensive Internal Object Relations

At the neurotic level of personality organization, in areas of conflict, the internal object relations that are closest to consciousness and come to organize self experience can be seen to serve defensive functions. These internal object relations tend to have the qualities of being relatively realistic, well integrated, and ego-syntonic; they exclude conflictual motivations, and often also include a self representation that is in some way childlike. Defensive internal object relations will be enacted in settings that might stimulate conflict, in this process supporting repression of more threatening internal object relations closer to the expression of conflictual motivations.

From the perspective of the subject, this process is automatic, habitual, and seamless. From a structural perspective, this process can be thought of in terms of a *layering* of internal object relations; those internal object relations at or close to the conscious surface serve defensive purposes, protecting against activation of underlying layers of unconscious (repressed) mental contents that are more highly conflictual and remain inaccessible to consciousness. Thus, in the TFP-E model, repression is not simply a defense mechanism, but rather corresponds to the enactment of a defensive object relation that functions to keep more conflictual object relations outside awareness. In sum, in the setting of a neurotic structure, defensive internal object relations will be enacted in a stable and predictable fashion, organizing the individual's self experience in an area of conflict while supporting repression of more conflictual internal object relations.

To illustrate how enactment of defensive object relations in NPO supports repression of more conflictual object relations, we consider a female patient with conflicts around sexual expression. The therapist might see a defensive object relation composed of a nonsexual, childlike self in relation to a caring, parental male figure, associated with feelings of happiness and closeness. In settings that might stimulate sexual interest, either on her part or on the part of a man, this internal object relation would be activated, and the patient would enact this relationship pattern; she would be unaware of any sexual feelings as she comfortably enjoyed the care and companionship of a male friend or confidant. Alternatively, were this same woman to have conflicts around aggression and authority, she might defensively experience herself as a compliant, pleasing, childlike self in relation to an approving parental authority, associated with feelings of security—enacted, for example, in relation to her superiors at work. As long as this patient sees herself as nonsexual and childlike or as compliant and pleasing, conflictual motivations remain repressed and she is protected from anxieties associated with expression of conflictual sexual or aggressive motivations, respectively.

Rigidity and Character Defenses

As we have described, repression wards off anxiety and conflict associated with the expression of conflictual motivations, but at the expense of introducing rigidity into personality functioning. The therapist can anticipate that whenever the female patient in the immediately preceding example enters a setting that might stimulate sexual or competitively aggressive motivations, she will automatically and involuntarily find herself acting either in a nonsexual, friendly fashion or in a pleasing, compliant manner, respectively. This will be the case even in settings where she might want to be flirtatious or competitive. In fact, in such settings, she may find herself becoming *even more* exaggeratedly childlike or compliant, perhaps despite determined efforts to behave otherwise.

Thus, activation of defensive object relations is highly motivated, and behaviors associated with their enactment are difficult to change, even with effort and practice. In sum, the rigidity that is the hallmark of NPO can be conceptualized in terms of the habitual, automatic, and involuntary enactment of defensive object relations in settings that might stimulate activation of conflictual motivations and associated anxieties.

Up to this point in our discussion, we have been focusing on enactment of defensive internal object relations in focal areas of conflict. However, defensively motivated attitudes and behaviors often generalize; for example, the above patient's stance of being childlike and nonsexual, or compliant and pleasing, though initially functioning to defend against focal conflicts in relation to sexuality or aggression, may come to characterize her way of moving through the world in general, extending beyond sexual or competitive settings. In this case, her defensive attitudes and associated behaviors would be described in terms of *character defenses*. In TFP-E, character defenses refer to a constellation of behaviors, attitudes, and ways of being in the world that come to characterize an individual independent of the setting, in essence constituting a "personality style." In the above example, the patient would present herself as girlish and nonsexual, or pleasing and compliant, regardless of the setting, and likely without full awareness of doing so. Character defenses are not only habitual and automatic; they are also typically ego-syntonic—that is, relatively seamless and inconspicuous to the individual—although they are typically more visible to others. In NPO, character defenses may be relatively adaptive, but ultimately the rigidity that they confer can cause problems for an individual and/or for the people with whom he interacts.

Layering of Conflictual Internal Object Relations

Before moving on to compare the defensive layering of object relations that characterizes NPO with the defensive dissociation, or splitting, of internal object relations seen in BPO, we want to add a caveat about repressive mechanisms in NPO. As we have discussed, the internal object relations enacted defensively in NPO are not only well integrated but are also typically quite removed from conflictual motivational systems. However, this is neither a fixed rule nor a static situation. Just as in the example of the woman for whom internal object relations characterized by nonsexual love function to support repression of internal object relations associated with expression of other motivations that are more highly conflictual, at times enactment of a particular, relatively conflictual motivation can support repression of even more threatening motivational systems. This serves to highlight that *any* internal object relations can potentially serve defensive purposes, and it is therefore important clinically to maintain a flexible attitude as the therapist listens and tries to make sense of patients' communications.

In the treatment setting, as a particular conflict is worked through, conflictual motivations become better integrated and less threatening. In this setting, a change in function may occur: enactment of what had previously been a conflictual motivation can come to serve defensive functions, supporting repression of more conflictual object relations. For example, if the earlier female patient with hypothetical conflicts around aggression and authority were to successfully address and work through these conflicts, the therapist might see a change in function such that enactment of aggressive internal object relations, previously defended against, could come to serve defensive functions supporting repression of, for example, sexual or dependent motivations and anxieties that might be more conflictual. As these aggressive internal object relations are enacted defensively, this patient might find herself, for example, repeatedly becoming irritated with her boss, or her husband, or perhaps her therapist. In this context, her irritation might come to be seen as the defensive enactment of contentious internal object relations, functioning to ward off either sexual feelings that are beginning to emerge or her wishes to be taken care of—both of which are currently more threatening than aggressive motivations.

Thus, in NPO, the therapist thinks in terms of layering—from the conscious or enacted "surface" to the unconscious "depth"—with whatever is at the enacted surface functioning, in a relatively stable and predictable fashion, to support repression of more highly conflictual and threatening internal object relations.

Summary of Defensive Internal Object Relations and Defense

In NPO, enactment of defensive internal object relations—relatively well integrated, realistic, and ego-syntonic—functions to support repression of more highly charged internal object relations that are closer to the direct expression of conflictual motivations. Although this process prevents anxiety and keeps conflictual motivations out of conscious awareness, it introduces rigidity into personality functioning. NPO patients come to treatment unable on their own to modify rigid defensive behaviors and attitudes that represent the enactment of defensive internal object relations and associated character defenses.

Internal Object Relations and Defense in the Borderline Level of Personality Organization

Splitting and Mutual Dissociation of Internal Object Relations

In BPO, as in NPO, internal object relations are organized to serve defensive functions. However, in contrast to what is seen in NPO, in BPO, the therapist does not see relatively well-integrated and realistic defensive internal object relations that stably defend against activation of more highly charged, impulsive internal object relations that remain out of conscious awareness. Rather, what the therapist sees is enactment of mutually dissociated, highly charged internal object relations, one idealized and the other paranoid, each defending against enactment of the other, with both having full access to consciousness but at different times.

In BPO, the internal object relations serving defensive functions and the internal object relations defended against are *both* poorly integrated and highly charged motivational structures, each associated with specific anxieties; describing these internal object relations as *mutually dissociated* refers to the observation that in BPO, *defense* and conflictual motivation are essentially interchangeable, and in fact are an easy exchange of functions. As a result, the relatively stable defense-impulse constellation that typifies neurotic conflict does not apply. Instead, what the therapist sees is a rather fluid (or, to be more accurate, unstable) situation, such that whichever internal object relation is least threatening in the moment will be enacted, while that which is more conflictual will be dissociated. If an idealized internal object relation is currently organizing subjective experience while defending against activation of a paranoid object relation, that configuration can easily flip, so that the paranoid internal object relation is organizing subjectivity while defending against enactment of the corresponding idealized object relations. At the level of subjectivity, this results in unstable, shifting views of self and other that are mutually dissociated and contradictory.

To illustrate how enactment of a particular internal object relation supports dissociation of corresponding object relations of opposite valence, we consider a female patient organized at the high borderline level with conflicts around dependency and aggression. The therapist might initially see defensive activation of an idealized internal object relation composed of a perfectly cared-for self in relation to an ideal and attentive caretaker, with the entire object relation associated with feelings of perfect security. In settings that might stimulate dependent wishes and associated anxieties of being mistreated or exploited, this patient will enact the defensive, ideal version of the relationship, enabling her in the moment to split off and deny the dangers of dependent relations. At another time, perhaps in response to frustration of dependency needs, the exact opposite configuration would occur—the enactment of a paranoid object relation (e.g., a mistreated and exploited self in relation to a cruel and callous caretaker) associated with hostility and sadism. Enactment of this object relation functions to support the dissociation of dependency needs, with the patient essentially adopting the stance that "Everyone is cruel and out for themselves; I trust no one and therefore don't have to fear being mistreated or exploited." Enactment of both paranoid and idealized object relations defends against anxieties associated with expression of the other, whereas ongoing splitting operations defend against the overriding anxieties characterizing BPO, associated with simultaneously experiencing idealized and paranoid sectors.

In patients organized at the high borderline level, idealized internal object relations often color the patients' experience early in treatment, while the dangers of dependency and the associated paranoid internal object relations are dissociated and denied. It may be only with time, and often as a result of increasing intimacy, vulnerability, or conflict, that paranoid internal object relations begin to emerge in the treatment. In patients organized at the middle and low borderline levels, in contrast, the therapist initially tends to see the paranoid sector more consistently activated, with the idealized sector actively walled off and denied, protected by the dominance of paranoid object relations. In treatment, it can take time to identify the idealized aspects of a patient's experience, which may remain largely hidden, only to make transient appearances with a rapid return to a paranoid orientation.

Rigidity and Character Defenses

In BPO, splitting is both highly motivated and rigidly maintained. Mutual dissociation of idealized and paranoid object relations functions to ward off overwhelming anxieties but at the cost of introducing severe rigidity into personality functioning. The individual is left with fixed—albeit unstable, unrealistic, grossly distorted, and concretely experienced—views of self and other that organize his subjectivity in areas of conflict. When conflicts are activated, it can be nearly impossible for the individual to see past distortions and override pressures to action, virtually guaranteeing inappropriate or maladaptive responses to circumstances in the environment; the fixed, concrete, and highly charged quality of split internal object relations often compels the individual to respond to internal cues, resulting in flagrantly maladaptive actions and destructive interpersonal behaviors.

Summary of Internal Object Relations and Defense

In BPO, enactment of defensive internal object relations—made up of mutually dissociated, poorly integrated, and highly affectively charged, idealized, or paranoid internal object relations—supports dissociation of equally highly charged, split internal object relations of the opposite valence. This process wards off powerful anxieties associated with approximating the paranoid and idealized sectors of experience, but introduces severe and highly maladaptive rigidity into personality functioning. Idealized views of self and others are created, sequestered, and protected, but at the cost of introducing and maintaining a distorted and highly affectively charged subjectivity, and of interfering with processes of psychological integration that would lead, in the long term, to a tempering of aggression through the simultaneous experience of positively colored object relations and affect states. BPO patients come to treatment in great distress, typically entrapped in a repetitive cycle characterized by negative affect, maladaptive behaviors, and interpersonal failures that they are unable to modify.

Defense Within a Single Object Relation: Neurotic Projection, Projective Identification, and Role Reversals

Thus far we have described how, in both NPO and BPO, enactment of one object relation can function to defend against enactment of another. One internal object relation serves a defensive function, while another serves an impulsive one. In NPO, the distinction between defense and impulse is quite stable, whereas in BPO, the two are more or less interchangeable.

At this point, we turn to another way in which internal object relations can serve defensive functions, with a focus on the defenses that can be embedded in expression of a *single* impulsive object relation. This group of defensive operations can be understood in terms of different forms of projection. In the TFP-E approach, the forms of projection supported by repression in NPO are referred to as *neurotic projection*, and the forms of projection supported by splitting and dissociation in BPO are described in terms of *projective identification*. We also discuss how on close examination, dissociation and role reversal, integral to projective identification, can also be seen to play a role in projective defenses in NPO.

Neurotic Projection

In a neurotic structure, at times the therapist sees within a single impulsive internal object relation the attribution of a conflictual motivation to an object representation, coupled with dissociation of the conflictual motivation from the self representation (e.g., a sexually naive self representation in relation to a sexually stimulating object representation; a self representation entirely stripped of all aggression in relation to an aggressive object representation; a caretaking self representation in relation to a needy, dependent object). When this object relation is enacted, conflictual parts of the self are attributed to an object, while the subject represses any connection between the conflictual representation and the self ("You are sexual, or aggressive, or dependent, while I am not at all so"). This sort of defensive operation is different from repression proper (described earlier in this chapter) in terms of layering, in which a defensive object relation is enacted and a conflictual motivation and associated parts of the self are banished from consciousness. Instead, here is a defensive operation in which a conflictual motivation and associated parts of the self are banished not entirely from consciousness, but rather from *conscious self experience*. This process involves *projection*, insofar as a conflictual motivation and associated parts of the self have been split off or dissociated from self experience and attributed to an object, and *repression*, insofar as the subject has repressed all awareness of the connection between the self and the unacceptable mental representation.

As an example, we return to the female patient described earlier who presented with sexual conflicts. Instead of defensively enacting an object relation of a nonsexual, childlike self in relation to a caring, male parental figure, she might again enact an object relation in which the self representation is nonsexual, loving, and childlike, but now in relation to an object that is sexual and seductive. In this object relation, all sexual interest and seductiveness are attributed to the object representation, while the self representation has no connection to these motives (although all of this resides within the mind of the patient, she is ultimately identified with both self and object representation). This woman's conscious self experience is of love and sexual naiveté, associated with feeling herself in a childlike position. This self experience defends against awareness of her sexual feelings. Even though this woman is unable to keep her sexual desires entirely out of awareness, she is entirely unaware of her connection to them.

At the same time, embedded in the defensive object relation is an expression of the patient's sexual interest and her wishes to be seductive, although these are entirely dissociated from the loving, naive self and experienced as coming from the object. As a result, this internal object relation can be viewed as both a covert expression of and a defense against the patient's own sexual and seductive impulses. The patient defends against awareness of her own sexual interest, but at the same time remains in a universe where she is in contact with sexuality, albeit attributed to others; her sexuality is thus covertly expressed and perhaps partially gratified. This defensive construction, in which an impulse is simultaneously defended against and at the same time covertly or partially expressed is sometimes referred to as a *compromise formation.*

Initially in treatment, the patient organized at a neurotic level will be predominantly identified with one side of a given internalized relationship pattern. By the end of a successful treatment, the patient will come to tolerate awareness of her identification with both sides of the relationship. For example, in the foregoing illustration, the patient was initially identified with the naive, loving, childlike self representation; during the course of her treatment, she came to tolerate awareness of her identification with the seductive, sexual representation. In essence, identifying with the naive, loving child defended against anxieties associated with sexuality, whereas identifying with the sexual figure defended against anxieties associated with vulnerability and love. One patient will find one position more anxiety provoking, whereas another patient will find the other position more anxiety provoking.

Neurotic Dissociation and Role Reversals

The defensive operation just illustrated is typically conceptualized in terms of projection of unacceptable sexual needs and motivations, along with aspects of the self tied to erotic motivations; conflictual motivations are split off from the self and attributed to an object. However, on closer examination, this defensive strategy typically involves not only projection of unacceptable motivations and associated emotional states, but also the segregation, or dissociation, of different sets of motivations that are in conflict. This implies that in the example, the patient's problem is not simply an intolerance of her sexuality, needing to project sexual motivations; rather, her psychological situation is more complex, having to do with difficulty integrating sexual needs and relationships with dependent needs and relationships. Her defensive strategy is to ensure that sexual motivations remain segregated from dependent needs, both in the organization of her defensive internal object relations and in her daily functioning.

In treatment, what is typically seen is that as defenses become less rigid, the therapist first notes a *role reversal*—a shift from a naive, dependent patient in relation to a sexual object, to a sexual patient in relation to a naive object (Kernberg 1992). In the treatment of NPO patients, the emergence of role reversals typically represents a significant clinical development and a loosening of the patient's defenses. However, returning to the example, even though the patient is now better able to tolerate awareness of her own sexual needs, it is only safe to do so in a setting in which her sexual and dependency needs remain segregated. It is only after working through the patient's identifications with both sides of the split and with the manner in which one identification defends against the other—and also defends against the anxiety of simultaneously experiencing two conflicting sets of motivations—that increased personality integration and decreased personality rigidity occur, leaving the patient free to have a more varied and fluid self experience. The patient who presents as naive should be free to enjoy her sexual and seductive impulses, and she should no longer need to separate vulnerability and love from sexuality, lending her a greater capacity to experience and enjoy erotic love.

Projective Identification

In BPO, defense is seen within a single internal object relation, with attribution of a conflictual motivation to an object representation and directed toward a self representation. As in NPO, when this internal object relation is enacted, impulsive parts of the self are attributed to an object, while the subject experiences himself as the object of his projected, impulsive, self representation. (For example, in a setting stimulating hostility and activation of an internal object relation of a vengeful self representation in relation to a victimized object representation, a patient will attribute the aggressive self representation to another person, experiencing himself as victimized by—i.e., as the object of—his projected, aggressive self representation.)

However, in contrast to a neurotic structure, dissociation and projection occur without the support of repression, in the setting of a split and poorly integrated (paranoid or idealized) object relation under the umbrella of a single highly charged affect state. The individual organized at a borderline level is not able to repress the connection between projected mental contents and the self, but instead maintains an identification, albeit a dissociated one, with what has been projected. This *ongoing* identification refers to the observation that even though the subject does not experience himself as vengeful and aggressive, he maintains an emotional connection to the vengeful and aggressive parts of himself. This connection is dissociated and denied (whereas in NPO, it is repressed) and is typically expressed in behavior that is not part of the dominant self experience (Joseph 1988).

Because this process involves attribution, or *projection*, of a conflictual representation into an object, and at the same time an ongoing *identification* with the projected parts of the self, this process is referred to as *projective identification*. In projective identification, the subject 1) attributes a self representation and associated motivation (most frequently an aggressive one, but sexual, narcissistic, and dependent representations and motivations can also be involved) to another person, and as a result the subject 2) experiences himself as the object or victim of his projections. At the same time, the subject 3) maintains an identification with, or connection to, the projected mental content that is 4) dissociated and denied.

Such an identification is most typically expressed in the patient's attitude and behavior—most simply, the subject projects an aggressive object representation while behaving aggressively; however, because the identification is dissociated, the subject does not experience himself as aggressive, even though he is objectively behaving in an aggressive fashion. (If attention is called to his behavior, he is likely to see it as a justified response to an attack from the object.) Clinically, this leads to any of the following rather confusing situations in which, for example, a patient may aggressively accuse his therapist of being aggressive, criticize and attack the therapist for being critical and attacking, or behave overtly seductively while accusing the therapist of being a pervert.

Projective Identification and Role Reversals

In projective identification, because the subject retains emotional contact with *both* sides of the object relation, 1) self and object representations are experienced as only poorly differentiated from one another, and 2) rapid oscillation often occurs between identifications with contradictory representations: one moment the patient is victim, next victimizer, and what was a moment ago a victimized self representation is now a victimized object representation. Sometimes the two identifications may alternate: the patient consciously identifies alternately with the victim and the victimizer, reflecting the rapid exchange of self and object within a single object relation associated with a highly charged affect state. At other times, the two contradictory identifications may be simultaneously enacted: one may dominate conscious experience while the other is expressed in behavior, as described earlier in the subsection "Internal Object Relations and Defense in the Borderline Level of Personality Organization."

In treatment, a patient may feel criticized while behaving critically, or may at one moment feel criticized and at the next feel that she is justifiably criticizing the therapist (the first example illustrates the role of dissociation; the second, instability of identifications). In either case, the patient moves back and forth between identifications with two contradictory representations under the umbrella of a single affect state. Tracking these role reversals is a central strategy in transference-focused psychotherapy (TFP) and the dynamic psychotherapy of all BPO patients.

As an example, consider a BPO patient with conflicts around aggression and narcissistic vulnerability. In treatment, as he comes to feel reliant on his therapist, he might activate a paranoid object relation of a victimized and depreciated representation in relation to a powerful, critical, and superior representation, with the entire object relation associated with feelings of hostility and devaluation. The patient will attribute to the therapist the critical and devaluating representation, while identifying with the victimized, depreciated representation.

However, in contrast to NPO, when this object relation is enacted, the patient will not simply experience himself as victimized and depreciated, but will simultaneously mistreat and depreciate the therapist. In essence, the patient's behavior enacts the object relation with the patient in the role of victimizer at the same time that he consciously experiences the object relation with roles reversed (i.e., feels himself to be the victim of aggression). Alternatively, the patient's conscious identifications with victim and victimizer may rapidly alternate, with the patient at one moment feeling attacked, and at the next moment sadistically attacking the therapist.

Projective Identification, Actualization, and Action

At this point, we add a final—and essential—distinguishing feature of projective identification: projections tend to become *actualized*, played out in interpersonal reality, not just experienced within the mind of the subject.[1] Whereas neurotic projection relies on symbolic manipulation of representations within the mind of the subject, projective identification is more concrete and tends to lead to *actual* manipulation of the external object, so that the object takes on the feelings and thoughts that the subject is projecting. This is to say that in neurotic projection, as the individual projects her impulses, she will feel or believe that the other is behaving seductively, or that the other may be angry; however, this does not typically involve actually inducing sexual or angry feelings or behaviors in the

---

[1]Sometimes the word *identification* in *projective identification* is used to refer to the experience of the external object, who comes to identify with the subject's projected object representation (e.g., see Ogden 1993c).

other person. In contrast, in projective identification, the individual believes the other is seductive or hostile, and then the individual behaves in such a fashion as to unconsciously elicit seductive or hostile feelings in the other. Projective identification begins in the mind of the subject, then, but is played out interpersonally between two people, so that the subject often *actually* becomes the object of his own projected impulse. In sum, in projective identification, not only does the subject remain identified with both sides of an object relation and with his projected representation, but he also unconsciously pressures the external object to feel and ultimately act in accordance with what he has projected.

Returning to the recent example of the patient who feels victimized and depreciated while at the same time attacking and devaluing his therapist, we can add that in this setting, the patient felt ongoing pressure to relentlessly accuse and criticize the therapist, insisting that the therapist was abusive and depreciative. From the patient's perspective, it was as if the projected representation were a concrete thing that needed to be repeatedly and forcefully pushed into the therapist in an effort to distance it from the self.

In this setting, with time, a likely (and unfortunate) outcome of this extremely confusing situation is that the patient will induce in the therapist what may become an overpowering counterpressure to point out to the patient that it is actually the *patient* who is critical and attacking, and in this process to in fact criticize and attack the patient. Thus in an uncontained situation, what begins as an effort on the part of the patient to rid himself of aggression by projecting it leads first to the patient's experience of being attacked by the therapist, next to the patient's attacking the therapist, then the therapist's experience of being attacked by the patient, and finally to the therapist's actually in some way attacking the patient! This process, referred to as *induction*, is the cause of powerful and extremely challenging countertransference reactions in the treatment of BPO patients.

In the dynamic therapies of BPO patients, the therapist quickly sees the impact of projective identification on the patient's behavior and communications, typically played out between patient and therapist in the transference as well as in the patient's interpersonal life. Thus, in contrast to what is seen in the treatment of NPO patients, where role reversals are a midphase development reflecting the loosening of defensive rigidity, in the treatment of BPO the therapist can see role reversals from the earliest sessions, and they quickly become a focus of intervention.

Anxieties and Conflicts Central to the Treatment of Personality Disorders: Paranoid and Depressive Anxieties and Oedipal Conflicts

When it comes to understanding the relationship among psychological conflict, defense, and personality disorders, especially useful are the constructs of depressive and paranoid anxieties, along with the distinctions between dyadic and triadic, or oedipal, conflicts. These constructs provide a clinically near way to classify the psychological conflicts and anxieties that are the foci of clinical intervention in the psychotherapies of patients with personality disorders. Further, the therapist's understanding of the patient's paranoid and depressive anxieties and their interdigitation with oedipal conflicts forms the basis of the conceptualization of the relationship between psychodynamic exploration and structural change.

Paranoid and Depressive Anxieties: Melanie Klein

It was Melanie Klein (1935/1975) who first introduced this extremely influential and clinically useful approach to understanding and classifying psychological conflicts. Klein's theories focus to a large degree on the role of aggression in psychopathology and on the impact of conflicts between hateful and loving impulses in psychological development and pathology. Klein introduced the constructs of the more immature or primitive *paranoid-schizoid position* (1946/1975) and the more advanced *depressive position* (1935), understood as two distinct psychological organizations, each with its own characteristic patterns of object relations, anxieties, and defenses.

In Klein's model, the paranoid-schizoid and depressive positions represent sequential developmental phases for the young child, and also fundamental and enduring psychological organizations. Although Klein's theory has not held up empirically as a model of development, it remains extraordinarily powerful for understanding adult psychological functioning within a psychodynamic frame of reference. Contemporary Kleinian views of the paranoid-schizoid and depressive positions emphasize that these are two ways of organizing mental experience; the two positions are conceptualized as two different mental states that exist in a more or less stable equilibrium within all of us (Bion 1963; Ogden 1993a; Steiner 1992). Each position is associated with its own set of anxieties and defensive operations.

Klein's model of paranoid-schizoid and depressive positions is the basic framework out of which Kernberg (1975) developed his model of borderline and neurotic levels of personality organization.[2] In particular, the constructs of paranoid and depressive anxieties as developed by Klein not only are of historical significance but also remain central to our understanding of developments in the treatment of patients with personality disorders. For this reason, we briefly summarize Klein's theory here.

Paranoid-Schizoid Positions in Equilibrium

The Paranoid-Schizoid Position

For Klein (1946), the central anxieties of the paranoid-schizoid position reflect the impact of inborn, *primitive* aggression. Primitive aggression is poorly integrated and of catastrophic proportions. In the young child overwhelmed by his internal aggression, projection of primitive aggression creates paranoia and a world of "bad" external objects; these "bad" external objects may be *reintrojected* (defensively taken back inside), creating an experience of internal persecution. Projection of bad internal objects onto the mother in particular leads to the experience of an all-bad, frustrating, and persecutory mother, whereas projection of the child's loving impulses, seen initially as expressions of the child's inborn loving dispositions, leads to the experience of an all-good, gratifying mother. Internal objects, both all-good and persecutory ones, are built up through repeated cycles of projection and introjection, and in this process, the mother's loving and gratifying ministrations contribute further to the development of the all-good, or idealized, sector, while splitting serves to protect the good, pleasurable experiences with the mother from the bad, persecutory ones.

As a result of these inevitable processes, the child has two contradictory experiences with the mother: on the one hand, the experience of a

---

[2]While there is a great deal of overlap between Kernberg's model of levels of psychopathology and that of contemporary Kleinians, differences in the underlying psychoanalytic frames of reference—and in particular, a relative de-emphasis in the Kleinian frame of reference on identity formation and diagnostic considerations, as well as different conceptualizations of drives—account for fundamental divergences.

mother who is gratifying, who is felt to provide for his needs, and with whom he has an idealized relationship; and on the other hand, the experience of a mother who is frustrating, who is felt to be withholding and attacking, and with whom he has a persecutory relationship. The young child cannot manage this degree of complexity, instead maintaining these idealized and persecutory experiences as separate and distinct.

Klein called this psychological situation the *paranoid-schizoid position* because projection of aggression creates paranoia, and at the same time splitting of the object involves concomitant splitting in the self, creating a schism within the self. The fundamental anxiety in the paranoid-schizoid position is the destruction of idealized internal and external object relations by persecutory object relations and primitive aggression, and the dominant defenses are splitting and projective identification. In addition to paranoid anxieties and splitting-based defenses (referred to by Klein as *primitive defenses*), the paranoid-schizoid position is characterized by weak ego boundaries, omnipotent and concrete thinking, and so-called *part objects*.

Part and Whole Objects

In the paranoid-schizoid position, both external and internal objects are experienced as part objects. In this term, *part* refers to the young child's ability to experience the mother only as a part—as a feeding or withholding breast that either meets his needs or fails to do so. At this level of development or psychological organization, external objects are experienced entirely on the basis of the degree to which they do or do not meet the needs of the subject, and are not experienced as separate people who exist in their own right and have needs of their own that might warrant attention or concern.

In this context, *part* can also be understood to refer to the all-good or all-bad quality of objects in the paranoid-schizoid position, and is contrasted with the *whole*—that is, the ambivalent, better-integrated internal and external objects that characterize more advanced phases of development and psychological organization. *Whole objects*, in contrast to part, are neither all good nor all bad, but instead include both positive and negative attributes. The experience of a whole object implies the capacity to tolerate *ambivalence*—for example, to recognize that the mother who gratifies and the mother who frustrates are one and the same—and an appreciation of the other as separate and apart rather than as omnipotently controlled.

Klein makes a clear distinction between *idealized objects*, which are all-good part objects built up in the paranoid-schizoid position, and *good objects*, which are integrated and ambivalently held, seen to include both positive and negative attributes under the dominance of the positive. The establishment of good objects, internal and external, is for Klein a pivotal developmental achievement and marks the introduction of the depressive position.

The Depressive Position

In Klein's theory, in the paranoid-schizoid position, the gradual building up of a world of idealized internal objects helps mitigate the anxieties associated with the expression of primitive aggression and persecutory object relations. This partial security reduces to some degree the need for splitting, and in conjunction with cognitive development introduces awareness that the ideal mother and persecutory mother are one and the same: "The mother who feeds me is also the mother who frustrates; the mother whom I love is also the mother whom I hate and whom I attack in fantasy." This awareness heralds a new level of development and a shift from the paranoid-schizoid position to the depressive position, representing a qualitative transformation, and leading to a new level of psychological integration and a new set of anxieties, defenses, and object relations.

According to Klein, the initial awareness that the ideal and the persecutory object are one and the same causes acute anxiety. Whereas in the paranoid-schizoid position, anxieties were only about preservation of the self—with projection of aggression to off-load it into an object, and with no concern for survival of the object—now the child is worried about the state of the object, for the first time seen as separate and vulnerable. In the paranoid-schizoid position, if the object is frustrating in the mind of the child, it in essence becomes a bad object (this is an example of the omnipotence of thought characteristic of more poorly integrated mental states). Similarly, if the object is absent or unavailable, it also becomes bad. Thus, the child does not have the experience in the paranoid-schizoid position of directing aggression toward a good object or of missing or mourning the loss of a good object, and as a result is never compelled to take responsibility for his aggression, which within a paranoid-schizoid orientation is both projected (so that it is the object and not the self that is aggressive) and justified (the child's aggression is always directed at an object that is bad). As a result, in the paranoid-schizoid position, the child experiences no concern for the object, and the only anxiety is in relation to the child's own safety.

In contrast, with the introduction of the depressive position, for the first time the child has the experience of directing his aggression toward an object that is frustrating but is also good. Rather than fearing for his own safety, the child now fears for the safety of his object, now seen as at risk of being destroyed by the child's own sadism and aggression. This new fear is experienced as *depressive anxiety*, or guilt.

Klein (1935) described this organization as *depressive* because it involves the individual taking responsibility for his aggression rather than projecting it, leading to feelings of guilt and depression in relation to his destructiveness. The depressive position also initiates a process of depression and mourning in relation to loss of the idealized object, which is sacrificed and mourned in the process of integration, and also in relation to the newfound awareness of separateness from the object, with a capacity to pine for the object who is good but absent. The object is now understood as having a life of its own and its own needs, beyond the subject's control and with other objects (Ogden 1993b). This new awareness introduces the triangulation essential for the Oedipus complex.

Depressive Position and Psychological Growth

In depressive anxieties, the individual takes responsibility for his aggression directed at an object perceived as good, and blames himself, experiencing self-recrimination; thus, tolerating ambivalence, a capacity tied to integrative processes and psychological growth, leads initially to pain, depression, guilt, loss, and remorse, and ultimately the wish to make reparation. In this setting, the individual takes responsibility for and experiences regret in relation to the damage he has inflicted on his objects in fantasy as he comes to tolerate emotional awareness of the loss of ideal images of himself and his objects (Segal 1964). Contemporary Kleinians describe this process in terms of the subject's "working through of the depressive position" (Hinshelwood 1991).

In the Kleinian model, working through the anxieties of the depressive position is associated with a series of related and important psychological developments. Working through depressive anxieties enables the individual 1) to take responsibility for his own destructive, aggressive, and sexual impulses, while tolerating awareness of these impulses in others; 2) to establish mutually dependent relationships; 3) to feel love and concern for others, who are experienced as separate and complex; and 4) to tolerate loss and to mourn. Further, the capacity to experience others as separate is closely tied to 5) recognition of the internal world as distinct from the external world (i.e., with a shift away from concrete and omnipotent thinking) and to 6) the capacity for symbolic thought (Ogden 1993b; Spillius 1994).

In the object relations theory model elaborated in this book, all these capacities correspond with identity consolidation; they are the hallmarks of the normal personality. Thus, the process of working through depressive anxieties as described in a Kleinian model can be seen to facilitate the integrative processes that are the central objectives of transference-focused psychotherapy—extended.

Triangular Conflicts and the Oedipus Complex

When Klein introduced the depressive position, she was building on earlier seminal contributions of Sigmund Freud (1887–1902/1954, 1900/1964), who introduced the construct of the Oedipus complex, referring to the complexities of the child's relationship with the parents as a couple. To this point, our discussion of paranoid and depressive anxieties has focused on the relation between the child and the mother as the prototype for dyadic conflicts; now we focus on the child in relation to the mother in a triangular, or *triadic*, setting—one in which the mother is seen to have relations with others, needs of her own, and an internal life that does not revolve entirely around the child. Also, up to this point we have focused our discussion of depressive anxieties predominantly in relation to conflicts between love and aggression, but we now expand this discussion to include conflicts among the complex array of motivations and needs that come into play in the oedipal situation, and ultimately in all human relations.

For both Freud and Klein, the oedipal situation—the relationship between the child and two parents—is the prototypic triangular, or triadic, conflict. The hallmark of triadic conflicts, in contrast to dyadic ones, is that an individual's relation to a loved, desired, or needed person or source of gratification is inextricably tied, psychologically, to a third party. From the perspective of triangular conflicts, the developmental hurdles of the oedipal situation entail coming to terms with living in a world in which the people the individual loves and needs have relationships with others that exclude him (as well as needs of their own that do not involve him). The capacity to appreciate and grapple with this dilemma is predicated on the awareness of a self with a subjective inner life, of another person separate from the self and not controlled by the self, and of a third party. This constellation signifies a relatively mature level of psychological and cognitive development; it is compatible with what Klein described as the depressive position and is typically associated with the capacity for self-observation and self-reflection.

In oedipal conflicts, sexual, dependent, competitive, narcissistic, and aggressive wishes, needs, and fears are linked to childhood fantasies of breaking up the parental couple to possess the sole attention of one or both parents, excluding and triumphing over the other parent as well as over other members of the family. As a result, sexual, dependent, competitive, narcissistic, and aggressive wishes, needs, and fears, and the fantasies to which they are linked, are conflictual, and enactment of the object relations associated with these motivations will lead to feelings of guilt and loss (depressive anxieties), coupled with fantasies of feared retribution (paranoid anxieties).

For example, for the oedipal girl, fantasies of possessing her father as her own love object will also involve fantasies of displacing, triumphing over, and perhaps doing away with her mother. To the extent that the girl retains a positive image of her mother in the face of her rivalrous feelings, she is confronted with a painful conflict. Her wishes to gratify her sexual and sadistic impulses, along with her competitive and narcissistic desires to possess her father, are in conflict with her love for her mother, her dependency on her mother, and her fear of her mother's retribution. Alternatively, she can retreat to a paranoid orientation in which she projects her impulses onto her mother, the girl now feeling frightened and hostile, or devaluing and triumphant. In the adult, these conflicts can remain unresolved and buried. To the degree that this is the case, situations that stimulate oedipal conflicts, particularly sexual intimacy and competitive struggles, will stimulate anxiety, guilt, and fear. It is because of the unconscious link between sexual love and guilt-provoking childhood fantasies of incestuous triumph that NPO patients often have difficulty integrating passionate sexuality with tenderness and love.

Dyadic and triangular conflicts, conflicts in relation to depending on and trusting another person and those in relation to living in a world where an individual is mindful of the needs of those on whom she depends and from whom she wants things, are often condensed and may play off one another. Conflicts around dependency and trust make it difficult to negotiate triangular and oedipal conflicts. At the same time, experiencing a situation in terms of dyadic needs and conflicts can serve as a way to avoid anxieties associated with oedipal and triangular conflicts. As a result, the activation of dyadic object relations in treatment will at times reflect the dominance of dyadic conflicts, but at other times and as these conflicts are worked through, such activation of dyadic object relations will be used defensively to avoid oedipal-level conflict—just as the activation of oedipal-level material will at times be used to defend against the emergence of dyadic conflicts around dependency and trust. Triangular and oedipal conflicts tend to play a central role in the treatment of NPO patients, and often become a context for working through depressive anxieties in the treatments of these patients. In BPO patients, although oedipal issues may be evident even from early on, triangular conflicts tend to emerge as central in the middle or late phase of treatment, coinciding with the emerging centrality of depressive anxieties in the clinical process.

Level of Personality Organization and Paranoid-Schizoid, Depressive, and Oedipal Conflicts

The organization of anxieties, defenses, and object relations at a paranoid-schizoid versus depressive level differentiates patients with severe personality disorders from those with higher-level personality disorders, and also distinguishes these groups from individuals with normal personality. From a structural perspective, the psychological anxieties, defenses, object relations, and quality of thought that define the paranoid-schizoid position correspond with the internal world of the patient with severe personality pathology and identity diffusion, whereas those of the depressive position correspond with the internal world of the patient with higher level personality pathology and a consolidated identity.

Similarly, in more severe pathology, dyadic conflicts predominate, whereas in higher-level personality disorders, triangular and oedipal conflicts predominate. Thus, the overall trajectory from less well- to better-integrated psychological states traces a shift from the predominance of paranoid anxieties and dyadic conflicts to the predominance of depressive anxieties and triangular conflicts—and ultimately from depressive anxieties and triangular conflicts to a less anxious state characterized by comfort in the individual's own capacity to deal flexibly and morally with conflictual motivations. In the setting of a sense of the self as predominantly good, the individual is able to balance concern for others with the needs of the self, and forfeits projection, splitting, and repression, instead tolerating awareness of and taking responsibility for aggression and other conflictual motivations.

Although these are some clinically useful generalizations about the relationship between the paranoid-schizoid and depressive positions and different levels of personality organization, it is important to appreciate that at any given level of personality organization, paranoid and depressive anxieties exist in a state of equilibrium. Thus, from a dynamic perspective, the repeated working through of paranoid and depressive anxieties is seen as a universal feature of psychological growth at *all* levels of personality organization.

In the treatment of BPO patients, shifts between the paranoid and depressive *positions* and associated anxieties are central to the exploration and working through of core conflicts motivating splitting. In the treatment of NPO patients, temporary emergence of a paranoid-schizoid organization also may occur, with splitting predominating, as in the clinical illustration that follows of a patient who defensively retreats from the pain of depressive anxieties to the paranoid-schizoid position. More commonly and consistently in the treatment of NPO patients, in the setting of a neurotic structure and an overall depressive orientation, oscillation is seen between 1) paranoid anxieties (i.e., feeling persecuted by their projected impulses or by anxieties associated with the expression of their impulses, such as "He is angry at me"; "I will be punished because I am angry") and 2) depressive anxieties (i.e., feeling responsible for their impulses, such as "I am angry at him"; "I feel guilty, ashamed, or remorseful"). This dialectic may emerge in the NPO patient's attitude toward and expectations of the therapist; for example, such a patient may feel that the therapist is not sufficiently caring or interested and, paradoxically, may also feel undeserving of the therapist's help and care.

In sum, the psychodynamic treatments of patients with personality disorders across the spectrum of severity are characterized by repeated working through of both paranoid and depressive anxieties, each defending against the other. With each incremental step toward integration, these anxieties are activated, and the patient must be helped to tolerate them and ultimately to work through them. In the BPO patient, this process will be associated with identity consolidation; in the NPO patient, it will be associated with the integration of conflictual object relations into an already consolidated identity. In both settings but at different levels of integration, the individual will oscillate between the pain of taking responsibility for his conflictual motivations and the anxiety that results from projecting them, with a gradual shift toward responsibility and containment. When treatment is successful, repeated and progressive working through of cycles of paranoid and depressive anxieties occurs as the patient makes a gradual shift toward a more solidly depressive mode of functioning.

Clinical Illustration: Dynamic Relationship Between Paranoid and Depressive Orientations in a Patient Organized at a Neurotic Level

A middle-aged man has had a history of a long and troubled relationship with his domineering father, who is now elderly. A year into a very helpful but somewhat stormy therapy, the patient moved from high BPO to a predominately neurotic level of personality organization and functioning. However, after a 2-week break in treatment, the patient came into his session complaining angrily and bitterly about his father. His tone was rancorous; he described his father as being intractable, infuriating, selfish, undermining, and cruel. The patient went on to happily acknowledge, "I really let him have it this time!"

The therapist inquired about what had precipitated this marked change from the patient's recently more positive attitude toward his father, to which the patient angrily responded that he had been kidding himself, that a relationship with such a "self-centered, sadistic son of a bitch" was impossible. He then proceeded to criticize the therapist for seeming not to understand this.

The therapist noted to himself the rather striking return of the patient's polarized, poorly integrated view of his father (and though not affectively dominant in the moment, also of the therapist), colored by hostility. When the therapist inquired further about the circumstances of the argument, it emerged that the patient had become enraged that his father would not give him a large sum of money that he asked for, even though, at the same time, the patient understood that his father was concerned about maintaining a financial cushion for himself.

At this point, the therapist shared his impression with the patient, commenting that he was struck by the patient's current rather extreme attitude toward his father, noting that it felt to some degree like a return to an "all-bad" view of his father that he had entertained early in his treatment but that had been changing in recent months.

The patient at this point acknowledged the abrupt shift in his attitude and seemed thoughtful. The therapist suggested that perhaps, with his father aging and increasingly frail, the idea of the patient's own hostility and greed being directed toward someone whom he cared about and who seemed to care about him (even though this person may have been deeply flawed) was too painful; perhaps it was easier to see his father as undeserving of love. The patient began to weep silently.

This vignette illustrates the oscillation between depressive and paranoid anxieties, and in particular the defensive emergence of a paranoid orientation ("My father, who is all bad, wants to hurt me and is selfish, and I am justifiably angry") in a patient struggling predominantly at this point in his treatment with depressive conflicts: "I want to hurt and take advantage of my father, who is not all bad, and I feel guilty about that." The emergence of paranoid anxieties can be viewed as defensive, serving to avoid what are at this point in treatment more central depressive conflicts. This defensive emergence of paranoid anxieties as a retreat from the pain of depressive anxieties is sometimes referred to as *splitting of the depressive position.*

Ambivalence, Integration, and Structural Change

Ambivalence can be defined as the capacity to tolerate awareness of conflicting motivations simultaneously directed toward the same object. In our discussion of paranoid and depressive anxieties, we focused predominantly on the integration of aggressive and loving object relations. In our discussion of the Oedipus complex, and also of neurotic dissociation, we broadened that view to consider how integration not only of aggressive and loving motivations but also of sexual, narcissistic, and dependent motivations can pose a challenge, activating oedipal conflicts as well as depressive and paranoid anxieties.

In other words, we conceptualize integrative processes in TFP-E not only in the relatively simple terms of an individual simultaneously experiencing love and aggression, but also in terms of the difficulties integrating other motivations that for a particular individual may be in conflict (e.g., love and sexuality; dependency and aggression; narcissistic, self-serving motivations and love). Moving from least well-integrated to better-integrated personality structures, from low BPO through NPO, there is increasingly greater complexity of conscious motivational structures, and greater capacity to simultaneously activate, contain, and integrate motivational structures that are potentially in conflict with one another within any given object relation—and within an overall sense of self experienced as largely positive, moral, and able to contain and make reparation for conflictual motivations. These capacities correspond with increasing complexity in the sense of self and others and increasing depth in relations with others.

This transition—from splitting, repression, and dissociation to integration and containment of conflictual motivations within an overall positive sense of self—is illustrated in the following dream, reported by a patient toward the end of her treatment. In the dream, she was carrying a white bag. She realized that one side of the bag was dirty. But rather than panicking and feeling she had to run home, as would be usual for her, she felt relaxed. She could simply turn the bag around. She would still know the dirt was there, but it would not really show. And even if it did, it was okay; she could clean the bag when she got home.

Key Clinical Concepts

- A psychological conflict is organized in relation to a conflictual motivation ("impulse"), a defense against awareness or expression of the conflictual motivation, and a negative affect or "anxiety-motivating defense."
- In a neurotic structure, enactment of defensive internal object relations supports repression of impulsive object relations.
- In a borderline structure, defensive and impulsive object relations are mutually dissociated and interchangeable (idealized object relations defend against paranoid object relations, and vice versa).
- In the depressive position, the individual struggles with depressive conflicts, in which he takes responsibility for his impulses and experiences pain, guilt, and remorse in relation to whole objects.
- In the paranoid-schizoid position, the individual projects responsibility for her impulses and experiences fear in relation to "part" of split objects.
- The capacity to tolerate ambivalence is a marker of psychological integration and a cornerstone of healthy personality functioning.

References

Bion WR: Elements of Psycho-Analysis. London, Heinemann, 1963

Freud S: Letters to Wilhelm Fleiss (1887–1902). New York, Basic Books, 1954

Freud S: The interpretation of dreams (1900), in The Standard Edition of the Complete Psychological Works of Sigmund Freud, Vols 4–5. Edited and translated by Strachey J. London, Hogarth Press, 1964, pp 1–626

Hinshelwood RD: A Dictionary of Kleinian Thought. Northvale, NJ, Jason Aronson, 1991

Joseph B: Projective identification—some clinical aspects, in Melanie Klein Today, Vol 1. Edited by Spillius EB. London, Routledge, 1988, pp 138–150

Kernberg OF: Countertransference, in Borderline Conditions and Pathological Narcissism. New York, Jason Aronson, 1975, pp 49–68

Kernberg OF: Aggression in Personality Disorders and Perversions. New Haven, CT, Yale University Press, 1992

Kernberg OF, Caligor E: A psychoanalytic theory of personality disorders, in Major Theories of Personality Disorder, 2nd Edition. Edited by Lenzenweger MF, Clarkin JF. New York, Guilford, 2005, pp 114–156

Klein M: A contribution to the psychogenesis of manic-depressive states (1935), in Love, Guilt and Reparation and Other Works, 1921–1945. London, Hogarth Press, 1975, pp 262–289

Klein M: Notes on some schizoid mechanisms (1946), in Envy and Gratitude and Other Works, 1946–1963. New York, Free Press, 1975, pp 1–24

Ogden TH: Between the paranoid-schizoid and the depressive position, in Matrix of the Mind: Object Relations and the Psychoanalytic Dialogue. Northvale, NJ, Jason Aronson, 1993a, pp 101–130

Ogden TH: The depressive position and the birth of the historical subject, in Matrix of the Mind: Object Relations and the Psychoanalytic Dialogue. Northvale, NJ, Jason Aronson, 1993b, pp 67–99

Ogden TH: Projective Identification and Psychotherapeutic Technique (1982). Northvale, NJ, Jason Aronson, 1993c

Segal H: An Introduction to the Work of Melanie Klein. New York, Basic Books, 1964

Spillius EB: Development in Kleinian thought: overview and personal view. Psychoanal Inq 14:324–364, 1994

Steiner J: The equilibrium between the paranoid-schizoid and the depressive positions, in Clinical Lectures on Klein and Bion. Edited by Anderson R. London, Routledge, 1992, pp 34–45

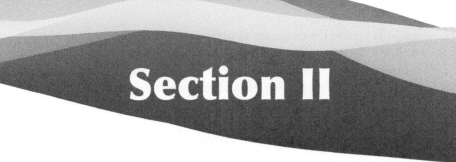

Section II

Overview of TFP-E

Basic Tasks,
the Therapeutic Relationship,
and Strategies of Treatment

HAVING PROVIDED A FOUNDATION FOR
conceptualizing and classifying personality disorders within the framework of object relations theory, we now provide a foundation for conceptualizing our approach to treatment. In the three chapters composing
Section II, we introduce the general clinical principles and basic constructs
that define transference-focused psychotherapy—extended (TFP-E).
Based on object relations theory, TFP-E is a flexible treatment model that
focuses on self and other functioning and the relationship between the patient's personality organization and treatment strategies:

- In Chapter 4, we introduce the basic tasks of the TFP-E therapist, as
  we provide an overview of the basic elements that make up the treatment and define essential terms.
- In Chapter 5, we discuss the therapeutic relationship; in TFP-E, the
  therapeutic relationship forms the matrix within which the treatment
  unfolds. In this chapter, we consider the attitude and stance of the TFP-
  E therapist, the therapeutic alliance, transference, and countertransference.
- We complete our overview of TFP-E in Chapter 6 with a discussion of
  the strategies of TFP-E. The strategies of treatment organize our clini-

cal approach to the treatment of patients across the entire range of personality disorders. Also in Chapter 6, we describe how basic strategies of treatment are modified to meet the varying clinical needs of patients with borderline personality organization and those with neurotic personality organization. In our discussion of strategies, we focus on our understanding of how the strategies of treatment support different psychological capacities in patients at different levels of severity, facilitating therapeutic change.

For an in-depth discussion of assessment, see Section III, "The Skillful Consultation," where we review our model of classification and its relation to patient prognosis and treatment planning.

Basic Tasks and
Elements of Treatment

IN THIS CHAPTER, WE INTRODUCE THE
basic therapeutic tasks of transference-focused psychotherapy—extended
(TFP-E), both to provide an overview of the treatment approach and to
introduce constructs that will be discussed in detail in the chapters that
follow. We define key terms and familiarize the reader with the basic elements that form the conceptual foundation and the technical building
blocks of the treatment. Our overall approach is to focus on promoting
the coalescence of conflictual object relations to foster identity consolidation and integration, which can take place at increasing levels of complexity. As we explain, integrative processes are different at different levels of
personality organization. At the same time, there are unifying objectives
and clinical principles that organize work across the spectrum of severity.
In this chapter, we review basic elements of the treatment while calling attention to how these elements may serve different functions or be subject
to differential implementation as a function of severity of personality pathology.

Basic Tasks

- The first task of the TFP-E therapist is to **create a setting that will facilitate the activation and enactment of conflictual object relations in**

the therapy, while at the same time ensuring that this occurs in a controlled and therapeutic fashion. This task is accomplished by creating a therapeutic relationship between therapist and patient that is safely contained within the boundaries established by the treatment frame and contract.

- The therapist's next task is to **identify a focus of intervention**. This task entails listening attentively as the patient speaks openly and freely, in order to identify the object relations that are affectively dominant in any given session while at the same time directing attention to developments in the patient's life outside the treatment.

- The therapist's third task is to **help the patient explore and work through core conflicts** as they are repeatedly activated and enacted in his current relationships and in his interactions with the therapist. This entails interpreting the anxieties motivating the defensive operations that interfere with integrative processes, while promoting self-observation and reflection. In the process of working through, the therapist emphasizes the link between the patient's core conflicts and the treatment goals.

Basic Elements of the Treatment

Task 1: Setting the Stage for Exploration— Bringing Conflictual Object Relations Into the Treatment

The treatment contract establishes the *treatment frame*, which defines the conditions for the treatment, including the respective roles of therapist and patient. Within the structure provided by the treatment frame, the therapist establishes the psychotherapeutic relationship. The therapeutic alliance developed between patient and therapist and the therapist's stance of therapeutic neutrality are central aspects of the psychotherapeutic relationship.

The Treatment Frame

The treatment frame is a defining feature of any kind of psychotherapy, creating the context within which therapeutic work can take place. The treatment frame defines the structure of the treatment and the respective roles of therapist and patient in the treatment. The frame establishes the frequency and duration of sessions, expectations about attendance, and arrangements about scheduling and payment. The treatment frame also establishes clear expectations about contact between therapist and patient outside regularly scheduled appointments hours, including face-to-face meetings, telephone calls, texting and e-mail contact, and handling of emergencies. The treatment frame is formally established and mutually agreed upon by patient and therapist before treatment begins and is tailored to meet the needs of each individual patient. It is the treatment frame that clearly distinguishes the relationship between therapist and patient from other relationships in the patient's past and current life.

Together, the treatment frame and the psychotherapeutic relationship establish a reality-based framework for the treatment, and enable patient and therapist to manage destructive and self-destructive behaviors on the part of the patient. The mutual agreement between patient and therapist that establishes the treatment frame is often referred to as the *treatment contract* (Etchegoyen 1991; Yeomans et al. 2015). In TFP-E, this is not a written contract but rather a clearly and specifically described agreement between patient and therapist outlining the necessary conditions for treatment.

In the treatment of patients with severe personality disorders, it often takes a number of sessions to establish a mutually agreed-upon treatment contract; thoughtfully and effectively negotiating this process can reduce the likelihood that the patient will drop out of treatment (Yeomans et al. 1994). Challenges to the frame are common when working with severe personality disorders, and the treatment contract provides a baseline of mutually agreed-upon expectations from which the therapist can make use of *limit setting* as needed. Contracting around destructive behaviors, be they self-destructive, destructive to others, or destructive to the integrity of the therapy, plays an important role in helping patients control maladaptive behaviors, and maintaining the frame is a focus of clinical attention, especially in the early phases of treatment.

In contrast, in the treatment of patients with higher level personality pathology, contracting around destructive behaviors is generally not needed. With these patients, the treatment contract and frame function largely to create a predictable and reliable setting within which the patient's internal object relations can safely unfold and be explored.

The Psychotherapeutic Relationship

Within the reliable structure provided by the treatment setting, the TFP-E therapist and patient establish a special relationship, referred to as the *psychotherapeutic relationship*. This relationship is a highly specialized relationship in which one party, the patient, is encouraged to communicate his inner needs as fully as possible, while the other participant, the therapist, refrains from doing so.

The role of the therapist is to use her expertise to broaden and deepen the patient's capacity for self-exploration and self-awareness. To this end, the therapist is fully engaged in ongoing efforts to understand the patient's internal experience as it is expressed in verbal and nonverbal communications and the countertransference. The psychotherapeutic relationship, with its relative lack of usual social conventions and its singular focus on the needs of the patient, stimulates activation of key motivational systems within the patient, and promotes the enactment of conflictual object relations. The psychotherapeutic relationship is established by the therapist during the opening phase of treatment and is the necessary context within which the psychotherapeutic technique described in this book can be implemented. The therapeutic alliance, transference, and countertransference are all embedded in the therapeutic relationship.

The Therapeutic Alliance

The *therapeutic alliance* is an important component of the psychotherapeutic relationship (Bender 2005). In a psychodynamic framework, the alliance is the relationship established between the self-observing part of the patient that wants and is able to make use of help and the therapist in the role of helpful expert. The alliance reflects, on the one hand, the patient's realistic expectations that the therapist has something to offer on the basis of training, expertise, and concern, and, on the other, the therapist's commitment to help the patient and make use of a developing understanding of the patient (Kernberg 2004).

Patients with higher level personality pathology are for the most part able to establish a relatively stable alliance in the early phases of therapy (Bender 2005). Initial difficulties or ruptures of the alliance that may arise over the course of treatment are relatively easily resolved and often serve, once worked through, to deepen the patient's self-understanding while further solidifying the working relationship between therapist and patient (Caligor et al. 2007).

In contrast, patients with more severe personality disorders often have difficulty establishing a therapeutic alliance, and the quality of the alliance is vulnerable to wide fluctuation across sessions and even moment to moment within a session (Yeomans et al. 2015). Efforts to establish an alliance rely on the therapist's ability to avoid taking sides in the conflict presently activated within the patient and in the treatment. Ruptures are common and inevitable, and may be accompanied by strong emotional re-actions on the part of the patient; not uncommonly, these may include hostility, accusations, and paranoia. Exploration of ruptures as they occur throughout the treatment is central to the psychotherapeutic process in TFP-E, especially in the treatment of severe personality disorders. In the successful treatment of patients with such disorders, a gradual consolidation of a stable therapeutic alliance develops over the course of the treatment.

Technical Neutrality and the Therapist's Stance

As the TFP-E therapist establishes a therapeutic alliance with the patient, she maintains what has been referred to as a *technically neutral* stance (Auchincloss and Samberg 2012; Levy and Inderbitzin 1992), in which *technical* refers to the techniques employed by the therapist. Although technical neutrality as a construct is a cornerstone of TFP-E, the term is rather problematic. *Technical neutrality* is sometimes mistakenly taken to mean that the TFP-E therapist is neutral in her attitude toward the patient, and the term may conjure up images of the caricature of a psychoanalyst, sitting impassively and inactively, listening to her patient and rarely intervening. In fact, technical neutrality does not imply that the therapist is unresponsive or indifferent to the patient's progress or that the therapist is passive. To the contrary, the TFP-E therapist is quite active, and her attitude toward the patient should reflect an interest in the patient's well-being and a willingness to help, combined with an attitude of warmth and concern (Schafer 1983).

When we speak of technical neutrality, we refer not to the therapist's attitude toward the patient but rather to the therapist's attitude toward the patient's conflicts; technical neutrality calls on the therapist to avoid actively getting involved in or taking sides in the patient's conflicts. With this objective in mind, the technically neutral therapist exercises restraint in relation to making supportive interventions, such as offering advice or attempting to intervene in the patient's life. Instead, the neutral therapist strives to be as open as possible to all aspects of the patient's conflicts and behaviors, and to maintain a commitment to understanding the patient's inner life as completely as possible. To this end, the neutral therapist allies herself with the part of the patient that has a capacity for self-observation (Kernberg 2004).

Technical neutrality is perhaps best understood in terms of *therapeutic neutrality*. The TFP-E therapist's neutral stance is an essential element in our understanding of the therapeutic process in TFP-E and is a defining feature of the therapist's stance within the psychotherapeutic relationship. At the same time, deviations from technical neutrality are inevitable. In the treatment of severe personality disorders, planned deviations are an essential part of psychotherapeutic technique, introduced most commonly in relation to limit setting to help the patient control destructive behaviors. In the treatment of healthier patients, it is easier to more consistently maintain a neutral stance. In addition to intentional or planned deviations from neutrality, countertransference pressures can lead to unintended deviations from our customary therapeutic stance.

Task 2: Establishing a Focus for Intervention — Identifying the Affectively Dominant Object Relations While Attending to External Reality and the Hierarchy of Therapeutic Priorities

As the patient speaks freely and openly, his internal world and his external difficulties begin to take shape in the treatment through his verbal communications, behavior, and interactions with the therapist, as well as in the countertransference. The therapist's task is to sort through and in her own mind organize the patient's various communications, focusing on the task of identifying the object relations that seem to represent the central theme in the session; we refer to these object relations as the *affectively dominant object relations* or simply the *dominant object relations*. Identifying these object relations points to an area of conflict and a focus of inquiry, and putting the dominant object relations into words begins to stimulate processes of self-observation and reflection in the patient, setting the stage for exploring and interpreting core conflicts. At the same time, on a parallel track, the therapist maintains a watchful eye on important developments in the patient's life outside the treatment, while attending to a hierarchy of therapeutic priorities and also to the integrity of the treatment frame.

Free and Open Communication

In TFP-E, the patient's role is to speak in an unstructured way, as freely and openly as possible and without a structured agenda, about whatever goes through his mind when he is in his therapy session. It is through this process that the patient's conflictual object relations begin to come alive in the therapy.

In the treatment of higher-level personality disorders, in which repression-based defenses predominate, this process is in many ways similar to the process of *free association* (Auchincloss and Samberg 2012) used in psychoanalytic treatments. The objective is to facilitate the emergence of conflictual, largely unconscious object relations and associated defenses in the treatment. Activation of conflictual object relations is stimulated by the invitation to communicate openly and freely in the psychotherapeutic relationship and other aspects of the setting. As conflictual and defensive object relations are activated and enacted in the treatment, they are expressed largely through the patient's thoughts, feelings, and associations as they are communicated verbally and through whatever difficulties he experiences (*"resistances"*[1]) in communicating openly and freely.

In the treatment of patients with more severe personality disorders, in which splitting-based defenses predominate, the therapist also asks the patient to speak openly and freely. With quite similar instructions to the patient, the therapist observes different developments than those described

---

[1]The term and concept of *resistance* are central to classical psychodynamic approaches to technique (Auchincloss and Samberg 2012), and *resistance* is used to refer to activation and enactment of a patient's defenses in relation to the treatment. In treatment settings where repression-based defenses predominate, the patient's defensive operations will frequently manifest as some sort of difficulty with ("resistance to") open communication or self-observation, often in the form of silences, noticeable omissions of specifics or particular content, or changes of subject. In treatment settings where splitting-based defenses are organizing the clinical material, "resistances" tend to be easier to identify, often taking the form of prolonged or even stubborn silences, discussion of trivial matters, or failure to bring important material into session (all reflecting the enactment of dissociative defenses in relation to the treatment), as well as challenges to the frame, such as persistent lateness or cancellation of sessions. In the context of TFP-E, the term *resistance* is somewhat problematic in that it implies that the patient is intentionally working against the treatment, when in fact activation of defenses is the cutting edge of the treatment. As a result, we have chosen to omit usage of the terms *resistance* and *analysis of resistance* in this volume. Within the object relations theory–based model employed in TFP-E, resistance can be more usefully and specifically understood in terms of activation and enactment of the patient's defensive object relations in the treatment, and analysis of resistance can be understood in terms of the identification, exploration, and interpretation of the impact and functions of these defensive object relations. For the reader interested in a contemporary discussion of resistance within the framework of ego psychology, we recommend the chapter "Resistance Analysis" Busch (1995) in *The Ego at the Center of Clinical Technique*.

in neurotic personality organization and that reflect the impact of dissociative defenses on communications of patients organized at a borderline level. In contrast with the setting of repression-based defenses, in which open communication leads to the unfolding of unconscious processes and defenses, in the setting of splitting-based defenses, efforts at free and open communication often result in discussion of trivial material—or in the patient's focusing on seemingly suitable content while splitting off and failing to bring into treatment important (and sometimes urgent) aspects of his own behavior and experience inside or outside the session. Often, the patient's behavior in session and the feelings he elicits in the therapist, rather than the content of his verbal communications, are the most useful channels of communication in the session.

Thus, rather than seeing *free association* in the setting of severe personality disorders, we see a process more accurately described as *free dissociation*, reflecting the impact of splitting-based defenses on the clinical process. When splitting-based defenses predominate, dissociative processes and their impact on the patient's verbal and nonverbal communications and his behavior are often the focus of clinical attention.

The Therapist as Participant Observer

In TFP-E, the therapist assumes a neutral stance when formulating an intervention. However, in her own internal reactions to the patient, rather than striving for neutrality, the therapist makes an effort to open herself up as fully as possible to the patient and to the thoughts and feelings stimulated within her by the patient. The TFP-E therapist's ability to maintain a technically neutral stance depends on her capacity both to open herself up to the patient and to observe her interactions with the patient, reflecting on the feelings that are stimulated in her by the patient's verbal and nonverbal communications. Thus, the TFP-E therapist is both participant and observer (Sullivan 1938/1964), interacting with the patient and allowing the patient to affect her internally, and then standing back and reflecting on what is happening in the session.

Therapeutic Listening and the Three Channels of Communication

In each session, the therapist strives to open herself as fully as possible to the patient's communications. It is helpful to think of these communications as coming through three channels (Yeomans et al. 2015):

1. **Verbal** content of what the patient has to say
2. **Nonverbal** communications embedded in the patient's behavior in session and in interactions with the therapist
3. Communications embedded in the feelings the patient elicits in the therapist as part of the **countertransference**

As the therapist listens, she tries to translate her cognitive and affective responses to what the patient is saying and doing, in order to imagine the object relations organizing the patient's communications. The therapist tends to focus particularly on descriptions of others and how the patient views himself in relation to others as she listens to the content of the patient's communications in the verbal sphere.

At the same time, the therapist attends closely to what the patient is doing, considering what is being enacted with the therapist in the telling of this particular material in this particular fashion, and contemplating what is embedded in the patient's tone of voice, body language, facial expressions, eye contact, and overall way of interacting with the therapist.

The therapist also observes her own internal reactions, or *countertransference*, and what is being stirred up in her by the patient. In the therapy of patients with higher level personality pathology, verbal communication, free association, and difficulties communicating openly and freely often form the dominant channel of communication. In the therapy of patients with increasingly more severe personality pathology, the dominant channels shift to nonverbal communications: *how* the patient is speaking with the therapist, what the patient is doing, and what is being stimulated in the countertransference (Kernberg and Caligor 2005).

Affective Dominance and Affectively Dominant Object Relations

The TFP-E treatment approach rests on the observation that conflictual object relations, and defenses in relation to these conflictual object relations, tend to be enacted in and to organize subjective experience, and that this process is magnified in unstructured interpersonal and attachment relationships. With this in mind, in each TFP-E session, the therapist works to identify the object relations that represent the most emotionally salient material in the session (Diener et al. 2007; Ogden 1989). We refer to these object relations as *affectively dominant*. The affectively dominant object relations are those images of self and other in interaction that can be seen to organize the rest of the clinical material and that serve as a marker of the central conflict currently activated in the session; once identified in the therapist's mind, these object relations typically become the focus of intervention.

Although heightened affectivity or emotional expression often leads the therapist to the dominant object relations, this is not always the case; sometimes affective dominance is marked by the absence of expected affect, signaling the activation of defenses such as suppression, repression, denial, or dissociation in relation to core conflicts. In addition, affective dominance is often expressed in the repetition of a particular relational pattern, communicated in the patient's verbal descriptions of interpersonal interactions and in nonverbal interactions with the therapist. In more severe personality disorders, the dominant object relations are most often (though not always) activated and enacted directly in the relationship with the therapist, whereas in higher-level personality disorders, affective dominance may frequently be located in extratransferential object relations, enacted in the patient's descriptions of his interpersonal life.

Attending to External Reality

In TFP-E, the therapist's focus is on identifying and exploring the object relations enacted in each session, attending to the patient's verbal and nonverbal communications and the countertransference. However, at the same time that the therapist focuses on identifying and exploring the dominant object relations enacted in the session, she is also keeping a "third eye" open to how the patient is conducting himself in his life outside the treatment. This awareness is necessary in the treatment of patients organized at a borderline level because dissociative defenses can easily result in discontinuity between what is discussed in the therapy and important (and at times urgent) developments in the patient's life. With a focus on exploration of the transference and the patient's internal life, there is always a risk that the treatment may become divorced from the rest of the patient's life, which continues separate from and unchanged (or at times is inadvertently disrupted) by the treatment. This possibility calls on the therapist to actively make whatever inquiries are necessary to maintain a clear view of the patient's current functioning. Interventions of this kind tend to be particularly central early in treatment, and may be organized around maintaining the treatment frame and contract. As dissociated aspects of the patient's life are identified and come into focus, the therapist will explore the dissociative defenses that have kept these developments out of the treatment, and will then link developments in the patient's life and current functioning to the transferences and conflicts currently being explored in the treatment.

In the treatment of patients organized at a neurotic level, dissociative defenses are not a central clinical issue, and there is less pressing need for the therapist to actively inquire about the patient's external life and functioning. Patients organized at a neurotic level tend to naturally bring relevant aspects of their day-to-day lives into the treatment, either purposefully or through their associations; typically, they do not engage in destructive behaviors that warrant inquiry. At the same time, the therapist does well to listen for chronic omissions of aspects of the patient's life that she would naturally expect to hear about in the course of an ongoing therapy. Typically, omissions of this kind reflect unconscious defensive maneuvers on the patient's part, although sometimes these omissions may represent purposeful skirting of material that the patient is reluctant to share.

Hierarchy of Therapeutic Priorities

In the treatment of patients with personality disorders, there is always a risk of the patient engaging in dangerous, self-destructive, or treatment-disrupting behaviors in life outside the treatment; often, but not always, these behaviors involve deviations from the treatment contract. To the degree that the patient is engaging in destructive behavior, addressing—and if need be, setting limits on—these behaviors becomes the highest priority in any given session. TFP-E provides a hierarchy of priorities that guides the therapist when determining which issues are of highest priority for intervention, as follows:

- Behaviors dangerous to the patient and to others
- Violations of the treatment contract and other threats to the treatment
- In-session and between-session acting out
- Life crises
- Destructive forms of communication in session

To the degree that any of these "emergency priorities" is an issue, they will supersede implementation of the basic strategies of treatment, which involve an exploration of the patient's internal world and focus on the patient's dominant object relations.

Task 3: Exploring, Interpreting, and Working Through Core Conflicts

In the absence of any superseding priorities, the therapist's central task is to identify, explore, and work through core conflicts linked to the dominant object relations. Exploratory interventions promote self-observation, self-awareness, and self-understanding on the part of the patient.

Describing the Dominant Object Relations

The first task in the exploratory process is to work with the patient to construct specific descriptions of the representations of self and other in interaction that are organizing the patient's communications, linking them to his current affect state. It is important to appreciate that the process of describing the dominant object relations does *not* entail exploring or commenting on unconscious conflicts or meanings; the task is simply to explore the specifics of the patient's *conscious* experience. Focusing on the specifics of the patient's experience in areas of conflict, while working with the patient to articulate and put words to his experience, serves the dual function of identifying a focus of exploration and promoting the patient's observational and reflective processes. The patient is invited to observe and describe his own thoughts, feelings, and behaviors, and in this process begins to develop a distance from his immediate experience, a requisite first step for reflective processes.

For patients with higher-level personality disorders, the process of describing the dominant object relations usually serves as a natural segue to the exploration of and reflection on internal meanings and motivations. In contrast, in more severe personality disorders, self-observation and reflection, and sometimes even cognition, may to some degree be compromised in an area of conflict; in such cases, specifying and describing the dominant object relations—putting words to thoughts and feelings—can introduce a greater level of coherence into the patient's experience, and provides cognitive containment of affect. The process of describing the dominant object relations, in addition, supports the patient's capacity for self-observation in areas of conflict, setting the stage for introspection and reflection. For all patients across the spectrum of severity, the process of describing the dominant object relations provides the patient with the experience of being understood and of the therapist as trying to understand.

The Interpretive Process

Once the dominant object relations have been identified and articulated, the next task is to explore the psychological conflicts embedded in those object relations, while at the same time helping the patient to tolerate awareness of threatening aspects of psychological experience that have been defensively warded off. This process involves gradually and tactfully bringing to the patient's conscious awareness conflictual aspects of experience that are repressed, split off and denied, or enacted outside his awareness. We organize our thinking about this approach under the heading of the *interpretive process* and conceptualize this process as a series of interventions that incrementally help the patient to expand his awareness to include conflictual aspects of experience, while promoting deepening levels of self-understanding.

The interpretive process can be conceptualized in broad strokes in terms of clarification, confrontation, and interpretation proper (Auchincloss and Samberg 2012):

- *Clarification* entails the therapist's seeking to clarify the patient's subjective experience. Areas of vagueness are addressed until both patient and therapist have a clear understanding of the patient's conscious experience, or until the patient feels puzzled by an underlying contradiction in his thinking that has been brought to light.
- *Confrontation* involves the therapist's pulling together clarified information, expressed in the patient's verbal and nonverbal communications, that is contradictory or does not fit together, and tactfully presenting the patient with the material that warrants further exploration and understanding. Confrontations implicitly point out activation of defenses and integrate both verbal and nonverbal communications (Etchegoyen 1991).
- *Interpretation proper* follows clarification and confrontation and involves generating a hypothesis about the psychological conflict that is being defended against.

Interpretation overall is best thought of as a process that begins by calling attention to areas of defense while encouraging curiosity about the underlying psychological fears that are motivating defensive operations. The therapist begins with object relations most accessible to the patient and then moves to explore those more threatening and less accessible to him. This trajectory corresponds with beginning with the exploration of defensive object relations and then exploring the object relations defended against. In this process, the therapist works with the patient to generate hypotheses about why it is that the patient organizes his experience as he does.

The aim of the interpretive process is not to "make the unconscious conscious" but rather to support self-observation and reflection, to generate curiosity on the part of the patient about his internal life, and ultimately to help the patient tolerate awareness of conflictual aspects of his experience (Caligor et al. 2007). To make use of interpretation to expand awareness, the patient needs to be in a frame of mind to observe and reflect on his internal and external experience. Patients with higher level personality pathology typically come to treatment curious about themselves and are able to observe themselves and to reflect; with this population, the therapist can often move quickly through the early phases of the interpretive process, and emphasis is placed on interpretation proper—that is, exploration of unconscious fears and conflictual motivations.

In contrast, in the treatment of patients with more severe personality disorders, clarification and confrontation play a more central role, especially in the early phases of treatment. With these patients, these interventions function to provide affective containment and to promote the patients' capacity for self-observation, self-awareness, and reflective processes in areas of conflict (Caligor et al. 2009). As discussed in Chapter 10, the effectiveness of interpretation in promoting both reflective processes and self-understanding rests on the principle of technical neutrality.

Analysis of the Transference

In TFP-E, interpretations are made predominantly in the here and now, focusing on what Joseph Sandler (1987) referred to as the *present unconscious*. This means that for the most part, the interpretive process focuses on the patient's current anxieties as they are presently activated in his daily life and in the treatment. Conflictual object relations will be enacted in the patient's current interpersonal relationships, including the relationship with the therapist. When conflictual object relations are enacted and interpreted in relation to the therapist, the therapist makes a *transference interpretation* (Auchincloss and Samberg 2012).

In the treatment of patients with severe personality disorders, the affectively dominant expression of conflictual object relations in a therapy session will often occur in relation to the therapist; as a result, these treatments tend to be *transference focused*. Transference interpretation provides the therapist with an opportunity to interpret the link between the patient's conflictual internal object relations, his current difficulties, and the transference. In contrast, in the treatment of healthier patients, conflictual object relations may be most accessible in relation to the patient's significant interpersonal relationships, while remaining largely unconscious in relation to the therapist for much of the treatment.

In general, the more severe the pathology, the more central the role played by transference interpretation in the patient's treatment. However, we see this as a flexible and shifting distinction. Rather than conceptualizing a given treatment as transference focused or not, we think of our overall approach as *object relations focused*. Intervention will be organized in relation to the dominant object relations in the session, which may or may not be enacted in relation to the therapist at any given moment in a treatment.

Genetic Interpretations

Interpretations that make links between the patient's early history and the object relations enacted in a therapy session have historically been referred to as *genetic interpretations* (Auchincloss and Samberg 2012). When treating patients with higher level personality pathology, it is often easy to make these links, even during a consultation or in the opening phase of treatment. In contrast, in the treatment of patients with more severe personality disorders, the patient's descriptions of important early figures are often inconsistent and unstable, making it less tempting to make links to the past. We have found, however, that with both groups of patients, early focus on linking current conflicts to the past is best avoided. Early focus on the past can lend an overly intellectualized quality to sessions and may protect the patient from experiencing conflicts in an immediate and affectively meaningful fashion. It is helpful to keep in mind that the goal is not to understand the patient's past, but to make sense of and modify the patient's current psychological experience and behavior.

Thus, early on, the therapist is more likely to characterize the patient's experience "as if in relation to a negligent maternal figure," for example, than to characterize the patient's mother as negligent. However, as an understanding of the patient's current experience and conflicts becomes to some degree elaborated, and as customary defensive views of self and other are no longer convincing to the patient, connections to the past become useful. As part of the process of working through, interpretations that make connections between the patient's early history and his current difficulties and conflicts serve an important function, further deepening the patient's emotional experience and promoting his capacity to tolerate awareness of conflictual object relations.

Support and Supportive Interventions

In psychotherapy, *supportive interventions* are interventions that directly fortify the patient's adaptive defenses and help him cope with environmental demands (Rockland 1989). Providing direct advice, teaching coping skills, supporting reality testing, and making environmental interventions are examples of supportive techniques. Supportive techniques form the backbone of supportive psychotherapy (Rockland 1989; Winston et al.

2012)[2] and of cognitive-behavioral therapy, and can be especially helpful to patients with acute or chronic major psychiatric disorders. In contrast, in TFP-E, supportive techniques do not play a central role and in fact represent a deviation from the therapist's customary technically neutral stance.

When supportive interventions are introduced in TFP-E, it is done judiciously—for example, to limit destructive behaviors in the setting of severe personality pathology, to provide referral or advice in the setting of an acute medical problem, or to provide direct emotional support in the setting of a personal crisis. This approach, although different from what many others recommend (e.g., Gabbard 2010), is both reasonable and useful when flexibly implemented within the therapeutic frame of TFP-E. In essence, to the degree that the therapist is able to limit the use of supportive interventions, he sacrifices the short-term benefits of providing the patient with help or relief, in the service of promoting the longer-term treatment goals of promoting self-awareness and reflective processes.

Having said this, we want to make clear the distinction between a patient's feeling emotionally *supported* by a therapist and a therapist's making use of *supportive techniques*. Even though the TFP-E therapist does not typically make use of supportive techniques, she creates an environment that is intrinsically supportive of the patient—of his inner needs and of his wish to be understood and to obtain help—by providing a consistent and reliable treatment frame; demonstrating commitment, warmth, interest, and concern; and adopting an accepting and nonjudgmental attitude toward the patient.

Insight

The interpretive process helps a patient become aware of and make sense of some aspect of his inner life that he has been keeping out of awareness. As the TFP-E therapist interprets conflicts that are currently being enacted or are actively being defended against, the interpretations help the patient make sense of something he is actively experiencing (or trying not to experience) in the moment. This combination of emotional experience and

---

[2]For the reader interested in learning more about supportive therapy, we recommend *Supportive Therapy: A Psychodynamic Approach* (Rockland 1989), which provides a sophisticated, psychodynamically informed description of the treatment while comparing and contrasting supportive and exploratory psychotherapy, and also *Learning Supportive Psychotherapy: An Illustrated Guide* (Winston et al. 2012) for a more integrative approach.

intellectual understanding, in the setting of concern regarding what is newly understood, is referred to as *insight* (Auchincloss and Samberg 2012; Caligor et al. 2007). Insight brings with it the experience of deepening, of something falling into place in an affectively meaningful fashion, and is not to be confused with an individual's intellectual understanding of his history or dynamics. Although sometimes painful in stimulating feelings of personal responsibility or regret, insight often provides a feeling of relief coupled with deepening self-understanding. Even so, insight does not automatically bring about the structural and dynamic changes that are the goal of TFP-E. It is the process of *working through* that translates insight into personality change.

Containment

The term *containment*, introduced by Wilfred Bion (1962/1967), refers in a general sense to the capacity of thinking to temper affect states (Bion 1962, 1959/1967, 1962/1967). *Containment* implies that the individual can fully live through an emotional experience without being controlled by that experience or having to turn immediately to action; *containment* also implies both emotional freedom and self-awareness. In TFP-E, the therapist contains her own emotional reactions to the patient and to the transference, and in this process she helps the patient better contain the anxieties activated in the treatment. Containment on the part of the therapist is an essential component of the therapeutic process, promoting reflective processes in the patient and supporting the patient's own capacity to tolerate awareness of conflictual object relations, and ultimately to contain them within his dominant self experience (Joseph 1985).

In contrast to interpretation, which is an explicit process, containment is an implicit component of the interaction between patient and therapist as they explore and come to understand the patient's inner world. In TFP-E, the therapist helps the patient put highly affectively charged psychological experiences into words and reflect on them. The containing therapist emotionally responds, internally, to her interactions with the patient and then reflects on whatever the patient is communicating both verbally and nonverbally. In her response to the patient's communication, whether verbal or nonverbal intervention, the therapist helps the patient contain the anxieties stimulated in the therapy. The therapist accomplishes this by communicating that she is accurately registering what the patient is feeling and communicating, while at the same time maintaining the capacity to observe and reflect on her own and the patient's inner states (Fonagy and Target 2003; Kernberg 2004).

Working Through

The process of *working through* involves the repeated activation, enactment, containment, and interpretation of a particular conflict in a variety of different contexts over the course of time (Auchincloss and Samberg 2012). In fact, the bulk of any long-term therapy for personality disorders involves the process of working through; once core conflicts and associated object relations have been identified, they are enacted and explored over and over again throughout the course of treatment. The process of repeatedly activating, enacting, and interpreting a given conflict, and of linking the various object relations and interpersonal patterns associated with it, will help the patient gain a deeper and more emotionally meaningful understanding of himself. Further, we believe it is the process of working through that provides the link between insight and therapeutic change, creating new, more adaptive neural circuits and emotional experiences that organize the patient's experience and behavior in areas of psychological conflict.

Working through relies on the therapist's capacity to contain the paranoid and depressive anxieties activated in the transference-countertransference, and also on the patient's developing capacity to contain and emotionally experience the anxieties associated with activation of conflictual object relations and associated mental states. In this process, the patient will come to appreciate the role of his identifications with both halves of any particular object relation, as well as the ways in which activation of a particular internal object relation or conflict defends against others.

It is also during the process of working through that the therapist is able to most effectively link the patient's current difficulties to the past. Folding in a link to the past promotes further containment and symbolization of conflictual object relations; current experience is enriched as the patient develops a new and deeper appreciation of the role of his developmental past in his current experience. Ultimately, the patient will come to take responsibility for previously repressed and dissociated aspects of himself and of his internal objects, past and present.

Focusing on the Treatment Goals

In the process of working through in TFP-E, the therapist focuses on the patient's predominant areas of difficulty, identified in the presenting complaints and treatment goals. This means that while the patient is encouraged to communicate openly and freely without setting an agenda, the therapist keeps the treatment goals in mind. As conflictual object relations are enacted in the treatment and the patient's core conflicts come into focus, the therapist will be asking herself, "What is the relationship between the object relations currently being explored and the treatment goals?" Similarly, when a session seems unfocused or confusing, the therapist will ask herself, "How does this material relate to, or fail to relate to (i.e., represent avoidance of), the treatment goals?" In the process of working through, the therapist will focus her interpretations on the relationship between the conflicts currently being explored and the mutually agreed-upon treatment goals.

Key Clinical Concepts

- The first task facing the TFP-E therapist is to establish and maintain the treatment frame and the psychotherapeutic relationship, which together provide the setting within which the patient's experience and behavior can be explored.

- The second task of the TFP-E therapist is to identify a dominant issue in the session, which will become the focus of clinical attention.

- In deciding where to intervene, the therapist attends to the patient's verbal and nonverbal communications and the countertransference, while following a clearly specified hierarchy of priorities guiding intervention.

- The third task of the TFP-E therapist is to systematically explore the dominant issue in the session.

References

Auchincloss AL, Samberg E (eds): Psychoanalytic Terms and Concepts. New Haven, CT, Yale University Press, 2012

Bender DS: Therapeutic alliance, in The American Psychiatric Publishing Textbook of Personality Disorders. Edited by Oldham JM, Skodol AE, Bender DS. Washington, DC, American Psychiatric Publishing, 2005, pp 405–420

Bion WR: Learning From Experience. London, Heinemann, 1962

Bion WR: Attacks on linking (1959), in Second Thoughts. London, Heinemann, 1967, pp 93–109

Bion WR: A theory of thinking (1962), in Second Thoughts. London, Heinemann, 1967, pp 110–119

Busch F: Resistance analysis, in The Ego at the Center of Clinical Technique. Northvale, NJ, Jason Aronson 1995, pp 95–120

Caligor E, Kernberg OF, Clarkin JF: Handbook of Dynamic Psychotherapy for Higher Level Personality Pathology. Washington, DC, American Psychiatric Publishing, 2007

Caligor E, Diamond D, Yeomans FE, Kernberg OF: The interpretive process in the psychoanalytic psychotherapy of borderline personality pathology. J Am Psychoanal Assoc 57(2):271–301, 2009 19516053

Diener MJ, Hilsenroth MJ, Weinberger J: Therapist affect focus and patient outcomes in psychodynamic psychotherapy: a meta-analysis. Am J Psychiatry 164(6):936–941, 2007 17541054

Etchegoyen RH: Fundamentals of Psychoanalytic Technique. London, Karnac Books, 1991

Fonagy P, Target M: Psychoanalytic Theories: Perspectives From Developmental Psychopathology. London, Whurr Publishers, 2003

Gabbard GO: Long-Term Psychodynamic Psychotherapy: A Basic Text, 2nd Edition. Washington, DC, American Psychiatric Publishing, 2010

Joseph B: Transference: the total situation. Int J Psychoanal 66:447–454, 1985

Kernberg OF: The interpretation of transference (with particular reference to Merton Gill's contribution), in Contemporary Controversies in Psychoanalytic Theory, Technique, and Their Applications. New Haven, CT, Yale University Press, 2004, pp 232–245

Kernberg OF, Caligor E: A psychoanalytic theory of personality disorders, in Major Theories of Personality Disorder, 2nd Edition. Edited by Lenzenweger MF, Clarkin JF. New York, Guilford, 2005, pp 114–156

Levy ST, Inderbitzin LB: Neutrality, interpretation, and therapeutic intent. J Am Psychoanal Assoc 40(4):989–1011, 1992 1430771

Ogden TH: The Primitive Edge of Experience. Northvale, NJ, Jason Aronson, 1989

Rockland L: Supportive Therapy: A Psychodynamic Approach. New York, Basic Books, 1989

Sandler J: From Safety to Superego: Selected Papers of Joseph Sandler. New York, Guilford, 1987

Schafer R: The Analytic Attitude. New York, Basic Books, 1983

Sullivan HS: The data of psychiatry (1938), in The Fusion of Psychiatry and Social Science. New York, WW Norton, 1964, pp 32–55

Winston W, Rosenthal RN, Pinsker H: Learning Supportive Psychotherapy: An Illustrated Guide. Washington, DC, American Psychiatric Publishing, 2012

Yeomans FE, Gutfreund J, Selzer M, et al: Factors related to drop-outs by borderline patients: treatment contract and therapeutic alliance. J Psychother Pract Res 3(1):16–24, 1994 22700170

Yeomans F, Clarkin JF, Kernberg OF: Transference-Focused Psychotherapy for Borderline Personality Disorder: A Clinical Guide. Washington, DC, American Psychiatric Publishing, 2015

The Therapeutic Relationship

The Therapist's Attitude and Stance, the Therapeutic Alliance, Transference, and Countertransference

ALL PSYCHOTHERAPIES ARE DEEPLY embedded in the patient-therapist relationship, and it is generally agreed that this relationship serves not simply as context for the treatment but also as a central vehicle of change. With this in mind, in transference-focused psychotherapy—extended (TFP-E), the therapeutic relationship is structured in a very particular fashion that is closely linked to the overall treatment objectives and to our understanding of the processes that lead to clinical change. The therapist's attitude and stance are designed 1) to facilitate the development of a therapeutic alliance and at the same time to promote the unfolding of the patient's conflictual internal object relations in the treatment; and 2) to enable the therapist to intervene in a fashion that promotes the patient's ability to reflect on, and ultimately to explore, contain, and contextualize, these object relations within a progressively coherent and well-integrated self experience.

The therapist's attitude and stance are embedded in a matrix of ongoing transference-countertransference; attention to these processes organizes the therapist's understanding of the patient's current psychological situation, the clinical process, and the conflictual object relations activated in the clinical field. Exploration of the patient's conflictual object relations both depends on and further solidifies the therapeutic alliance developed between patient and therapist.

The Therapist's Attitude

In his attitude toward the patient, the therapist sets the emotional tone of the treatment. From the first consultative session, the therapist's attitude will impact the development of an alliance and potentially the therapeutic outcome. The objective for the TFP-E therapist is to make himself available as a person with whom the patient feels motivated to build a relationship while the therapist maintains the focus on the patient and her needs, protecting the therapeutic relationship as much as possible from intrusion by the therapist's needs or personal interests. This asymmetry, characterized by its singular focus on the patient's needs and experience, is a distinguishing feature of the therapeutic relationship and tends to activate central motivational systems, along with associated conflictual object relations.

The TFP-E therapist is active, collaborative, warm, and concerned—far from the outdated caricature of the dynamic therapist as relatively silent, anonymous, and abstinent in his attitude toward and interactions with the patient. The TFP-E therapist communicates empathy and the wish to understand and be of help. The therapist is emotionally responsive to the patient, and he does not try to hide his personality. At the same time, he does not speak at length about his personal life; he is professional and emotionally restrained in his interactions with the patient. In response to what the patient says and does, the therapist is tolerant, nonjudgmental, and flexible, communicating his openness to all aspects of the patient's internal situation, including those that the patient himself rejects (Schafer 1983). While sometimes difficult for inexperienced therapists to maintain, an attitude of competence and quiet self-assurance, combined with the capacity to tolerate and acknowledge not knowing, is the TFP-E therapist's goal.

Clinical Illustration 1: Expressing Empathy and Practicing Technical Neutrality

A middle-aged male professional presented with passivity, problems with self-esteem, and feelings of depression. He told his therapist that he had been hoping to be assigned to a new project at work but that it had been given to someone else. The patient looked extremely upset, perhaps on the verge of tears.

> Therapist: I can see that this is very upsetting. [*Patient remains silent but looks up at the therapist. The therapist feels encouraged to proceed.*]

The therapist first makes an empathic comment, communicating warmth and concern. She then goes on to invite the patient to take a step back and put current events into the context of his self representation and personal history.

> Therapist: You know, I think we can understand how this might be especially difficult.... We've been talking a lot about the negative view that you hold of yourself, that you feel things never go your way and it is because you are somehow deficient. Something like this must just feel like a confirmation.

This comment involves the implicit communication that even though the patient's current situation presents him with an objectively painful reality with which he will have to deal, the degree of anguish that the patient feels also reflects a more personal, subjective experience of the situation that can be reflected on, reframed, and eventually understood.

> Patient: But you can't possibly truly understand—this kind of thing doesn't happen to you.

The patient rejects the therapist's expression of concern and wish to help. At this point, the therapist has the option of correcting the patient's distortion by sharing that she also has recently suffered a major setback. For a moment, the therapist considers doing so, but on reflection she feels that this self-disclosure would do little to help the patient cope more effectively with his disappointment and would call unnecessary attention to the therapist and the therapist's needs.

Instead, the therapist chooses to point out to the patient that he is making an assumption, one that renders his current situation even more painful and that interferes with his experience of the therapist as helpful.

> Therapist: You see me as unable to understand or empathize with your situation?

> Patient: I do. Things obviously go much better for you than they do for me.
>
> Therapist: I can understand how seeing me as someone invulnerable to setbacks and disappointments might make it difficult to be here or to talk about these things with me, but I am curious why it is that you believe my experience must be so different from yours.

The therapist's attitude in this exchange is one of curiosity and ongoing concern for the patient. She is empathic and continues to make herself emotionally available without commiserating or sharing her personal experience, and without withdrawing. She keeps the focus on the patient's distress and attempts to help the patient take a step back to reflect on his painful and alienating assumption about the therapist (presumably one he habitually makes about others). At the same time, the therapist's response to the patient's difficulty in accepting her supportive presence implicitly communicates the therapist's availability and her comfort in tolerating the patient's rejection and potential hostility. All these behaviors set the stage for a collaborative exploration of the object relations activated in the session.

The Therapist's Stance

In the TFP-E approach, the therapist's stance refers to how the therapist positions himself in relation to the patient's conflicts and how he frames his interventions with this in mind. The therapeutic *attitude* is distinguished from the therapeutic *stance* (which may not be distinguished in other approaches) because of the intention to differentiate between 1) the therapist's attitude toward the patient from an interpersonal perspective and 2) the therapist's position in relation to the patient's internal needs and conflicts.

Within the TFP-E frame of reference, the therapist's attitude can be described as emotionally supportive, but the therapist's stance is quite different from that assumed in supportive psychotherapy (Rockland 1989), or in mentalization-based treatment (MBT; Bateman and Fonagy 2006), dialectical behavior therapy (DBT; Linehan 1993), cognitive-behavioral therapy (CBT; Beck et al. 2004), or even supportive-expressive therapy (Gabbard 2010; Luborsky 1984).

The supportive therapist actively allies himself with the most adaptive forces within the patient (Winston et al. 2012) and intervenes to directly encourage and support such adaptive functioning on the patient's part. The supportive-expressive therapist moves between the supportive stance of the supportive therapist and a more expressive stance, depending on the individual patient and clinical moment. CBT and DBT therapists assume the stance of a coach, teaching the patient skills to help her modify maladaptive thoughts and behaviors, whereas the MBT therapist assumes a mentalizing stance in which he does whatever he can to model and support an open, reflective attitude in the patient by assuming one himself.

For example, with a patient who has a disappointment at work, the supportive therapist might provide encouragement or advice, and might well share a relevant personal anecdote. The supportive-expressive therapist's initial response to the patient's disappointment might be similar, but with the expectation of shifting to a more exploratory approach as the patient comes to feel less acutely disappointed. The CBT therapist might make direct suggestions to the same patient about how to modify automatically negative thoughts about herself; the DBT therapist might reinforce skills for affect regulation; and the MBT therapist might directly communicate a stance of open-mindedness that considers alternative perspectives on the therapist's as well as the patient's experience, while avoiding excessive affective arousal.

In contrast to all of these possibilities, the TFP-E therapist takes a different approach, choosing not to make use of emotional support or directive interventions, or to model a mentalizing stance, but instead to position himself as someone able to tolerate the patient's pain and anger and motivated to help the patient observe and reflect on her experience.

In Clinical Illustration 1, when the therapist draws attention to the patient's assumption, the therapist is initiating an exploration of the patient's *internal* situation and underlying conflicts, rather than focusing directly on the patient's situation at work. The therapist's stance enabled the patient to gain some perspective on his situation and to appreciate that his pain went beyond the realities of the current situation and had much to do with his internal assumption of his own inferiority. The therapist's expectation is that such a shift in perspective might help the patient experience his situation as objectively dire, while laying the foundation for a process that could improve his professional performance over time.

The therapist in the vignette maintains an eye on the long-term objective of the treatment, which can be understood in terms of exploring the patient's defensive, devalued self representation. The therapist's interventions are designed not simply to provide perspective in the short term, but also to facilitate in the longer term the exploration and working through of underlying anxieties and conflictual object relations—for this patient, fears of other men and wishes to dominate and triumph over them. Meanwhile, in the immediate clinical situation, even though the therapist abstains from making supportive interventions, the patient is able to leave the session feeling supported by the therapist, and is now better equipped to cope with his disappointment and frustration.

Technical Neutrality

The classical description of the stance assumed by the TFP-E therapist and exemplified in Clinical Illustration 1 is one of *technical neutrality* (Auchincloss and Samberg 2012; Levy and Inderbitzin 1992). The word *technical* in this phrase is somewhat unfortunate insofar as it has cold, mechanical connotations. In fact, however, the word *technical* simply refers to the therapist's *technique*; it describes the TFP-E therapist's neutrality in his *interventions* but not in his attitude toward the patient. Another way to think about this is that the therapist attempts to be neutral in relation to the patient's *conflicts*, not in relation to the patient as a person.

In some clinical settings, the therapist can identify different motivations within the patient that are in conflict; in others, the therapist may see a conflict between a particular wish or desire and internal prohibitions, or between particular motivations and the demands of reality. Regardless of the nature of the conflict, the neutral therapist attempts to avoid allying himself with any particular side of the active conflict, but instead tries to ally himself with, and in this process support, what is sometimes referred to as the patient's *observing ego*—that part of the patient that is able to *stand back and observe* her own behavior, thoughts, and feelings. From an operational perspective, the neutral therapist attempts to identify all the conflicting forces within the patient without supporting or rejecting any particular side of those conflicts.

Neutrality implies that the therapist seeks to understand rather than to direct—and entertain all the conflicting forces in the patient, even those the patient is rejecting, while helping the patient do the same—thereby promoting self-observation and reflection on the patient's part. To facilitate this process, the neutral therapist generally refrains from providing advice or actively intervening in the patient's life, while monitoring his own impulses to do so. Instead of reflexively acting on his emotional reactions to the patient, the therapist first attempts to contain and reflect on them. We address this further near the end of this chapter, in the subsection "Countertransference Developments in the Setting of Consolidated Identity and Repression-Based Defenses," and in Chapter 12, in the section "Utilizing Countertransference."

The next two clinical illustrations highlight the therapist's professionalism, warmth, and concern while he maintains a technically neutral position in relation to the conflicts currently activated within the patient. The patient in Clinical Illustration 2 is organized at a borderline level, and the patient in Clinical Illustration 3 is organized at a neurotic level, with predominantly repression-based defenses.

Clinical Illustration 2: Assuming a Neutral Stance With a BPO Patient: Promoting Containment of Conflict Rather Than Supporting Splitting, Externalization, and Action

A 25-year-old single woman with a high borderline level of personality organization (BPO) and diagnosed with histrionic personality disorder with narcissistic features had a history of initiating various forms of treatment and then precipitously dropping out. During the consultation, the therapist discussed with the patient his assessment that the patient's treatment goals would be best addressed in twice-weekly, longer-term therapy, noting that less intensive approaches had apparently failed in the past. Patient and therapist agreed to work together on a twice-weekly basis as part of their treatment contract. Two months into the treatment, the patient began to complain about the frequency of sessions. There was a devaluing quality to her comments as she complained that coming to two sessions a week was inconvenient, given her work schedule; she wanted to cut back to weekly sessions.

In this familiar clinical situation, the supportive therapist might respond by encouraging the patient to stick with the plan, perhaps reassuring the patient that the treatment was worth the inconvenience and that if all else failed, the frame could be modified to meet the patient's demands. In this process, the supportive therapist would be actively siding with and attempting to support one part of the patient—the part wanting help—without addressing the other part of the patient—the part that rejects help and is motivated to disrupt the treatment.

In contrast, the TFP-E therapist would likely take a quite different approach, attempting to avoid taking a position in relation to the patient's conflict and instead working to address the clinical situation from a position of technical neutrality. To this end, he would refrain from cajoling the patient and instead encourage her to step back and look at both sets of motivations that were in conflict within herself and, in particular, to explore the more destructive or rebellious parts of herself that were motivated to disrupt the treatment.

The TFP-E therapist might begin by supporting the patient's observing ego, putting the current situation in context, by reminding the patient of their initial discussion and their agreement that twice-weekly treatment would be the best way to address the difficulties that had brought her to seek help and would therefore be most likely to meet her treatment goals. The therapist might remind the patient of the difficulties that had brought her to treatment and of her wish at that time to commit to a therapy that could address them in depth. Interventions of this nature call attention to the observation that the therapist's neutral stance does not preclude his actively calling the patient's attention to reality issues; to the contrary, calling attention to denied aspects of reality is an essential role of the neutral therapist. Interventions of this kind are especially central in the treatment of BPO patients, in whom dissociation and denial play such a central role in maladaptive functioning. In this setting, calling the patient's attention to denied aspects of her external as well as her internal reality is a central task for the therapist, and to fail to undertake it is in essence to side with the patient's denial and dissociative defenses.

After reminding the patient of their earlier discussions, the TFP-E therapist might then move on to say the following:

> I sense that there is a division within you; a part of you wants to be in treatment, and is committed to addressing the problems that brought you here and to pursuing the goals we established before we began. At the same time, there is another part of you that does not want help—that has, in fact, consistently rejected help in the past. This part is unconcerned about your self-destructiveness and it seems is now tempted to abort yet another effort to get help.

Throughout this exchange, the therapist continues to maintain a neutral stance. He takes a position in which he stands back, observing and describing the entire situation without siding with either position or passing judgment, and in so doing, he encourages the patient to do the same. In this process, attention is directed away from the decision to be made in the behavioral domain ("Do I quit or do I stay?"), in which the therapist is pressured to support a particular line of action. Instead, attention is focused on the patient's internal psychological situation ("What is going on inside me that I am talking about cutting back or disrupting my treatment?"), reinforcing that the therapist is there to help the patient stand back, observe her internal situation, and reflect on it. This reframing is compatible with the overall objectives of psychodynamic treatments, which focus not only on changing behavior but also on supporting the patient's capacity for self-observation and reflection in areas of conflict, with the longer-term objective of promoting integrative processes.

Looking in greater depth at the current clinical moment, we can say that from the perspective of the patient's psychodynamics, she is avoiding conflict by using splitting, denial, and projection. These defenses protect her from the anxiety to which she would be exposed were the therapist to be aware of both her wish to get help and her contrary wish to destroy all opportunity for help. The patient manages to keep apart her conflicting motivations, to experience only the wish to destroy the treatment, and externalizes into the therapist the parts of herself concerned about her destructiveness and motivated to protect the treatment. (This is an example of projective identification in the clinical setting.)

Thus, the patient is attempting to use the therapeutic setting and her relation with the therapist to support her defenses and externalize her conflict, but the therapist's overall objective is to promote the exact opposite process; rather than enabling the patient's use of splitting, projection, and action to deny conflict, the therapist's goal is to help the patient tolerate awareness of the conflict, to *contain* it. This is the first step in the integrative processes that promote personality integration. The therapist who communicates, for example, a personal wish that the patient stay in treatment, or who resorts to bargaining or cajoling, would be "going with" the patient's defensive strategy by enacting, or speaking for, one side of the patient's motivations. By doing so, he would enable the patient to further distance herself from those motivations and from any conflict she might feel about disrupting the treatment. In TFP-E, in contrast, the therapist would note internally in the *countertransference* his temptation, for example, to encourage the patient to stay or perhaps to express his frustration, and would instead work to contain and reflect on, rather than act on, those feelings.

Clinical Illustration 3: Assuming a Neutral Stance With an NPO Patient: Promoting Increased Self-Awareness Rather Than Supporting Repression

A 45-year-old married man with a neurotic level of personality organization (NPO) and diagnosed with obsessive-compulsive personality disorder described his wife as excessively critical, a character trait that he found particularly distasteful. He went on to say that while he loved her, he wished she were different in this regard. Several months into the treatment, after a 2-week break, the patient came in and described a dinner out with another couple in which the patient felt that his wife had been openly critical of him. The patient had been uncomfortable and felt that his wife had embarrassed herself. He denied any feelings of anger toward her.

After inquiring and hearing more about what transpired, the supportive therapist might respond by helping the patient be more assertive with his wife, perhaps explaining that he had a right to be angry, or coaching him with regard to how best to respond; the therapist might communicate sympathy for the patient's discomfort, or he might try to help him accept his wife's limitation. In pursuing any of these options, the therapist would be in essence siding with the patient in relation to his wife, while at the same time supporting the patient's view of himself as the unwitting and defenseless object of his wife's aggression.

In contrast, the TFP-E therapist would likely attempt to avoid taking a position in relation to the patient's criticism of his wife and would instead view the patient's comments as opening up an opportunity to explore his conflicts around hostility. The TFP-E therapist, like the supportive therapist, might begin by asking for a more detailed description of what happened at dinner—how the patient responded and what he was feeling at the time. The therapist might then move on to say the following:

> You describe a situation in which it seems it would be only natural for you to ask your wife to stop criticizing you or for you to feel angry with her. Yet it seems you did nothing to stop her and you experienced little anger, only embarrassment. In addition, I can't help noticing that even in telling me the story, your affect is muted, without the kind of emotional expression that might be expected. What are your thoughts about this?

In this intervention, the therapist has maintained a neutral stance. He has not sided with or criticized either the patient or his wife, or attempted to change the patient's behavior by suggesting a course of action, or tried to change the patient's feelings by giving him permission to feel anger. Rather, the therapist has invited the patient to stand back and look objectively at the situation, and from that perspective he has pointed out that something is missing, that expectable reactions are absent from the patient's narrative. In his intervention, the therapist has turned the patient's attention inward, to his feelings and motivations, rather than focusing on what happened at the dinner table; as in the example of the BPO patient (Clinical Illustration 2), the therapist is reframing the conversation, redirecting it toward the patient's internal experience and conflicts, and promoting self-observation, introspection, and reflection.

In terms of the patient's psychodynamics, we can say that regardless of his wife's motivations and behavior, in his interaction with her, the patient is enacting a defensive, ego-syntonic, albeit problematic and painful, view of himself as someone who stoically or passively tolerates criticism and devaluation. This view protects him from awareness of any critical or hostile feelings that he might have but that he deems unacceptable or in some way threatening. In a neurotic organization, these feelings and the associated object relations are largely repressed and/or projected. In essence, the patient's wife can be seen as speaking for a part of the patient outside his awareness, while the patient uses his interactions with his wife to further shore up his defenses against awareness of critical or hostile feelings within himself.

The objective in dynamic treatment is to create the opposite situation, one in which the patient comes to be aware of his conflictual motivations rather than repressing and projecting them, but in a tolerant, neutral atmosphere in which the patient can be helped to accept that these motivations are a part of himself and can be contained within his overall conscious self experience. To the degree that the therapist criticizes or expresses disapproval of the patient's wife, or even simply assumes that the problem at hand is the wife's aggression, the therapist is implicitly taking a critical stance in relation to the wife's aggression while supporting the patient's defensive view of himself. On both counts this non-neutral stance would make it more difficult for the patient to become conscious of or tolerant of his own critical feelings. Instead of supporting the patient's defenses and the assumption that aggression is unacceptable, the neutral therapist positions himself to best help the patient forfeit his rigidly held defenses and broaden and deepen his self experience.

The TFP-E Therapist's Stance Does Not "Go With" the Patient's Defenses

In our discussion thus far, we have focused on how the TFP-E therapist's technically neutral stance facilitates emergence in the treatment of the patient's conflictual, defended-against object relations. In the setting of splitting, this process entails bringing to awareness at the same time the contradictory motivations and views of self and other, both of which are conscious but have been defensively dissociated or split apart (in Clinical Illustration 2, the help-seeking part of the patient and her destructive, treatment-rejecting part). In the setting of repression, this process entails facilitating the emergence into consciousness of conflictual, largely repressed motivations and internal object relations (in Clinical Illustration 3, the patient's critical and devaluing feelings toward his wife). In both cases, the therapist's neutral stance facilitates the patient's increased awareness of conflict as the therapist fails to support the patient's defenses as they might be supported in other relationships. (For example, a friend might insist that our man stand up to his wife, or a family member might beg our treatment-refractory patient to remain in treatment.)

Technical Neutrality, Therapeutic Alliance, and Flexible Implementation

When the TFP-E therapist assumes a stance of concerned neutrality, this is not something he does rigidly or blindly. The experienced therapist maintains neutrality in a flexible fashion, tailoring his stance as he deems most useful, weighing the costs and benefits of doing so at a particular moment in the treatment. The overall objective is not to rigidly maintain a neutral stance but rather to be aware when intervening in a neutral fashion or when intervening from a position that deviates from neutrality, and to have an understanding of why one is doing so. This entails the therapist's measured consideration—in advance, if possible, or if not, after the fact—of whether his choice, be it to deviate from neutrality or to maintain a neutral stance, is being driven by countertransference pressures or by sound clinical judgment based on what he deems best for the overall trajectory of the treatment. In sum, rather than a monolithic and rigid description of the therapist's position, technical neutrality is a conceptual framework against which the therapist can organize interventions and understand how psychodynamic therapy works to promote integrative processes in patients with personality pathology.[1]

The Therapeutic Alliance

The *therapeutic alliance* (Bender 2005) is an important component of the psychotherapeutic relationship. In contrast to the therapist's attitude and stance, which are characteristics of the therapist and can be seen as tactics of the treatment, the alliance requires the participation of both therapist and patient; it is jointly established between them. Most of the psychotherapy outcome literature has focused on three related components of the alliance—shared goals, clearly defined tasks, and the patient-therapist bond (Bordin 1979)—and has found the alliance to be a relatively robust predictor of outcome in a variety of forms of psychotherapy, predicting

---

[1]A variety of clinical situations call on the therapist to temporarily deviate from technical neutrality; for further discussion, see Chapter 12, "Intervening III."

approximately 15% of variance in outcome (Horvath et al. 2011; Orlinsky et al. 2004).

In a psychodynamic framework, the alliance can be understood as the working relationship established between the self-observing part of the patient that wants and is able to make use of help and the therapist in his role as helpful expert (Gutheil and Havens 1979). Operationally, the therapeutic alliance reflects, on the one hand, the patient's realistic expectations and experience of the therapist as having something to offer on the basis of training, expertise, and concern—and, on the other hand, the therapist's commitment to helping the patient by making use of his expertise and his developing understanding of her.

Establishing a therapeutic alliance is a central task of the opening phase of treatment (see Chapter 13), and maintaining an eye on and managing the alliance remains a task for the therapist throughout the course of the therapy. In fact, the building of an alliance begins in the consultation phase. Formulating the presenting problems, identifying shared goals, and explicitly discussing treatment procedures and the specific tasks of patient and therapist in the treatment (see Chapter 7) all contribute to the development of a therapeutic alliance (Hilsenroth and Cromer 2007).

The development of the bond between patient and therapist is facilitated by the therapist's nonjudgmental and accepting attitude, his attentiveness and interest, and his warmth, concern, and communication of empathy. In supportive therapies and cognitive-behavioral therapies, the therapist also relies on encouragement, advice, and praise to solidify an alliance and to manage negative feelings that the patient may experience toward the therapist, but typically does not explore idealization of the therapist (Winston et al. 2012). In contrast, the TFP-E therapist relies on exploration of negative feelings about the treatment and the therapist to support the developing alliance; more extreme idealization of the therapist is seen as an indication of underlying negative feelings, potentially disruptive to the alliance, that are best explored rather than buried.

Patients with higher level personality pathology are for the most part able to establish a relatively stable alliance in the early phases of therapy (Bender 2005; Connolly Gibbons et al. 2003; Marmar et al. 1986; Piper et al. 1991). Initial difficulties, or ruptures of the alliance should they arise over the course of treatment, are relatively easily resolved and often serve, once worked through, to deepen the patient's self-understanding while further solidifying the working relationship between therapist and patient (Caligor et al. 2007; Safran and Muran 2000; Safran et al. 2011).

In contrast, patients with more severe personality disorders typically have difficulty establishing a stable therapeutic alliance, and the quality of the alliance is vulnerable to wide fluctuation across sessions and even moment to moment within a session (Levy et al. 2015; Wnuk et al. 2013; Yeomans et al. 2015). Ruptures are common and inevitable, and may be accompanied by strong emotional reactions on the part of the patient, which not uncommonly include hostility, accusations, devaluation, and even paranoia. In this setting, the alliance can be operationalized in terms of the patient's capacity to maintain some trust in the therapist while experiencing and openly expressing aggression, and in light of the therapist's capacity to see something positive in the patient and maintain an attitude of wanting to help while confronting the patient's aggression. In the successful treatment of patients with severe personality disorders, the therapist sees the gradual consolidation of a stable therapeutic alliance over the course of the treatment and developing facility on the part of the patient to tolerate challenges to the alliance and to repair ruptures.

Transference and Countertransference

A defining feature of the TFP-E therapist is his attention to transference and countertransference. The construct of transference has been a cornerstone of dynamic treatments since Freud's development of psychoanalytic technique in the early twentieth century (for excellent reviews and citations, see Auchincloss and Samberg 2012 and Høglend 2014).[2] Views of countertransference have developed in tandem. An in-depth consideration of transference and countertransference and their roles in clinical process must be embedded within the framework of a particular model of the mind and treatment. In this chapter, we define transference and countertransference within the framework of contemporary object relations theory, and then discuss the clinical presentation of transference and countertransference in TFP-E, focusing on how the nature of these developments differ across the spectrum of severity of personality pathology.

In Chapter 11, we elaborate on how to explore transferences in TFP-E, discussing how work with transference presents different challenges and rewards in the treatment of patients with personality disorders at different levels of severity. In Chapter 12, we cover how to make use of countertransference to "listen" to patients' verbal and nonverbal communications.

---

[2]See also works by Etchegoyen (1991), Harris (2005), Joseph (1985), Sandler (1976), Smith (2003), and Westen and Gabbard (2002) for views on transference within different psychodynamic frames of reference.

Transference

Defining Transference Within the Framework of Object Relations Theory

In the model of object relations theory, early, significant, and emotionally charged interactions, colored by genetic and temperamental factors as well as fantasies, defenses, and developmentally based distortions, come to be organized in the mind in the form of memory structures or internalized relationship patterns that are referred to as *internal object relations* (see Chapter 1). These psychological structures, organized as neural networks, function as latent schemas—ways in which the individual can potentially organize her experience—that will be activated in particular contexts (Kernberg and Caligor 2005; Westen and Gabbard 2002). Once activated, internal object relations will color the individual's subjective experience, and will lead her to act and feel in ways that correspond with these internal object relations.

We think of this process in terms of the individual's "enacting" or "living out" her internal object relations in her daily life and, in particular, in her interpersonal relationships; when internal object relations are enacted, psychological structures are actualized. As we use the term *enactment*, it does not necessarily imply action. Rather, *enactment* implies *that a particular setting has led to the activation of a particular object relation (or neural circuitry), and that this object relation has come to organize or impact the individual's experience or behavior*. Thus, enactment may be reflected in behavior, but it is equally likely to be expressed primarily in the subjective experience of the individual.

For example, if a patient with conflicts around competition experiences a success but then finds himself feeling inferior to his brother, his therapist, or someone else, we would say that his subjective state in the moment reflects enactment of a defensive object relation of an inferior self and a superior other. For this process, whereby internal object relations are enacted in interpersonal relations, we use the term *transference*. Thus, *transference* can be defined as the *playing out, or enactment in the present, of patterns of interaction derived from significant relationships in the past* (Auchincloss and Samberg 2012).[3]

The term *transference* is most commonly used to refer to enactment of a patient's internal object relations *in relation to the therapist*, and for purposes of clarity, we restrict our use of the term to this more specific meaning. However, it is widely accepted that transference to the therapist is just an example of a more general process wherein internal object relations tend to become actualized, or enacted, in the patient's interpersonal life and subjective experience (Høglend 2014). Thus, transference constitutes a specific example of the routine ebb and flow of day-to-day experience; in treatment, this experience then becomes a jumping-off point for exploration of the subject's internal object relations. In particular, it is conflictual object relations that tend to be enacted or defensively externalized in the treatment setting (Kernberg and Caligor 2005), bringing to life processes underlying the maladaptive character traits, interpersonal difficulties, and subjective disturbances that bring patients with personality disorders to treatment.

When we define *transference* as the enactment of an internal object relation, we highlight that it is an *entire object relation* or relationship schema that is activated, not simply a particular representation of another person; any transference disposition will be defined by both a self and an object representation, as well as by a particular affect state. Thus, for example, if a relationship with a rejecting father is enacted in the transference, it is not simply the image of a rejecting father that is activated; it is also, for example, a corresponding view of an inadequate self and the associated affect.

Further, it is extremely important to keep in mind that in this setting, the patient is ultimately identified not only with the self representation (a rejected, inadequate self) that has been activated in the transference, but also at some level with what is currently projected and experienced as an object representation (e.g., the rejecting father). In the setting of BPO, the patient's identification with one side of any particular object relation tends to be unstable, and the therapist may see role reversals in which the patient identifies with both self (inadequate self) and object (rejecting father) representations. Identifications with the two representations may both be consciously experienced but at different times, or identification with one side may at any moment dominate conscious experience, while identification with the other side is simultaneously expressed in behavior but dissociated from dominant conscious experience. In contrast, in the setting of higher level personality pathology, the patient's conscious identification with a particular self representation (inadequate self) is often

---

[3]Conceptually, we can make a distinction between *enactment* and *acting out*. Enactment of internal object relations is a universal and ubiquitous property of mental functioning. In contrast, the term *acting out* is applied to situations in which a patient turns to *action* specifically to block awareness of internal object relations currently activated in treatment.

stable, while his identification with the object relation (rejecting father) may be stably repressed and experienced only in projected form (self as victim of critical father), with the patient's identification with the object representation (the rejecting father) coming to light only gradually during the course of treatment.

In psychotherapy, the patient's relationship with the therapist often offers a special opportunity for patient and therapist to explore, in their immediate here-and-now interactions, the ways in which the patient's conflictual object relations are enacted in her interpersonal relationships. Transference manifestations differ according to the nature of the patient's psychopathology and, in particular, the patient's level of personality organization. Further, any given patient will have many different transference dispositions, and the quality and content of a patient's transferences will shift over the course of treatment.

Transference and the Developmental Past

The example of a rejecting father in interaction with an inadequate self also calls attention to the degree to which transference developments can be seen to reflect and shed light on a patient's early significant relationships with parents and other important figures. Classical approaches to transference focused on "reliving" the past in the present, and considerable attention was directed toward exploring the relationship between childhood experience and current relational patterns (Auchincloss and Samberg 2012). Our understanding of and approach to this important issue is somewhat different, and flows naturally from the object relations theory model of psychological functioning; our focus is not on the past as relived in the present but rather on *information processing in the here and now*. We are interested primarily in elaborating how the patient's current psychological organization impacts her present subjectivity and behavior. This approach is compatible with that of Høglend (2014), who defines *transference* as follows:

> The patient's patterns of feelings, thoughts, perceptions, and behavior that emerge within the therapeutic relationship and reflect aspects of the patient's personality functioning (regardless of the developmental origin of these patterns). (p. 1057)

Having said this, we would also like to point out that in the setting of consolidated identity, transferences can often be understood quite readily in terms of the activation of aspects of the patient's internalized early relationships with parental objects, where we see derivatives of actual aspects of that relationship as well as representations colored by defense and fantasy. In contrast, the poorly integrated object relations characteristic of patients organized at a borderline level are activated in the transference in ways that do not permit the reconstruction of childhood conflicts with parental objects. Rather, the transference reflects a multitude of internal object relations of dissociated or split-off aspects of self and objects, often of a highly fantastic and distorted nature. It is only in the advanced stages of treatment of patients with identity disturbance, when internal object relations are better integrated, that we see the kinds of more advanced transference developments that shed light on early childhood conflicts.

In sum, within the framework of contemporary object relations theory, any given transference development will reflect a combination of early developmental experiences with attachment figures, fantasized and wished-for experiences, and defenses against both—all experienced and organized in the context of underlying genetic and temperamental factors. So, for example, at the beginning of this subsection, the rejecting father and inadequate self may reflect the individual's actual developmental experiences with a powerful, rejecting father, but could equally well reflect defensive needs, perhaps in relation to anxieties about having an inadequate father or in relation to feelings of hostile rejection of the father. This object relation might at the same time reflect the impact of constitutional predispositions to aggression and/or rejection sensitivity on psychological structures. It follows that any given patient will have a spectrum of transferences, and these transferences, as well as the patient's image of his important attachment figures, will change and evolve through the course of treatment.

Transference and the Therapeutic Setting

While patients come to treatment with a circumscribed group of conflicts and potential transference dispositions, the specifics of the clinical setting will have an impact on which conflicts and transferences are activated and in what order. In general, coming to a professional for help tends to stimulate childhood feelings and associated conflicts in relation to important attachment figures, as well as related anxieties and defenses. In addition, depending on a patient's particular conflicts and developmental history, a variety of factors tend to trigger conflicts in relation to sexuality, trust, dependency, autonomy, competition, and aggression, such as the following: the intimacy of the treatment setting, the therapist's singular focus on the patient's needs, and/or the hierarchical imbalance of power in the relationship.

In addition to the more generic features of the treatment setting, specific and idiosyncratic aspects of the therapist's person, behavior, and attitudes will also influence transference developments (Høglend 2014). The following, for example, will have some impact, at least initially, on the object relations activated and enacted in the treatment: the therapist's gender, age, and personality style; the degree to which he openly demonstrates warmth versus restraint; his use of humor; and his level of activity and responsiveness. Therefore, we recommend that the therapist maintain an attitude of restrained concern coupled with persistent attention to the effects of the therapeutic setting and the therapist's interventions on the patient's experience of the therapist and the relationship.

We are in no way suggesting that the therapist can erase the impact of his personality on the interpersonal field or that it would necessarily be desirable if he could. The therapist's personality and behavior always serve as an anchor point for the transference as well as of the alliance. Mindful of this, the TFP-E therapist behaves in role, accepting the impact on transference developments of those aspects of his personality that are commensurate with an ordinary professional relationship. In this setting, it becomes possible to explore transference developments for what they reveal about the patient's internal difficulties, even though they may be organized superficially in relation to aspects of the therapist's personality or behavior. Thus, while we appreciate that the transference-countertransference represents a complex intersubjective field molded in an ongoing fashion by the therapist's interactions with the patient, we also believe that transference-countertransference can be used by a responsible, reflective, and adequately trained clinician to explore the patient's internal world.

Clinical Manifestations of Transference

In TFP-E, there are many different ways in which transference may manifest in the clinical setting. In the most straightforward case, transference developments manifest in the form of conscious thoughts and feelings that the patient has about the therapist, either inside or outside the treatment hours. Transference thoughts of this kind may be fleeting and vague, so much so that the patient does not think to mention them, or they may be repetitive, even intrusive, and highly charged. Thoughts about the therapist often manifest initially as curiosity—for example, "Why did he say that?" "Does she think I'm attractive?" "Is he a good father?" "Can he understand my religious beliefs?"—or they may manifest as convictions— for example, "He doesn't like me"; "She is flirting with me"; "He wants to get rid of me."

At other times, transference developments may first become evident in the patient's nonverbal communication and behavior in session, rather than in direct verbal communication of conscious thoughts and feelings about the therapist. For example, object relations activated in the transference may be expressed in how the patient sits in her chair, in whether or not she makes eye contact, or in her tone of voice. The patient may convey a particular attitude toward the therapist—for example, seeming anxious, threatening, obsequious, imperious, or seductive—or she may convey an attitude toward the treatment as a whole—for example, by being reluctant to come to sessions or, conversely, seeming overly eager. When the transference is initially identified in the patient's nonverbal communication, it is often only after the therapist calls attention to the patient's behavior that the patient becomes aware of it and is able to reflect on underlying transferences that are organizing her behavior.

It is not uncommon in the treatment of patients with personality pathology for developing transferences to first become evident in a patient's attitudes and behavior in relation to the treatment frame. For example, the patient may demonstrate resentment in relation to scheduling, frequently missed appointments, chronic lateness, delay or withholding of payment, frequent phone calls, failure to communicate openly and freely, or violation of the treatment contract. In TFP-E, once the frame has been clearly established, deviations from or challenges to the frame are seen as expressions of an underlying attitude or relationship pattern that has been activated in the transference. In an analogous fashion, transferences may be first expressed in acting-out behavior outside the sessions.

Clinical Manifestations of Transference Across the Spectrum of Severity

The nature, quality, and course of transference developments in TFP-E will differ radically, depending on the type and in particular the severity of various patients' personality pathology. These differences, which reflect each patient's defensive style and the nature and organization of the patient's conflictual object relations, guide psychotherapy technique, leading to important differences in treatment strategies in the setting of borderline levels of personality organization, in contrast to strategies used with higher level personality pathology. Understanding of the patient's level of personality organization and of the structural and dynamic features of personality pathology at different levels of severity enables the clinician to anticipate transference developments and to structure the treatment and clinical technique accordingly.

In TFP-E, we always focus on the *affectively dominant* object relations (see Chapter 9), but depending on the patient's level of personality organization, we see variation in 1) the degree to which these object relations are likely to be affectively dominant in relation to the therapist in the transference versus affectively dominant in the patient's interpersonal life and 2) the degree to which transference developments are affectively charged, extreme, and unstable versus affectively well modulated and relatively realistic and stable.

In the setting of clinically significant identity pathology with a predominance of splitting-based defenses, transference developments tend to occur rapidly and to be relatively highly affectively charged; they typically lead to overt, if at times subtle, distortions of the relationship between patient and therapist. In this setting, object relations enacted in the transference tend to quickly assume affective dominance. It is for this reason that clinical interventions in the treatment of patients with severe and moderately severe personality disorders tend to emphasize exploration of the transference (i.e., tend to be "transference focused").

In contrast, in the setting of consolidated identity and repression-based defenses, transferences tend to develop gradually, to be relatively realistic, and to be relatively stable over time. In this setting, it is not uncommon for conflictual object relations enacted in the patient's interpersonal relationships to assume affective dominance much of the time, rather than being activated in the transference; such conflictual object relations may remain repressed (i.e., they are enacted and come to life outside the transference). As a result, in the treatment of higher level personality disorders, the focus of exploration and intervention is often *not* the transference, with primary attention aimed instead on the object relations emerging in the patient's interpersonal life, subjective experience, and free associations.

Table 5–1 summarizes transference developments across the level of personality organization, discussed further in the following sections on transference developments.

Transference Developments in the Setting of Identity Pathology and Splitting-Based Defenses

In the treatment of patients with severe personality disorders, the patient's conflictual, paranoid, and idealized object relations tend to emerge vividly in the transference. Enactment of poorly integrated object relations tends to lead to transference developments that are *concretely experienced*, lacking the "as-if" quality that tends to characterize the transferences of patients with higher level personality pathology. Often such transferences are initially communicated in the patient's behavior and in the countertransference, rather than in the patient's verbal communications. When in the grasp of concretely experienced transferences, the patient is typically

TABLE 5–1.　Level of personality organization and transference developments

Typical transference developments	Borderline level of personality organization	Neurotic level of personality organization
Overall organization	Polarized, idealized and paranoid	Integrated
Quality of representations	Poorly differentiated, caricature-like	Well differentiated, complex
Quality of affect	Poorly integrated, poorly modulated	Well integrated, well modulated
Distortion of relationship	Gross	Subtle
Rate of development	Often rapid	Typically gradual
Stability	Largely unstable	Highly stable
Sequence	May be chaotic	Systematic
Quality of experience	Concrete	Symbolic, "as if"
Major channels	Patient's behavior and countertransference	Patient's verbal communication
Observing ego	Weak, easily compromised	Relatively stable
Alliance	Weak, easily compromised	Relatively stable
Clinical focus	Often	Sometimes
Clinical challenge	Contain, reflect	Identify, explore

unable in the moment—and indeed sees no need—to step back and observe or reflect on what is transpiring; whatever she is feeling in the immediate moment monopolizes her subjectivity and is experienced as a material fact. Experiences of this kind often leave the patient with tremendous pressure to act, to get away from painful affect states stimulated in the treatment. This can lead to acting-out behavior, both in the session and in the patient's external life, including dropping out of treatment. Managing developments of this kind presents a central challenge in the psychodynamic therapy of patients with severe personality disorders.

In the treatment of high-BPO patients, transferences also tend to emerge rapidly and are characterized by paranoid and idealized representations that may be concretely experienced. However, high-BPO patients are typically better able, with help from the therapist, to reflect on experience and more easily entertain alternative perspectives in relation to their experience in the transference than are patients with more severe pathology.

The paranoid object relations that may come to dominate the treatment setting with high-BPO patients tend to be less extreme, less aggressive and paranoid, and less rigidly concrete than transferences characteristic of the severe personality disorders, and idealization plays a more central role. In fact, high-BPO patients may activate relatively stable idealizations of the therapist that function to keep paranoid object relations out of the treatment. With patients in this group, the therapist may see extended periods of superficially smooth collaboration in the treatment, which often entails a somewhat intellectualized or superficial exploration of the patient's life problems. This exploration may be accompanied by more or less subtle forms of acting out, or it may be dissociated from the treatment, and it will inevitably be interrupted by the breaking through of more highly charged hostile, paranoid, devaluing, or erotized transferences.

In sum, transference developments, especially in the early phase and early part of the middle phase of treatment of low- and middle-BPO patients, are predominantly paranoid, although paranoid transferences may at times be warded off by fragile idealization of the therapist and of the therapeutic relationship. In contrast, high-BPO patients frequently present with idealizing as well as paranoid transferences. Transferences in BPO patients are often concretely experienced, and may lead the patient to action, either in the session or outside. When patients respond to transference developments with action rather than reflection, we speak of *acting out*; in this setting, the patient resorts to action to replace awareness of painful emotional experiences stimulated in the treatment.

Clinical Illustration 4: Transference Developments in a Low-BPO Patient: Acute, Concretely Experienced Paranoid Transference Leads to Acting Out

A patient with a paranoid personality disorder with antisocial features insists, in his first phone contact with a prospective therapist, that the therapist promise to treat him during their phone conversation, before arranging a consultation. When the therapist explains that he will be happy to meet with the patient but can agree to work with him only after they have the opportunity to meet, the patient becomes enraged, accusing the therapist of being dishonest and wanting to get rid of him. He questions whether he can work with a therapist whom he cannot trust.

Object relation: An untrustworthy, dishonest, and rejecting therapist in relation to a mistreated and mistrustful patient, associated with suspicion and rage.

This vignette illustrates the extreme, highly charged, and concretely experienced paranoid transferences that can be rapidly activated in patients with severe personality disorders. In this case, the overwhelmingly paranoid transference activated during the initial phone call makes it impossible for this patient to begin treatment.

Clinical Illustration 5: Transference Developments in a Middle-BPO Patient: Chronic, Concretely Experienced Paranoid Transference Leads to Acting Out

A patient diagnosed with borderline personality disorder avoided all eye contact with her male therapist, recently out of training. This was the situation from their first meeting and persisted over time. As a child, the patient had been the victim of sexual abuse at the hands of her grandfather. What emerged with time was the patient's conviction that were she to look at her therapist, he would become overwhelmed by sexual excitement and would not be able to control himself. From the patient's perspective, this was the inevitable outcome of her holding the therapist's gaze, an experience that left her feeling unbearably powerful and afraid.

Object relation: An impulsive, sexually driven, and sexually preoccupied therapist in relation to a controlling, extremely powerful, and stimulating patient, associated with intense fear and sexual excitement.

This vignette illustrates that in the setting of more severe pathology, the patient's nonverbal communication is often the earliest indication of transference developments. This example also illustrates the impact of role reversal in the transference and its defensive functions; in this case, the patient's experience of herself as powerful, controlling, and sexually exciting to a sexually out of control therapist protected her from the experience of a powerful and controlling therapist in relation to a sexually overstimulated and powerless self. Both configurations were associated with painful degrees of sexual excitement and with fear, each mutually defending against the other.

Clinical Illustration 6: Transference Developments in a High-BPO Patient: Long-Standing, Idealizing Transference Cannot Withstand Frustration

A patient with histrionic personality disorder was anxious, idealizing, and eager to please in interacting with her therapist. Things proceeded smoothly, and the therapist felt they were developing a solid working alliance, with the patient at first focusing in session on conflicts in her marriage, and then reporting that things had greatly improved in her relations with her husband.

Six months into the treatment, the patient called her therapist to cancel a session at the last minute so she could take her young son to the pediatrician. The patient asked to reschedule, but the therapist explained that she had no open hours that week. The phone call struck the therapist as unremarkable. When the patient came to her next session, however, she was hostile and cold—a dramatic change from her usual demeanor. She accused the therapist of not trusting her and of having made a decision to punish the patient by refusing to reschedule, because the therapist assumed that the patient was being manipulative and lying about her son's being ill. The therapist was totally taken by surprise.

Object relation: A suspicious, punitive, callous therapist in relation to a dependent patient, associated with rage.

This vignette illustrates the rapid emergence of a paranoid object relation in the transference in response to frustration. Until that point, the patient had been able to anxiously sustain a rather fragile idealization of the therapist as caring and of the patient as special, warding off the paranoid experience of the relationship. When the therapist was unable to reschedule, the underlying paranoid transference, which expressed the patient's hostility and mistrust, came to dominate her experience of the therapist.

Clinical Illustration 7: Transference Developments in a High-BPO Patient: Narcissistic Transference Leaves No Room for the Therapist

A high-BPO patient with narcissistic personality disorder spent many sessions talking about problems getting along with others that had interfered with his performance at work and prompted him to seek treatment. He spoke steadily throughout the sessions, seemingly communicating that he needed the therapist to hear every detail, but rarely giving the therapist opportunity to comment or interject.

After several failed attempts, the therapist finally tried more forcefully to explore the patient's behavior in the session. She suggested to the patient that they reflect on his apparent need to keep her "out of the conversation." When the patient essentially ignored her comment, the therapist remarked on his failure to acknowledge her words, citing this as an example of exactly what she had been attempting to understand with him.

At this point, the patient refused to speak. What emerged was an experience in the transference of the therapist as condescending, as "preaching" but not listening, and as demonstrating a dismissive attitude toward the patient's need to be heard.

Object relation: A grandiose, condescending therapist who does not listen in relation to a patient who is depreciated and ignored, associated with feelings of humiliation, envy, and rage.

The preceding vignette illustrates the mobilization and enactment of narcissistic defenses in the transference. As long as the patient controlled the session and the therapist, he was able to ward off the experience of humiliation (a form of paranoid transference) connected in his mind with being in treatment. When the therapist called attention to the patient's behavior, at the same time failing to enact the defensive object relation, the roles reversed and the patient felt ignored and depreciated.

Role Reversals and Splitting in the Transferences of BPO Patients

The transference developments that characterize the treatments of BPO patients reflect the impact of splitting-based defenses on the clinical field—in particular, splitting proper, projective identification, omnipotent control, and denial. These developments mirror the difficulties that characterize the interpersonal lives of these individuals. We have attempted to illustrate the intrinsically confusing and often chaotic quality of these transferences, which are characterized by both role reversals and what can be abrupt shifts between contradictory and mutually dissociated, idealized, and persecutory experiences of the relationship. In particular, the impact of projective identification on the patient's experience of the therapist and on the patient's behavior in session can be extremely confusing to therapist and patient alike. When this occurs, as in several of our examples, the patient projects an object representation into the therapist, while remaining identified with that object representation (e.g., the patient experiences herself as having been deceived when she herself has deceived the therapist).

The impact on the transference is to create a situation—that we refer to as a *role reversal*—in which a relationship pattern is being enacted, with the patient either behaving under the influence of both sides of the object relation or rapidly oscillating between two contradictory positions (e.g., deceiver and deceived, dominant and depreciated). See Chapter 3 for further discussion of the concept of projective identification.

Transference Developments in the Setting of Consolidated Identity and Repression-Based Defenses

In higher level personality pathology (i.e., NPO and personality disorders falling on the continuum between NPO and high BPO), transference developments initially reflect the impact of defensive object relations on the therapeutic relationship, while more conflictual, impulsive object relations remain stably repressed, emerging only later and as a result of exploration of the patient's defenses.[4] Further, very much in contrast with what is seen in the setting of more severe personality disorders, many NPO patients are able to maintain a relatively stable, benign relationship with the therapist, relatively free of impingement by conflictual object relations. Even though on close observation conflictual (predominantly defensive) object relations are often identifiable in the patient's experience of the therapist, these transference manifestations are often subtle and ego-syntonic. As a result, in the treatment of patients with higher level personality pathology, as conflictual object relations unfold, they are often affectively dominant predominantly in the patient's interpersonal life rather than in the transference.

In the treatment of patients with higher level personality pathology, when transferences do emerge and assume affective dominance, they tend to develop gradually, to be relatively stable, and to evolve slowly over time. First, the therapist sees the impact of ego-syntonic, defensive object relations as they organize the patient's experience of and interactions with the therapist, and only later does the therapist observe the effects of underlying conflictual object relations. In this setting, when transferences become a clinical focus, they often present as mirroring experiences that have already been explored in relation to the patient's interpersonal life.

Patients with higher level personality pathology are for the most part able, with the therapist's help, to stand back, observe, and reflect on their view of the therapist, appreciating that there may be other ways to look at things and to understand their experience. In other words, healthier patients tend to retain the "as-if" quality of the transference, which is a major distinction between transference developments in this group and those seen in severe personality disorders. As a result, neurotic transferences are

---

[4]This is in contrast to the situation with middle- and low-BPO patients, in which defensive and impulsive object relations are interchangeable and often interchange in the transference.

relatively easy to work with and, when affectively dominant, can function as a useful entry point for exploration of the patient's internal world and conflictual object relations.

Clinical Illustration 8: Transference Developments in an NPO Patient: Gradually Evolving Negative Transference Does Not Interfere With Reflective Capacities

After being in treatment for 6 months with a male therapist with whom he had felt a solid sense of collaboration and mutual respect, a male patient began to have the uneasy feeling that perhaps his therapist did not really approve of him. The patient began to worry that the therapist, as a nationally recognized lecturer and author, might secretly be feeling critical of the patient's lack of professional ambition and his choice to become the primary caretaker for his children while his wife worked in a high-powered job.

Object relation: An ambitious, demanding parental object in relation to an inferior, passive self, associated with feelings of disappointment and disapproval.

This vignette illustrates the gradual emergence, over the course of many months, of transferential anxieties that impinged on the patient's benign, collaborative experience of the therapist. As the patient began to share his concerns with the therapist and to explore them, the two were able to elaborate a rather specific, well-differentiated and well-integrated object relation. This vignette highlights that although there may be a subtly concrete quality to their experience in the transference, most of the time, NPO patients remain able to step back, reflect, and consider the possibility of alternative perspectives. Even if he experienced his own viewpoint as "real," the patient was able to wonder whether his perception was realistic and to feel that even if it was, it might at the same time say something about his own internal motivations. This capacity to consider the transference as symbolic, in conjunction with a stable observing ego and a strong therapeutic alliance that can weather the intrusion of transference distortions, characterizes transference developments in the treatment of patients with higher level personality pathology.

This vignette also serves to illustrate the role of the developmental past in transference developments with healthier patients. On the one hand, this transference could easily be linked to the patient's relationship with his father, himself a highly ambitious man whom the patient experienced as profoundly invested in his children's academic and professional accomplishments. On the other hand, what emerged over time was that embedded in this object relation enacted in the transference, there was an expression of the patient's own ambivalence about competition and achievement. The patient's perception of disappointment and disapproval by the therapist was an expression of a part of the patient that was not fully comfortable with the path he had taken, and at a deeper level, the patient was managing this conflict by projecting into the therapist his own wishes to compete.

Clinical Illustration 9: Transference Developments in an NPO Patient: Slowly Emerging Negative Transference Leaves Patient Reluctant to Attend Sessions

A patient with depressive-masochistic personality, who had previously enjoyed her therapy sessions and looked forward to them, suddenly started to feel reluctant to come to sessions. As these feelings were explored, it became clear that the patient was feeling frustrated with the treatment and with the therapist. She wondered why things were not moving more quickly. As the patient and the therapist continued to explore the patient's frustration, the object relation emerging in the transference and organizing that frustration was elaborated.

Object relation: An inadequately attentive parent-therapist in relation to an angry-neglected child self.

This vignette illustrates emergence of initial transferences in relation to the patient's attitude toward the treatment. In addition, it demonstrates the gradual emergence of stable and well-organized transferences typical of NPO patients.

Clinical Illustration 10: Transference Developments in an NPO Patient: Premature Attention to the Transference Alienates the Patient

A patient in treatment for mild chronic depression in the setting of obsessive-compulsive personality disorder had conflicts in relation to authority. He described being unable to assert himself, even at times when he understood it would be appropriate to do so. In the early weeks of treatment, the therapist was able to help the patient become aware of the repeated enactment in the patient's interpersonal relationships of a passive, dependent self in relation to a needed but critical and potentially rejecting caretaker (an example of character defenses), and they explored its pervasive impact on his experience and behavior.

However, when the therapist attempted to point out the same dynamic as it was subtly played out between the two of them, the patient politely rejected the therapist's suggestion, commenting that he understood it was the therapist's job to be nonjudgmental, so he did not worry about being rejected or criticized. When the therapist persisted, the patient quietly withdrew and commented that the therapist did not seem to understand him.

Object relation: A demanding, critical authority in relation to a dependent, eager-to-please self, associated with fear of rejection.

The preceding vignette illustrates the relatively common situation in the treatment of NPO patients in which defensive and impulsive object relations are enacted and productively explored in the patient's interpersonal life while the transference remains protected, with the patient maintaining a stable, positive relation with the therapist as a professional provider of help. Although in this example the therapist is correct in her understanding that the object relations explored outside the treatment were also active in relation to the therapist, the patient was able to actively repress awareness of them. The therapist's efforts to "push" exploration of the transference in this setting did not promote the clinical process and served only to put a strain on the alliance. In many cases, as the patient becomes more comfortable with himself and more self-aware, he will become cognizant of the way that material initially explored in relation to his day-to-day functioning is subtly mirrored in the transference.

Character Defenses and Transference Developments

Initial transference developments in the treatment of higher level personality pathology typically reflect enactment of the defensive object relations that make up the patient's *character defenses* (see Chapter 3). These object relations organize the patient's behavior and subjective experience in his day-to-day life across all or most domains of functioning; even relatively self-aware and reflective patients may have a great deal of difficulty appreciating that character defenses are anything more than "just who I am." Initial transferences and associated defensive object relations represent the patient's habitual ways of viewing himself and of interacting with others. Character defenses and the object relations that organize them account for the patient's personality *style*, and at the same time introduce rigidity into personality functioning.

Transferences corresponding with the enactment of character defenses are typically identifiable (at least in retrospect) from the get-go, as they are in all the patient's interpersonal relationships. These early transferences tend to be fixed, relatively neutral, socially appropriate, and ego-syntonic. They may be quite subtle, identifiable perhaps only in the patient's interactions with the therapist, especially in his nonverbal communication and his attitude toward the treatment. Patients are highly invested in maintaining the views of self and other embedded in their character defenses, insofar as character defenses ward off awareness of underlying conflictual object relations. This remains true even though these views of self and other may be painful and are often to some degree maladaptive.

Clinical Illustration 11: Transference Developments in an NPO Patient: Ego-Syntonic Character Defenses Subtly Color the Therapeutic Atmosphere

A single, professional man in his late 30s sought treatment for difficulties establishing a satisfactory relationship with a woman and sexual inhibitions in the setting of neurotic personality rigidity and hysterical conflicts. The treatment began smoothly, with the therapist finding the patient pleasant and easy to work with. However, over time, she noted that she felt somewhat bored as the therapy took on a bland, rather superficial quality. This alerted the therapist to the degree to which the patient was actively keeping all potentially aggressive, sexual, and competitive object relations out of his discourse, and also provided a window into why women seemed to quickly lose interest in him, despite his intelligence and attractiveness.

Object relation: A compliant, bland self in relation to a pleasant but unengaged parental figure, associated with the absence of anxiety.

This vignette is an example of enactment of a character defense in the transference. The patient's unexamined, ego-syntonic self-presentation was that of a compliant and pleasant but bland childlike person, whose relationships with men and women alike were free of any sexual or competitive tensions. This defensive object relation persistently and pervasively organized the patient's experience and behavior across a variety of settings, impacting all his relationships in a manner of which he was unaware.

Countertransference

A defining feature of the therapeutic relationship in TFP-E is the therapist's ongoing attention to his emotional reactions to the patient. The ability to monitor and contain these reactions enables the TFP-E therapist to maintain an attitude of authentic warmth and concern toward the patient in the face of clinical challenges that may arise, while sustaining a neutral stance in relation to the patient's conflicts.

We consider the therapist's emotional reactions to the patient under the umbrella concept of *countertransference* and his ability to make use of these feelings in terms of *containment* (Bion 1962) of countertransference. As further discussed in Chapters 9, 10, and 11, countertransference analysis focuses the therapist's attention as he listens to the patient's verbal and especially nonverbal communications, and informs the therapist's understanding of the object relations organizing the patient's experience and behavior. At the same time, uncontained countertransferences can cause blind spots in the therapist and can make it difficult for him to understand and/or empathize with particular aspects of the patient's conscious and dissociated or unconscious experience (Racker 1957).

Defining Countertransference Within the Framework of Object Relations Theory

Within any TFP-E session, the therapist will experience a steady flow of emotional responses to the patient. We describe these reactions under the broader term *countertransference*. Although there are a number of ways to define and understand *countertransference* (Auchincloss and Samberg 2012), we use the term in its broadest sense, to include all the therapist's emotional responses to the patient (Kernberg 2004), regardless of their origins.

In the same way that we think of transference as reflecting enactment of the patient's internal object relations in her relationship with the therapist, so we think about the therapist's countertransference in terms of the object relations activated within the therapist as a result of his interactions with the patient. These reactions will always be codetermined, to a greater or lesser degree, by the therapist's internal and external situation and the patient's internal and external situation.

Some countertransferences emerge largely from within the therapist, reflecting the therapist's conflicts and personal needs—that is, representing the *therapist's transference to the patient*. For example, a middle-aged therapist finds that a particular patient reminds him of his beloved, elderly mother and realizes that this has interfered with his exploring her sexual conflicts. Another therapist is having financial difficulties and finds himself feeling envious of his wealthy patients. Countertransferences of this kind tell us more about the therapist than they do about the patient.

Other countertransferences may originate largely within the patient; in such a situation, the *therapist is reacting to the patient's transference.* For example, a patient, a well-known television personality who relied heavily on narcissistic defenses, left his highly accomplished therapist feeling diminished and envious. This countertransference may have more to do with the patient's conflicts and defenses than the therapist's. The first form of countertransference, the therapist-centered one, reflects how different therapists might respond differently to the same patient, whereas the second, the *patient-centered countertransference*, reflects how different therapists might respond similarly to the same patient.

In sum, within an object relations theory frame of reference, countertransference will be codetermined by 1) the patient's transferences to the therapist, reflecting the patient's defensive style and the quality of her internal object relations; 2) the realities of the patient's life situation; 3) the therapist's transferences to the patient, as determined by the therapist's internal world and conflicts; and 4) the realities of the therapist's life situation.

In TFP-E, as the therapist monitors his reactions to the patient, he maintains an open attitude toward exploring the source of his reactions. Specifically, the therapist will always be asking himself to what degree his reactions to the patient provide data about the patient's internal world, and to what degree the therapist's reactions say more about the therapist's current needs and conflicts than they do about the patient's.

Regardless of the source, it is the therapist's task to monitor, register, and reflect on his reactions to the patient—that is, to contain them. This process will enable the therapist to make use of countertransferences to learn about the patient's internal situation while minimizing the likelihood of countertransferential interference in his ability to attend openly and impartially to the patient's verbal and nonverbal communications. Containment of the countertransference enables the therapist to intervene from a position of technical neutrality and minimizes the risk of countertransference acting out on the part of the therapist (see Chapters 9 and 10).

Concordant and Complementary Identifications in the Countertransference

Within the framework of object relations theory, countertransference can be classified as either *concordant* or *complementary* identification in the countertransference (Racker 1957). When identifications in the counter-transference are *concordant*, the therapist identifies with the current sub-jective experience of the patient—that is, the therapist identifies with those parts of the patient's internal object world that the patient is presently ex-periencing as parts of himself (i.e., when countertransference is concordant, the therapist's internal experience parallels that of the patient). For exam-ple, if a patient says, "My wife is always critical when I am even a little bit late; it's as if she holds me accountable for traffic patterns," then the ther-apist might share the patient's feeling of being criticized unfairly by a loved one. In other words, in concordant identification, the therapist dips into the patient's current self state, learning how the patient currently feels.

In contrast, when identifications in the countertransference are *com-plementary*, the therapist identifies with the object representation that is paired with the representation with which the patient is currently identi-fied. If the patient is identified with a self representation, the therapist is identified with the corresponding object representation. Complementary identifications typically provide information about aspects of the patient's current subjective experience that he is experiencing as coming toward him from outside himself rather than as emerging from within him. Re-turning to our example, the therapist might find himself feeling critical of the patient, thinking about how the patient has been consistently 5 min-utes late for his sessions and thereby essentially identifying with the pa-tient's wife and with the patient's own critical internal objects.

Clinical Illustration 12: Concordant Identification in the Countertransference: Vicariously Sharing in Patient's Pride and Joy

Toward the end of a long and successful therapy, a middle-aged male pa-tient with obsessive-compulsive personality disorder with depressive fea-tures described his youngest son's college graduation the previous week. Both his older children were in attendance, his eldest son with his fiancée, and the family had a wonderful weekend together. The patient shared with the therapist how proud of his family he had felt and how the weekend had filled him with joy.

He then went on to reflect on how far he had come from his own col-lege graduation, which he had experienced as joyless and lonely, with only his mother begrudgingly attending; and he reflected on how far he had come from the tension that had characterized his relations with his sons in the past. As the therapist listened to the patient, she found herself ex-periencing feelings of pride and joy, vicariously sharing in her patient's pleasure while implicitly identifying with him as a generative father; in this

instance, the therapist occupied the role of the patient's father in the transference-countertransference.

Clinical Illustration 13: Complementary Identification in the Countertransference: Identifying With Patient's Wife

A patient with dependent personality disorder came to his therapy session
in the midst of a fight with his wife. He complained that his wife criticized
him and put him down incessantly, and that she had "no empathy"; all he
did was try to please her and make her love him, while all she did was find
fault. As he listened, the therapist noticed within himself rising feelings of
irritation, and he found himself feeling critical of the patient, with fantasies of pointing to his failure to take any responsibility for his wife's experience of him.

In this example, the patient was experiencing himself as an unfairly
criticized person in relation to a partner who was critical and rejecting. In
the complementary countertransference that emerged, the therapist found
himself feeling critical and rejecting, identifying on the one hand with the
patient's wife as he experienced her, and on the other with a critical, rejecting internal object that the patient projected onto his wife.

In sum, as a consequence of *concordant identification*, the therapist
identifies with the patient's central subjective experience. This is the source
of ordinary *empathy*, in which the therapist is able to put himself in the patient's shoes and imagine feeling what the patient is consciously experiencing. In contrast, under conditions of *complementary identification*, the
therapist identifies with the patient's objects. As a result, in the case of complementary identifications, the therapist is empathizing with aspects of the
patient's experience that are currently dissociated, projected, or repressed.
The overall empathy of the therapist is both with the patient's subjective
experience and with what the patient cannot tolerate experiencing (in the
example above, the critical, rejecting parts of himself). This view of the
therapist's empathy exceeds ordinary empathy in the social sense.

Acute and Chronic Countertransference

Countertransference reactions can be acute or chronic (Kernberg 2004).
Acute countertransferences affect the therapist from moment to moment
and mirror developments in the transference. Typically, acute countertransferences are relatively easy to identify. They are consciously experienced by the therapist, and in some settings may be felt with an intensity

or a kind of urgency that makes them difficult to contain. In Clinical Illustration 13, presented in the previous section, the therapist's mounting irritation in response to the patient's complaints about his wife illustrates a fairly typical instance of acute countertransference.

In contrast, *chronic countertransferences* affect the therapist over periods of time, represent a stable attitude on the part of the therapist toward the patient, and reflect the therapist's characteristic responses to the patient's transferences and/or life situation. Chronic countertransferences may be subtle or preconscious and are typically not highly affectively charged. Chronic countertransferences are often expressed in the therapist's maintaining a particular attitude toward or feeling about a patient over time. Common examples are patients whom therapists see as special in some way—for example, as particularly needy or vulnerable or desirable. Chronic countertransferences may be ego-syntonic for the therapist and are often so for the patient as well. As a result, chronic countertransference reactions may be enacted without their being noticed by the therapist, and if they remain unresolved can lead to stalemates in the form of repeated transference-countertransference enactments.

Clinical Illustration 14: Acute Countertransference: Feeling Acutely Helpless and Frustrated

In a particular session, a patient with narcissistic personality disorder consistently either disregarded or misrepresented her therapist's comments, leaving the therapist feeling frustrated, dismissed, and helpless. This experience represented activation within the therapist of an object relation of a helpless, frustrated self in relation to a devaluing, dismissive object. The therapist's experience represented an acute complementary countertransference as she identified with the patient's projected dependent self, while the patient enacted her identification with a frustrating, dismissive parental object. These feelings were fully conscious on the part of the therapist, who had to make a focused effort to avoid getting sucked into a power struggle with the patient.

Clinical Illustration 15: Chronic Countertransference: Retrospectively Identifying a Long-Standing Blind Spot

A therapist was treating a patient who had been sexually molested as a child. The treatment had initially been productive, with the patient maintaining a mildly idealizing relation to the therapist, but after a year, the therapy seemed to founder. In consultation with a colleague, the therapist came to recognize the extent to which she had been excessively passive in the treatment from the outset, reflecting a view of the patient as a vulnerable child who needed to feel in control and should not be intruded upon. This attitude interfered with the therapist's ability to notice and explore the meaning of the patient's need to control the therapist.

It was only after the therapist reflected on the sources of her passivity that she was able to be more active. In this setting, the patient quickly came to experience the therapist as an intrusive enemy, which left the patient feeling fearful and self-righteously enraged. As this relational theme was explored in the transference, it became clear that activation of this relational pattern had routinely disrupted the patient's intimate relations.

Clinical Manifestations of Countertransference Across the Spectrum of Severity

The nature and quality of countertransference developments, and the relative centrality of countertransference as a channel of communication, typically vary according to the nature and severity of the patient's personality pathology (Colli et al. 2014). These differences parallel differences in transference developments across the spectrum of severity outlined in the earlier section "Transference," and in particular reflect the impact of the patient's defensive style on the therapist's experience. Table 5–2 summarizes countertransference developments across the level of personality organization, discussed further in the following sections on countertransference developments.

Countertransference Developments in the Setting of Identity Pathology and Splitting-Based Defenses

As a general rule, as personality pathology becomes more severe, countertransference analysis becomes increasingly central to the therapist's clinical work, from the perspectives both of identifying the object relations that are affectively dominant in the session and of organizing the patient's experience in the transference at any given moment, as well as from the perspective of minimizing countertransference acting out. Countertransferences in the treatment of BPO patients often reflect the therapist's responses to patients' transferences (what we refer to as *patient-centered countertransferences* in the earlier subsection "Defining Countertransference Within the Framework of Object Relations Theory") and the impact of splitting-based defenses on the clinical process. At times, the situation is compounded by what can be relatively extreme circumstances in a patient's life in the setting of more severe pathology. In this setting, counter-

TABLE 5–2.   Level of personality organization and countertransference developments

Typical countertransference developments	Borderline level of personality organization	Neurotic level of personality organization
Quality of affect	Highly charged, intense	Well modulated, subtle
	Poorly integrated	Well integrated
	Unfamiliar range of affective experience for therapist	Familiar range of affective experience for therapist
Quality of experience	Experienced as "alien," imposed on therapist	Experienced as coming from within the therapist
Challenge for therapist	High level of discomfort	May be ego-syntonic
	Difficult to contain	Easy to miss
Centrality in therapist's clinical process	Major channel of communication	Less central channel of communication
Typical source	Patient's transference to therapist	Variable combination of patient and therapist factors
Nature of identification in countertransference	Usually complementary	May be concordant or complementary

transference comes to serve as a central source of information about the object relations organizing the patient's experience in the moment.

Along the BPO spectrum, as pathology becomes more severe, countertransferences become increasingly affectively charged and not infrequently uncomfortable for the therapist. In the treatment of severe personality disorders, countertransferences may leave the therapist feeling pressured to act or compelled to "do something," mirroring the pressure to action often experienced by BPO patients in the transference. In essence, in the treatment of patients with severe personality disorders, the therapist's affective experience in the countertransference can mirror the affects activated in the patient, taking the therapist outside his typical range of affective experience; these countertransferences can be extremely uncomfortable for the therapist, can be difficult to contain, and are often experienced as imposed on, rather than coming from within, the therapist. It is as if the therapist is controlled by and driven to action to rid himself of alien affective experiences and associated object relations that have been activated within him by the patient's projective defenses.

In contrast, in the treatment of high-BPO patients, countertransferences tend to be somewhat more subtle and less highly affectively charged, leaving the therapist feeling less controlled and with more psychological space in which to reflect.

Clinical Illustration 16: Acute Countertransference: Feeling Aggressively Controlled

A patient with borderline personality disorder and paranoid features organized at a middle borderline level experienced her therapist as a dangerous and controlling enemy (a paranoid transference). From her perspective, this justified her attacking and aggressively shutting down her therapist whenever he attempted to say anything, making it virtually impossible for him to speak. The therapist was left feeling that if he were to be active in any fashion, he would be attacked, and that he had no alternative but to fall mute.

Countertransference: The clinical situation left the therapist feeling controlled by the patient, frustrated, and ultimately helpless.

In this clinical situation, the therapist's countertransference was powerfully determined by the patient's behavior and by the patient's transference to the therapist. Although this therapist's psychology and conflicts likely contributed to some degree to his reactions to the patient, most therapists, regardless of their personal conflicts, would likely respond similarly to a patient's persistent attacks. At the same time, the countertransference can be seen as mirroring the patient's experience of herself as controlled and helpless in the hands of a frustrating enemy. This is an example of the impact of projective identification and omnipotent control on the clinical process; the patient aggressively controlled the therapist while simultaneously experiencing herself as aggressively controlled.

Clinical Illustration 17: Acute Countertransference: Feeling Extreme Anxiety and Pressure to Act on Behalf of the Patient

A 20-year-old patient organized at a high borderline level and diagnosed with an unspecified personality disorder, with sadomasochistic, narcissistic, and borderline features, spoke about upcoming deadlines at school.

She told the therapist that she saw little hope of being able to mobilize herself within the necessary time frame, and the threat of failing to graduate hung over her head. As she reported on her dismal academic situation, the patient sat back in her chair, seemingly relaxed, her attitude and behavior discordant with the level of anxiety that would befit her situation. The therapist started to feel anxious for the patient, worrying that she was about to undermine herself. He felt an urge to do something to get the patient to mobilize herself to complete her class work.

Countertransference: The clinical situation induced in the therapist feelings of anxiety for the patient, along with feelings of responsibility and a pressure to act.

In this example, the therapist's experience in the countertransference can be seen as reflecting the part of the patient, disavowed and projected, that would feel anxious about her imminent dismissal from school. The therapist became aware that his own anxiety and wish to rescue the patient sharply contrasted with the patient's attitude toward her academic situation. It was as if the patient were communicating, "This is not my problem; it is yours." In the countertransference, this interaction left the therapist feeling anxious, pressured to do something to remedy the situation, while the patient seemed perfectly comfortable, able to happily sabotage herself and remain free of all anxiety.

Clinical Illustration 18: Acute and Chronic Countertransference: Feeling Acutely Devalued and Retrospectively Identifying Chronic Feelings of Coldness Toward Patient

A high-BPO patient with narcissistic personality disorder and a history of bulimia maintained an attitude of manifest idealization toward her therapist. She never found fault with the therapist, but whenever the therapist made a comment, the patient described being unable to retain the therapist's words, finding herself struggling to hang on to them, and expressing great frustration with her inability to control what she experienced as her "dissociation." The therapist attempted to explore the patient's behavior, but the patient was aware only of her frustration with her own inability "to think right," while she continued to manifestly idealize the therapist and to make conscious efforts to grasp the therapist's words as she spoke.

Acute countertransference: The clinical situation left the therapist feeling devalued and frustrated, given that she experienced the patient as totally unreceptive and unreachable.

This situation persisted for many months. Despite the therapist's ongoing efforts to "get through" to her patient, nothing changed. The therapist presented the case to a colleague, and as she described the clinical situation, she came to recognize that she had gradually and quietly settled into an attitude toward the patient that was characterized by a kind of coldness, manifested in subtle but persistent feelings of devaluation. She did not believe that she had betrayed her attitude to the patient but nevertheless felt bad about the possibility of having appeared cold.

Chronic countertransference: The clinical situation left the therapist feeling a coldness toward her patient—an attitude reflecting a combination of hostility, contempt, and unreceptiveness—after which she felt concerned and guilty.

In this example, the therapist's countertransference reactions again seem to be largely determined by dissociated aspects of the transference. In this case, it was by attending to the countertransference that the therapist was best able, over time, to identify the cold, unmovable aspects of the patient that were dissociated from her superficial idealizing and collaborative relationship with the therapist. The therapist was a warm and giving person; the blanket coldness she experienced toward this patient was highly uncharacteristic for her, both in her clinical work and in her interpersonal life. In this situation, the therapist came to appreciate that her attitude toward the patient was the same attitude that the patient acknowledged she sometimes secretly maintained toward others, including her husband, friends, and colleagues. The patient was not aware, however, of harboring these feelings toward the therapist, and it did not occur to her that the therapist might harbor such feelings toward her.

Through exploration of her countertransference, the therapist was able to identify the object relation organizing the patient's behavior in session and unconscious attitude toward the therapist: that of a devalued and shut-out therapist in relation to a hostile, depreciative, and unreceptive patient.

Projective Identification and Omnipotent Control in Countertransference With BPO Patients

Splitting-based defenses—in particular, projective identification and omnipotent control—are interpersonally based defenses; they typically involve inducing feelings in others (Kernberg 1975). In the setting of projective identification, the patient does not simply *experience* the therapist in a particular way in the transference; she interacts with the therapist interpersonally in ways that pull for the therapist's participation in enacting or playing out the transference (Britton 1998; Ogden 1993).[5] It is for this reason that in the setting of BPO, countertransference reactions tend to be especially useful, both in terms of understanding the patient's transference and in getting a clearer read on chronic problems in the patient's interpersonal relationships. Countertransference reactions with BPO patients are also especially challenging to manage. In many of the examples we have discussed, the patient can be seen to make use of projective identification, resulting in specific countertransference responses in the therapist that directly relate to the transference. In each case, the therapist was aware of needing to reflect on what he was feeling and to restrain himself from immediately acting—that is, to "contain" countertransference (see Chapter 12).

It is helpful to be aware that in the setting of projective identification, countertransferences are by definition complementary; in projective identification, the patient induces feelings in the therapist that correspond to a projected part of the patient that the patient is denying (as in Clinical Illustration 17, in which the therapist felt anxious on behalf of the patient while the patient felt calm). As clearly described in Clinical Illustration 18, in which the therapist came to feel a certain coldness toward her patient, this process can easily compromise the therapist's ability to empathize with the patient's internal situation.

Similarly, in Clinical Illustration 16, the example in which the therapist felt attacked and controlled, it would be easy to lose sight of the fact that the patient felt precisely the same way, despite her attacking and controlling behavior. When patients use projective identification in the transference, it often feels as though the patient is forcing something onto or into the therapist, and because whatever the patient projects is closely tied to the patient's internal experience, projective identification can expose the therapist to unfamiliar and highly unpleasant affective experiences in the countertransference. It is only by containing, restraining action, and reflecting on his own internal situation and that of the patient that the therapist can use the countertransference to gain a fuller and deeper appreciation of the object relations organizing the patient's behavior and experience.

-----

[5]This process is what Thomas Ogden (1993) refers to as *induction*: the patient interacts with the therapist in such a way as to induce within the therapist countertransference feelings corresponding to the patient's projections. For example, the patient projects a critical parent, anticipating criticism from the therapist, and then the patient behaves in ways that leave the therapist feeling acutely critical of the patient.

For example, in Clinical Illustration 16, in which the patient left the therapist feeling attacked and controlled, the therapist's ability to reflect on this reaction enabled him to empathize with the part of the patient that felt as though in the hands of a dangerous enemy, controlled and helpless.

Countertransference Developments in the Setting of Consolidated Identity and Repression-Based Defenses

In the psychotherapeutic treatment of patients with higher level personality pathology, the dominant channel of patient communication is verbal. As a result, countertransference plays a less central role in the therapist's understanding of the clinical picture for these patients than for BPO patients. Nevertheless, it remains a central operating principle that feelings elicited in the therapist by the patient are as important as anything the patient may communicate in words about her internal experience.

Mirroring the transference, countertransferences with NPO patients tend to be relatively well integrated, emerging in the form of thoughts or associations, or as feelings experienced as responses *to* or at most pressures *from* the patient, rather than emotional states *forced on or into* the therapist by the patient. These countertransferences typically do not leave the therapist feeling pressured to act.

Patients with higher level personality pathology can affect their therapists in subtle and socially appropriate ways to meet defensive needs. The therapist's attunement to and monitoring of his countertransference can help identify defensive object relations, which are often linked to character defenses that may be subtly enacted in session. These enactments can result in countertransferences that may be almost imperceptible at first. The patient will generally be unaware that she is "doing something," and it may take the therapist some time to catch on as well.

For example, as illustrated earlier in this chapter, a patient afraid of being criticized may be quietly ingratiating or behave in ways that are pleasing to the therapist, attempting to avoid any hint of conflict (Clinical Illustration 3), or a patient afraid of erotic feelings might induce boredom on the part of the therapist, enacting a sexless child in relation to a parent who does not see him as stimulating or interesting (Clinical Illustration 11). These countertransferences reflect the patient's defensive efforts to keep conflictual object relations out of the relationship with the therapist.

Alternatively, a patient may, as we commonly see with BPO patients, use the relationship with the therapist to off-load or project conflictual emotional states. One example is the patient we describe in our example of chronic countertransference (Clinical Illustration 20); this patient gradually induced the same feelings of irritation in the therapist that he did in his wife, while the patient remained calm himself.

Clinical Illustration 19:
Acute Countertransference: Feeling Tempted To Be the Supportive Parent

A depressive patient who presented with problems of self-esteem and a chronic low mood criticized herself at every turn. Hardworking and earnest, she never seemed to allow herself to take a break or to give herself credit for the fruits of her labors. Listening to her berating herself for not "doing more" in relation to a particular situation in her workplace, her therapist found himself wanting to encourage and praise her, to point out her very positive attributes, and to share with her his admiration of her work ethic. He found himself thinking fondly of his eldest daughter.

Countertransference: The therapist felt protective of the patient; he had the fantasy of supporting her and telling her how admirable he found her, much as a loving parent would do.

This vignette illustrates the relatively well-integrated quality of countertransference responses to NPO patients, and also the ways in which a therapist's personal wishes and conflicts may come into play. Rather than seeming to be feelings forced on the therapist, these countertransference reactions are often experienced as reactions or associations to the patient's situation and communications, and may, as in this example, initially be expressed in fantasies or private associations on the therapist's part. As the therapist in the vignette became attuned to his feelings and wishes in the countertransference with the patient, he wondered if his fantasy of encouraging and sharing his admiration for the patient spoke largely to his own desire to feel like a loving and beloved parent. He could not initially feel certain, but with time he came to believe that much as the countertransference reflected his own personal wishes, it had at the same time tapped into buried wishes of the patient, wishes she viewed as shameful: to be a favored and admired child in relation to a beloved paternal object.

Clinical Illustration 20:
Chronic Countertransference: Experiencing Patient as Emotionally Detached

An obsessional patient who presented with marital problems described his relationship with his wife in intellectualized and emotionally distant terms. Initially, the therapist identified with the patient and had difficulty understanding why the patient's wife "had to be" so impatient and critical. Though the therapist had noted the patient's intellectualized style in their first meeting, with time, he gradually came to feel increasingly impatient and put off by the patient's overly detailed, almost robotic discourse; he found himself feeling sympathetic toward the patient's wife, who complained, according to the patient, "incessantly" about the patient's emotional distance.

Countertransference: The therapist felt critical and impatient, experiencing the patient as emotionally detached and unavailable.

This complementary identification on the part of the therapist in the countertransference provided a window into the patient's marital difficulties. In noting his own irritation, the therapist could see how the patient's stance served to subtly express repressed feelings of hostility (an example of a compromise formation; see Chapter 3, section "Neurotic Projection") that the patient could not comfortably incorporate into a dependent relationship.

Key Clinical Concepts

- The psychotherapeutic relationship provides the context within which the patient's internal world is enacted and can be explored.

- The therapist's attitude toward the patient is nonjudgmental and communicates a wish to understand and a concern for the patient's well-being, forming the basis of the therapeutic alliance.

- The therapist's attitude of interest and concern is complemented by a stance of technical neutrality in which he avoids taking sides in the patient's conflicts, instead observing the conflicting forces within the patient.

- The therapist's neutral stance and his ongoing attention to transference and countertransference enable him to become aware of and to empathize with all aspects of the patient's internal situation, including those that the patient rejects, and to help the patient to do so as well.

References

Auchincloss AL, Samberg E (eds): Psychoanalytic Terms and Concepts. New Haven, CT, Yale University Press, 2012

Bateman A, Fonagy P: Mentalization-Based Treatment for Borderline Personality Disorder. New York, Oxford University Press, 2006

Beck AT, Freeman A, Davis DD, et al: Cognitive Therapy of Personality Disorders, 2nd Edition. New York, Guilford, 2004

Bender DS: Therapeutic alliance, in The American Psychiatric Publishing Textbook of Personality Disorders. Edited by Oldham JM, Skodol AE, Bender DS. Washington, DC, American Psychiatric Publishing, 2005, pp 405–420

Bion WR: Learning from Experience. London, Heinemann, 1962

Bordin ES: The generalizability of the psychoanalytic concept of the working alliance. Psychotherapy (Chic) 16:252–260, 1979

Britton R: Naming and containing, in Belief and Imagination. London, Routledge, 1998, pp 19–28

Caligor E, Kernberg OF, Clarkin JF: Handbook of Dynamic Psychotherapy for Higher Level Personality Pathology. Washington, DC, American Psychiatric Publishing, 2007

Colli A, Tanzilli A, Dimaggio G, Lingiardi V: Patient personality and therapist response: an empirical investigation. Am J Psychiatry 171(1):102–108, 2014 24077643

Connolly Gibbons MB, Crits-Christoph P, de la Cruz C, et al: Pretreatment expectations, interpersonal functioning, and symptoms in the prediction of the therapeutic alliance across supportive-expressive psychotherapy and cognitive therapy. Psychother Res 13:59–76, 2003

Etchegoyen RH: Fundamentals of Psychoanalytic Technique. London, Karnac Books, 1991

Gabbard GO: Long-Term Psychodynamic Psychotherapy: A Basic Text, 2nd Edition. Washington, DC, American Psychiatric Publishing, 2010

Gutheil TG, Havens LL: The therapeutic alliance: contemporary meanings and confusions. Int Rev Psychoanal 6:447–481, 1979

Harris A: Transference, countertransference, and the real relationship, in The American Psychiatric Publishing Textbook of Psychoanalysis. Edited by Person ES, Cooper AM, Gabbard GO. Washington, DC, American Psychiatric Publishing, 2005, pp 201–216

Hilsenroth MJ, Cromer TD: Clinician interventions related to alliance during the initial interview and psychological assessment. Psychotherapy (Chic) 44(2):205–218, 2007 22122211

Høglend P: Exploration of the patient-therapist relationship in psychotherapy. Am J Psychiatry 171(10):1056–1066, 2014 25017093

Horvath AO, Del Re AC, Flückiger C, Symonds D: Alliance in individual psychotherapy. Psychotherapy (Chic) 48(1):9–16, 2011 21401269

Joseph B: Transference: the total situation. Int J Psychoanal 44:447–454, 1985

Kernberg OF: Object Relations Theory and Clinical Psychoanalysis. New York, Jason Aronson, 1975

Kernberg OF: Acute and chronic countertransference reactions, in Aggressivity, Narcissism, and Self-Destructiveness in the Psychotherapeutic Relationship. New Haven, CT, Yale University Press, 2004, pp 167–191

Kernberg OF, Caligor E: A psychoanalytic theory of personality disorders, in Major Theories of Personality Disorder, 2nd Edition. Edited by Lenzenweger MF, Clarkin JF. New York, Guilford, 2005, pp 114–156

Levy SR, Hilsenroth MJ, Owen JJ: Relationship between interpretation, alliance, and outcome in psychodynamic psychotherapy: control of therapist effects and assessment of moderator variable impact. J Nerv Ment Dis 203(6):418–424, 2015 25988432

Levy ST, Inderbitzin LB: Neutrality, interpretation, and therapeutic intent. J Am Psychoanal Assoc 40(4):989–1011, 1992 1430771

Linehan MM: Cognitive-Behavioral Treatment of Borderline Personality Disorder. New York, Guilford, 1993

Luborsky L: Principles of Psychoanalytic Psychotherapy: A Manual for Supportive-Expressive Treatment. New York, Basic Books, 1984

Marmar CR, Horowitz MJ, Weiss DS, Marziali E: The development of the Therapeutic Alliance Rating System, in The Psychotherapeutic Process. Edited by Greenberg LS, Pinsof WM. New York, Guilford, 1986, pp 367–390

Ogden TH: The depressive position and the birth of the historical subject, in Matrix of the Mind: Object Relations and the Psychoanalytic Dialogue. Northvale, NJ, Jason Aronson, 1993, pp 67–99

Orlinsky DE, Ronnestad MH, Willutzki U: Fifty years of psychotherapy process-outcome research: continuity and change, in Bergin and Garfield's Handbook of Psychotherapy and Behavior Change, 5th Edition. Edited by Lambert MJ. New York, Wiley, 2004, pp 307–390

Piper WE, Azim HFA, Joyce AS, et al: Quality of object relations versus interpersonal functioning as predictors of therapeutic alliance and psychotherapy outcome. J Nerv Ment Dis 179(7):432–438, 1991 1869873

Racker H: The meanings and uses of countertransference. Psychoanal Q 26(3):303–357, 1957 13465913

Rockland L: Supportive Therapy: A Psychodynamic Approach. New York, Basic Books, 1989

Safran JD, Muran JC: Negotiating the Therapeutic Alliance. New York, Guilford, 2000

Safran JD, Muran JC, Eubanks-Carter C: Repairing alliance ruptures. Psychotherapy (Chic) 48(1):80–87, 2011 21401278

Sandler J: Countertransference and role responsiveness. Int Rev Psychoanal 3:43–47, 1976

Schafer R: The Analytic Attitude. New York, Basic Books, 1983

Smith HF: Analysis of transference: a North American perspective. Int J Psychoanal 84 (Pt 4):1017–1041, 2003 13678504

Westen D, Gabbard GO: Developments in cognitive neuroscience, II: implications for theories of transference. J Am Psychoanal Assoc 50(1):99–134, 2002 12018876

Winston A, Rosenthal RN, Pinsker H: Learning Supportive Therapy: An Illustrated Guide. Washington, DC, American Psychiatric Publishing, 2012

Wnuk S, McMain S, Links PS, et al: Factors related to dropout from treatment in two outpatient treatments for borderline personality disorder. J Pers Disord 27(6):716–726, 2013 23718760

Yeomans F, Clarkin JF, Kernberg OF: Transference-Focused Psychotherapy for Borderline Personality Disorder: A Clinical Guide. Washington, DC, American Psychiatric Publishing, 2015

Strategies of Treatment and Mechanisms of Change

strategies of transference-focused psychotherapy—extended (TFP-E); these are the basic principles that organize the treatment as a whole, with the goal of promoting identity consolidation and psychological integration. The strategies of TFP-E define the overarching approach employed by the therapist throughout the treatment and in each session, and are closely linked to the understanding of how the treatment promotes integrative processes in patients. The strategies of TFP-E are embedded in the object relations theory model of psychological functioning and personality disorder presented in Chapters 1–3 and in the model of the therapeutic relationship described in Chapter 5. The strategies of TFP-E presented in this chapter function as the scaffolding for the in-depth description of the treatment in the chapters to come.

In Part I, we first present the basic strategies of TFP-E, which organize the overall TFP-E clinical approach to treatment of all personality disorders, across the spectrum of severity. In Part 2, we provide an in-depth discussion of the functions of these strategies. In Part 3, we discuss how this general TFP-E approach is modified to meet the clinical needs of patients with pathology at different levels of severity and with different presentations. In particular, in Part 3 we outline more specific aspects of strategies for patients at a borderline level of personality organization (BPO) and those at a neurotic level of personality organization (NPO). We emphasize how the strategies of treatment reflect the patient's defensive organization and the impact of defenses on subjectivity in individuals at different levels of personality organization, and we focus in particular on our understanding of how the strategies of treatment support different psychological capacities in patients at different levels of severity, facilitating therapeutic change.

Part 1

Overview of the Basic Strategies of TFP-E

THE CENTRAL STRATEGY OF TFP-E AT ALL PHASES of treatment is to focus attention on the object relations enacted in each session. As the patient speaks openly and freely in his therapy session or finds himself having difficulty doing so, the therapist should be able to identify one or two relationship patterns that are salient. These object relations are referred to as the *dominant object relations*. The dominant object relations are the *surface*, or most accessible, expression of the conflict currently active in the session; when the therapist identifies the dominant object relations, she identifies an area of conflict, and focusing on the dominant object relations initiates a process that involves exploring the currently active conflict.

In Strategy 1 of TFP-E, the therapist identifies the dominant object relations in any given session, and then works with the patient to describe the dominant object relations in words. In Strategy 2, the therapist calls the patient's attention to the ways in which enactment of the dominant object relations is organizing his experience and the clinical material in a repetitive and rigid fashion. This focus leads naturally to Strategy 3, in which the therapist explores and then interprets the relationship between object relations currently enacted and those defended against, focusing on the anxieties motivating splitting- or repression-based defenses.

In Strategy 4, identification, exploration, and interpretation of the conflictual object relations linked to core conflicts, repeated over time and in different contexts—that is, the working through of central conflicts—promotes the containment of conflictual internal object relations and the integrative processes that are the goals of TFP-E. In the process of working through, the therapist focuses on the treatment goals and also make links to the patient's developmental history.

The strategies of treatment lead the therapist to approach the clinical material through the patient's subjective experience, and then to gradually broaden and deepen the patient's view of his behavior and of his internal life, fostering first self-awareness and next self-understanding. The therapist first helps the patient attend to and elaborate his dominant conscious experience (Strategy 1); the therapist then helps the patient broaden his view to include, in the case of the BPO patient, the instability introduced by splitting-based defenses, and in the case of the NPO patient, the rigidity introduced by repression (Strategy 2).

The impact of repeatedly calling attention to and describing the repetitive, predictable quality of the patient's experience, insofar as it is organized by the patient's defenses, and inviting the patient to observe and reflect on what has been described, is that defenses become ego-dystonic and less effective, and the patient becomes more reflective. At this juncture, the therapist shifts the emphasis from simply observing and describing the patient's behavior and experience to exploring the anxieties and conflicts that might explain why the patient experiences things as he does (Strategy 3). Finally, the therapist helps the patient fully appreciate the impact of his conflicts and defenses on his experience and behavior in various domains of functioning (Strategy 4).

Table 6–1 provides an overview of the four basic strategies of TFP-E and their functions. In the next parts of this chapter, we discuss further the strategies of treatment and their functions (Part 2), as well as how we tailor the strategies of treatment for BPO and NPO (Part 3).

TABLE 6–1. Basic strategies of transference-focused psychotherapy—extended and their functions

---

Strategy 1. Defining the dominant object relations

    1a. Identifying the dominant object relations

        Function: Narrows the focus to an area of conflict

    1b. Describing the dominant object relations in words

        Function: Supports the patient's capacity for self-observation in an area of conflict and provides affect containment

Strategy 2. Calling attention to the repetitive, rigid, and/or contradictory nature of the patient's experience and behavior

    2a. Calling attention to the repetitive nature of the patient's experience and behavior as dominant object relations predictably organize the clinical material under the impact of repression or splitting-based defenses

        Function: Promotes self-observation and reflection

    2b. Focusing on role reversals and the impact of splitting and repression on the patient's experience and behavior

        Function: Introduces alternative perspectives, further promoting self-observation and reflection while supporting awareness of the internal, subjective nature of experience

Strategy 3. Exploring the anxieties and conflicts embedded in the dominant object relations and introducing hypotheses about underlying wishes, fears, and personal meanings

        Function: Supports the capacity to tolerate awareness of anxieties driving defensive operations, introducing greater flexibility into defensive functioning; broadens the patient's perspective to appreciate the constructed, symbolic nature of subjectivity and, ultimately, the impact of psychological conflicts on his experience and behavior

Strategy 4. Working through identified conflicts as they are activated in different contexts across time while making links to the treatment goals and the patient's developmental history

        Function: Enables the patient to contain conflictual internal object relations and associated anxieties and to relinquish maladaptive defenses, promoting integrative changes, contextualization of experience, and flexibility of functioning

---

Part 2

Basic Strategies of TFP-E and Their Functions

Strategy 1: Defining the Dominant Object Relations

1a: Identifying the Dominant Object Relations

This process narrows the focus to an area of conflict.

The first strategy of TFP-E is to identify the dominant internal object relations active in the session. Internal object relations are the mental representations that organize a person's experience of himself and of his internal and external reality. Although mental representations cannot be directly observed, the nature of the representations of self and other that are active at any given moment can be inferred from the ways in which they shape a person's thoughts, feelings, and behaviors. We refer to this process as the *enactment* of internal object relations.

In TFP-E, the therapist makes inferences about the internal object relations organizing the patient's experience in the moment on the basis of the patient's communications to the therapist, focusing on the patient's verbal and nonverbal communication and the countertransference. As the therapist works to define the self and object representations currently dominant, she pays special attention to the patient's descriptions of his interpersonal interactions, listening for the relationship patterns activated in the patient's interactions with others and in the current therapeutic relationship. In particular, the therapist listens for relationship patterns that present themselves repeatedly in the clinical process.

As described in Chapter 5, in the setting of more severe personality pathology, the dominant object relations and related conflicts tend to become affectively dominant in the transference; in the dynamic treatment of severe personality disorders, the transference-countertransference typically comes to dominate the clinical process, becoming the therapist's primary window into the patient's internal world. As pathology becomes less severe, the centrality of the transference in clinical process is more variable, and the patient's interactions with the therapist may not be the focus of clinical attention. In this setting, the therapist pays relatively greater attention to the patient's descriptions of his interactions with others, as well as of self states.

As the therapist listens to the patient with the objective of identifying the dominant object relations, she attends to what we refer to as the *three channels of communication*. The therapist makes inferences about the patient's internal object world on the basis of not only his *verbal communications* but also his *nonverbal communications*, attending both to the patient's behavior in session and also to what he is stimulating in the *countertransference*—that is, in the therapist's private reactions to the patient. The relative importance of each of the three channels is variable and tends to track with severity of pathology, reflecting the impact of defensive style on clinical process.

In work with an NPO patient, verbal communications, including his free associations and his difficulties communicating openly or freely, tend to be a major source of information about unconscious conflict and defense. What this patient is able to communicate through verbal channels is supplemented by nonverbal communication and the countertransference. In contrast, in work with a patient who has more severe personality pathology, behavior tends to be a more central source of information about the object relations enacted in the session, and the patient's verbal communications may be dissociated from his emotional experience and less helpful. Further, in work with a patient who has splitting-based defensive operations, the emotional reactions that the patient invites in the therapist become a central source of information about the object relations currently organizing the patient's experience; in fact, it is not unusual for the countertransference to become at times the most useful channel of communication, reflecting the impact of projective identification on the clinical process.

As the therapist listens to and interacts with her patient, she will be able to construct hypotheses about the internal object relations currently being enacted. At this stage, it can be helpful for the therapist to imagine, quite literally, two people in interaction, each playing a particular role. Typically, the patient will be identified predominantly with one particular role in any given relationship pattern, although at times his identification with both sides of a relationship pattern (or with all three, in the case of triadic relationship patterns) may be quite close to consciousness. For example, the therapist might see the patient as a dependent, gratified self in relation to an attentive provider; an angry, demanding, and childlike self in relation to a rejecting parental figure; a devalued, inferior self in relation to a powerful, demeaning other; or an abused victim self in relation to a sadistic persecutor.

When the therapist feels that a certain object relation is starting to come into focus, she will ask for additional details about the patient's experience of the interactions that the patient is describing or enacting with the therapist. Because, by definition, the dominant object relations are the most accessible expression of a conflict currently active in the treatment, by identifying the dominant object relations, the therapist is also beginning to focus clinical attention on an area of conflict.

1b: Describing the Dominant Object Relations in Words

This process supports the patient's capacity for self-observation in an area of conflict and provides affect containment.

After the therapist formulates in her own mind what she imagines to be the dominant object relations, the next task is to develop and share a description of these object relations with the patient. This description can be conceived of in terms of two actors, the patient and either the therapist or another person in the patient's life, each playing a particular role. By imagining and articulating the role that the patient is playing and the role attributed to the therapist or other person, the therapist can acquire a vivid sense of the patient's internal world.

The process of developing and presenting such a "description of the actors" typically begins with the therapist asking for clarification of the material, either focusing directly on the patient's experience of the therapist or asking for further details about interactions with others that the patient has been describing. When the therapist moves on to offer a description of the dominant object relations, it is always presented as a hypothesis, with the expectation that the therapist's understanding can be modified, depending on the patient's reactions. The following is an example:

> Therapist: As you tell the story, it seems as though your boss was trying to put you down in front of the group. Do you think that he did it on purpose?
> Patient: He loved every second!
> Therapist: So, if I hear you correctly, you see your boss as taking pleasure in putting you down and making you feel inferior, while you feel that you can't push back. Does that seem accurate?
> Patient: Yes. He's just a son of a bitch.
> Therapist: It sounds like all of this leaves you feeling powerless and humiliated.

Thus, as the therapist presents her current hypothesis about the dominant object relations, it is often helpful for the therapist to share with the patient his internal process leading up to the formulation, so the patient can understand that the therapist's suggestion is not a magical or arbitrary assessment, nor a condemnation, but rather an effort to understand. In this regard, it is especially helpful, if possible, for the therapist to use the patient's words, as in the following:

> When I asked about your getting here late, you responded that my question seemed "callous"—that I seemed not to understand, or even worse, not to care about how hard it is for you to get out of bed to get here. Since then you've been weeping. It's as if you view me as a callous taskmaster who is making impossible demands, while you feel helpless and overwhelmed, unable to stand up for yourself, able only to sit here and weep. Does what I am saying ring true?

It is best to name the actors when the patient is affectively involved but not so swept away in emotion that he is unable to consider what the therapist is suggesting. Sometimes, when emotion runs high, putting words to the patient's experience in the form of naming the actors can provide some degree of affective containment, leaving the patient feeling less affectively swamped and better able to step back, observe his experience, and think about what he is feeling. This is especially true with BPO patients, and in general when the dominant object relations are being enacted in the transference.

Strategy 2: Calling Attention to the Repetitive, Rigid, and/or Contradictory Nature of the Patient's Experience and Behavior

2a: Calling Attention to the Repetitive Nature of the Patient's Experience and Behavior as Dominant Object Relations Predictably Organize the Clinical Material Under the Impact of Repression or Splitting-Based Defenses

This process promotes self-observation and reflection.

After identifying and describing the dominant object relations, the therapist will bring to the patient's attention the rigid, repetitive, and predictable fashion in which particular relationship patterns present themselves, within a single session and across multiple sessions. This process involves the therapist's pointing out that the patient tends to experience the same relationship patterns in different settings and across time, as in these examples:

> You know, as I listen to what happened with your brother last night, it strikes me that your experience was similar to how you've described your interactions with your boss. Once again, you find yourself in the familiar position of feeling publicly put down, while he acts like a superior son of a bitch. It seems that this pattern keeps coming up.

> When I asked about your drinking, once again I seemed like a controlling and critical taskmaster, forcing you to think about things that you feel unable to manage. It seems that this relation comes up over and over, whenever I say or do something that you don't like.

2b: Focusing on Role Reversals and the Impact of Splitting and Repression on the Patient's Experience and Behavior

This process introduces alternative perspectives, further promoting self-observation and reflection while supporting awareness of the internal, subjective nature of experience.

Once the patient is familiar with the dominant object relations that tend to organize his experience from session to session, the therapist expands her interventions to address the relationship between the dominant object relations and other aspects of the patient's experience. At this stage, the therapist puts the relationship pattern currently organizing the patient's subjectivity into a broader perspective, exploring the relationship between the object relations currently enacted and those defended against by splitting- or repression-based defenses. In implementing this strategy, the therapist calls attention to the impact of splitting- and repression-based defenses on the patient's subjective experience.

When splitting-based defenses predominate, the therapist looks for opportunities to point out the impact of projective identification manifested as role reversals, and of splitting proper manifested as dissociation of idealized and persecutory aspects of experience. The therapist typically begins with role reversals, emphasizing either that she is seeing the same relationship pattern elaborated in Strategy 2a again enacted, but this time with the patient in the complementary position, or that the patient who is consciously identified with one side of an object relation is at the same time behaviorally enacting an identification with the other side in a dissociated fashion.

In calling attention to role reversals, the therapist asks the patient to step back and observe his behavior, often denied or dissociated, and to entertain alternative perspectives, as in this example:

> At the same time that you see me as controlling, it seems that you control me when you insist I not raise topics that you don't want to think about. What are your thoughts about this?

The therapist next focuses on the unstable and contradictory nature of the patient's experience as he moves between dissociated and contradictory, or idealized and paranoid, views of self and other. In this situation, in contrast to role reversals, which involve identifications with two sides of the same object relation, the therapist is broadening the patient's perspective to bridge two separate object relations, and also to span across time.

> In the beginning of the session, you described feeling safe and happy to be back here, but as soon as I raised the issue of your drinking, it was as if I became in your eyes rejecting and critical, like a cold mother who leaves you feeling criticized and uncared for.

In the setting of repression, after calling attention to the repetitive and rigid quality of the patient's experiences, which reflect the relatively fixed, repetitive, and predictable activation of defensive object relations, the therapist calls attention to inconsistencies and systematic distortions in the patient's view of self and other in interaction, which reflect the rigidity of defensive object relations and the impact of repression-based defenses on the patient's subjectivity.

> Once again you describe feeling humiliated at work, as if you feel yourself to be an ineffectual loser surrounded by competent men who take pleasure in putting you down. This is a familiar pattern, but I am struck by how it comes up just now, on the heels of your recent promotion. It seems that your real-life successes and the recognition you receive have no impact on how you view yourself; it is almost as though you are invested in holding on to this painful view of yourself.

In contrast to typical clinical developments when splitting-based defenses predominate, in the setting of repression-based defenses, role reversals may or may not be accessible, especially early in treatment.

In the treatments of both NPO and BPO patients, the outcome of the second strategy of treatment is that the defensive object relations organizing the patient's experience and behavior gradually become *ego-dystonic*, which is to say that from the patient's perspective, they are no longer seamless; the BPO patient becomes cognizant of how his experience is unstable and contradictory, and the NPO patient of how he rigidly holds on to particular views of himself and others. Further, interventions pointing to the rigid and repetitive nature of the patient's experience invite the patient to step back and observe himself—both his behavior and his internal experience. This stance enables the patient to entertain alternative perspectives; rather than taking his customary perspective for granted, the patient is now able to look at his view, entertain other views, and reflect.

Entertaining alternative perspectives in an area of conflict represents an essential shift, promoting the BPO patient's capacity to contextualize his experience and calling into question the NPO patient's defensive views of self and other. This shift also enables the patient to more fully appreciate that the focus of exploration is the patient's *internal, subjective experience*, in contrast to actual external events or material reality. Although many NPO patients may come to treatment with this capacity, the ability to appreciate the subjective and internal nature of experience is an especially important development in the treatment of BPO patients, many of whom have difficulty relinquishing a more concrete view of their experience in areas of conflict.

In work with either a BPO or an NPO patient, interventions that make up the second strategy of TFP-E focus the patient's attention on exploration of his internal experience and invite curiosity about why he might organize his experience as he does, laying the groundwork for exploration of the anxieties and conflicts associated with the dominant object relations while supporting reflective capacities in areas of psychological conflict and defense.

Strategy 3: Exploring the Anxieties and Conflicts Embedded in the Dominant Object Relations and Introducing Hypotheses About Underlying Wishes, Fears, and Personal Meanings

This process supports the capacity to tolerate awareness of anxieties driving defensive operations, introducing greater flexibility into defensive functioning; this process also broadens the patient's perspective to appre-

ciate the constructed, symbolic nature of subjectivity and, ultimately, the impact of psychological conflicts on his experience and behavior.

Strategy 3 involves exploring and interpreting conflicts linked to the dominant object relations. Up to this point, interventions have focused on descriptive features of the patient's psychological functioning and behavior, with emphasis on calling attention and putting words to aspects of the patient's experience of himself and others. With the third strategy, the therapist further expands her interventions to include exploration of anxieties and conflicts—that is, motivations for defense that in essence address the question "What would motivate the patient to organize his experience as he does?" The therapist pursues this line of inquiry only after earlier interventions have left the patient aware that the focus of exploration is on his *internal* experience and how it is organized, and the therapist offers interpretations only at those moments when the patient is capable of feeling curious about why he organizes things as he does.

In work with BPO patients, Strategies 1 and 2, which precede exploration of conflict, play an especially central role by supporting reflective capacities that can be easily compromised in areas of conflict in BPO patients. These capacities need to be in place, moment to moment, for the BPO patient to engage in exploration of internal motivations and conflicts in a meaningful and productive fashion. In NPO patients, reflective capacities are as a rule more stable, and patients in this group move more quickly and readily than those in the BPO group to explore internal motivations and meanings.

As the therapist explores and ultimately interprets core conflicts, she suggests possible ways to understand the repetitive and rigid activation of dominant object relations. These suggestions are offered in the form of interpretations of motivations for defense (see Chapter 10). For example, in the context of splitting-based defenses, the therapist might say, "Perhaps you revert to the more negative, critical view of me to protect the more positive, hopeful view of our relationship, to keep it in a safe place, safe from attack or disappointment." In the setting of repression-based defenses, the therapist might say, "Painful as it is, perhaps in some way it feels safer to see yourself as ineffectual and childlike in the workplace, as if this allows you to avoid the possibility of seeing yourself as in any way competitive or aggressive—as if any shred of competitive feeling on your part would in your mind turn you into a son of a bitch just like your boss." Exploration and interpretation of core conflicts help the patient tolerate awareness of anxieties motivating defense, the first step in the integrative processes supported by working through. We describe the interpretive process, as well as our understanding of the ways in which it promotes integrative changes, in Chapters 10 and 11.

Strategy 4: Working Through Identified Conflicts as They Are Activated in Different Contexts Across Time While Making Links to the Treatment Goals and the Patient's Developmental History

This process enables the patient to contain conflictual internal object relations and associated anxieties and to relinquish maladaptive defenses, promoting integrative changes, contextualization of experience, and flexibility of functioning.

As conflicts are enacted, explored, and interpreted repeatedly over time, the object relations associated with these conflicts become more familiar and less threatening; it is in the process of working through identified conflicts that the patient develops greater capacity to tolerate awareness of conflictual object relations and associated anxieties, to take responsibility for them, and ultimately to contain them within his dominant sense of self, leading to integrative changes. In this process, it is necessary that the patient have the experience of enacting and exploring the object relations that represent the defenses and anxieties associated with expression of a particular conflict from a variety of perspectives and in a variety of contexts; part of working through involves the patient's "trying on" new ways of behaving, thinking, and feeling, both in the treatment and in his daily life.

The process of working through a particular conflict takes place over the course of months, only to be followed by intermittent reactivation and further working through of the same cluster of internal object relations at a later time. In this process, patients move between paranoid and depressive anxieties as they struggle to tolerate, manage, take responsibility for, and contain conflictual object relations. In the process of working through, the therapist looks for opportunities to make a link between dominant conflicts and the difficulties that brought the patient to treatment and which contributed to the treatment goals determined at the initiation of treatment. It is also in the process of working through that the therapist is most likely to bring in material from the patient's developmental past and to consider ways in which the patient's current internal world and difficulties reflect important early experience. Links to the developmental past emerging during the process of working through function to deepen and contextualize current experience, while helping the patient develop a coherent, internal self-narrative across time.

Part 3

Tailoring TFP-E Strategies to the Individual Patient

IN THE FOLLOWING TWO SECTIONS OF THIS chapter, we present two variations to our preceding basic outline of strategies of treatment, highlighting differential implementation of core strategies in the treatment first of BPO patients and then of NPO patients. The differences between the two approaches reflect the impact of splitting- versus repression-based defenses on the patients' psychological functioning, subjective experience, and reflective capacities.

The following summarizes the strategies of treatment: The therapist tracks the impact of defenses on the patient's subjectivity and behavior, starting with the object relations that are most accessible and affectively dominant, and moving toward aspects of experience that are more conflictual and highly defended against. During this process, the therapist's focus is on the patient's moment-to-moment subjective experience. The therapist tailors her strategic approach to meet the needs of the individual patient at any point in treatment and in time; as the patient progresses or temporarily regresses in treatment, the therapist shifts her approach accordingly (Joseph 1989).

We illustrate our strategies of treatment in the therapies of BPO and NPO patients using two extended clinical vignettes. It is important to appreciate that over the course of treatment, strategies are implemented repeatedly over many weeks, months, and years to result in therapeutic change. Typically, early in treatment, it may take many sessions to move from Strategies 1 and 2 to begin exploration and working through of conflicts associated with the dominant object relations. As treatment progresses, the therapist can typically move through the strategies more quickly, sometimes many times in a single session, and ultimately the treatment comes to focus predominantly on working through core conflicts that have been elaborated earlier.

By necessity, the illustrations we provide telescope clinical developments; in our vignettes, we focus on one or two core conflicts, but of course in any treatment, strategies will be implemented in relation to a number of different conflicts and dominant object relations over the course of time, often simultaneously, depending on the patient's defensive structure.

Patients Along the Borderline Spectrum of Personality Organization

The overall psychotherapeutic strategy for the treatment of patients with severe personality disorders (low and middle BPO), as well as for those at a high borderline level of personality organization, is conceptualized in terms of the four overall sequential tasks outlined in the previous section, but with each task tailored to address the specific clinical needs of the BPO patient, focusing on the impact of splitting-based defenses on the patient's experience and behavior. Table 6–2 outlines the TFP-E strategies of treatment for BPO patients.

Clinical Illustration of Treatment Strategies in the Setting of BPO

When Ms. M presented for treatment, she was 30 years old, single, and unemployed. She had recently moved back to her mother's home from out of state, having been fired from her job as a waitress. She had become embroiled in an argument with a customer whom she felt had "disrespected" her, and she had ultimately threatened to throw a steaming-hot pizza pie in his face.

Socially isolated, Ms. M had had no long-term relationships outside her immediate family. She described a series of either superficial or short-lived stormy friendships with men and women, and had no history of dating or intimate relations. She was referred by her mother, who made being in treatment a condition for her living in her home.

Ms. M was a large, overweight, and overbearing woman, overtly hostile, rarely making eye contact except to glare at Dr. C. Her responses to

TABLE 6–2.   Strategies of transference-focused psychotherapy— extended and their functions, modified for borderline level of personality organization

Strategy 1. Defining the dominant object relations

    1a. Identifying the dominant object relations

        Function: Helps the therapist to better contain her own affects while narrowing the clinical focus to an area of conflict

    1b. Describing the dominant object relations in words

        Function: Supports the patient's capacity for self-observation and provides containment of highly charged affect states

Strategy 2. Calling attention to the repetitive, rigid, and/or contradictory nature of the patient's experience and behavior

    2a. Calling attention to the repetitive nature of the patient's experience and behavior as a single object relation predictably organizes the clinical material under the impact of splitting-based defenses

        Function: Promotes self-observation and reflection

    2b. Focusing on role reversals

        Function: Introduces alternative perspectives, promoting reflection and self-awareness by focusing on the impact of projective identification on the patient's subjective experience and behavior

    2c. Focusing on dissociation of idealized and persecutory object relations

        Function: Promotes reflection on internal states by highlighting the impact of splitting on the patient's subjective experience and behavior while inviting the patient to contextualize idealized and paranoid experiences across time

Strategy 3. Exploring the anxieties and conflicts motivating splitting and organizing the dominant object relations, and introducing hypotheses about underlying wishes and fears

        Function: Promotes the capacity to tolerate awareness of anxieties driving the mutual dissociation of idealized and paranoid object relations, introducing greater flexibility into defensive functioning; broadens the patient's perspective to appreciate the constructed, symbolic nature of subjectivity and, ultimately, the impact of psychological conflicts on his experience and behavior

---

TABLE 6–2. Strategies of transference-focused psychotherapy— extended and their functions, modified for borderline level of personality organization *(continued)*

Strategy 4. Working through identified conflicts

   4a. Working through identified conflicts and associated anxieties as they are enacted in different contexts across time while making links to the treatment goals and the patient's interpersonal relationships

   Function: Enables the patient to contain anxieties associated with the expression of aggression and to relinquish splitting-based defenses, promoting integration of idealized and persecutory internal object relations and leading to a gradual process of identity consolidation while improving interpersonal functioning

   4b. Linking identified conflicts to the patient's developmental history

   Function: Deepens the patient's level of self-understanding while further promoting containment of anxieties motivating defense, supporting contextualization of experience across time and the process of identity consolidation

---

Dr. C's efforts to obtain a history were curt and incomplete, nonverbally communicating that Dr. C's questions were alternatingly intrusive or idiotic. At the same time, Ms. M managed to communicate that she saw herself as "a useless, hopeless piece of shit."

After seeing the patient in consultation, Dr. C made the diagnosis of borderline personality disorder with paranoid and narcissistic features, organized at a middle borderline level. The patient's profile on the Structured Interview of Personality Organization—Revised (STIPO-R; Clarkin et al. 2016) had prominent scores for poor object relations and high levels of aggression.

Strategy 1: Defining the Dominant Object Relations

Although Ms. M initially agreed to the treatment contract, including twice-weekly sessions, she quickly experienced difficulty complying with the treatment frame. The trip to Dr. C's office was objectively inconvenient, but also, complying with the treatment frame that Ms. M felt Dr. C imposed upon her left Ms. M feeling quite paranoid. Ms. M was often late for sessions, at times stormed out early, and often sat in silence; she was "on strike." She would glare at Dr. C in silence or complain about how self-serving and unfeeling Dr. C was to insist that Ms. M come in twice a week; Ms. M accused Dr. C of caring only about rigidly sticking to the treatment model while caring nothing about how difficult all this was for Ms. M.

Often, when Dr. C attempted to speak, Ms. M would cut her off, interrupting her, arguing with her, or simply sitting forward in her chair, opening and closing her fists and glaring. In the countertransference, Dr. C felt frustrated, controlled, helpless, and at times also frightened.

1a: Identifying the Dominant Object Relations

This process helps the therapist to better contain her own affects while narrowing the clinical focus to an area of conflict.

Making use of her countertransference and Ms. M's verbal and nonverbal communications, Dr. C pulled together in her own mind a hypothesis about the dominant object relation organizing Ms. M's experience of the relationship in the moment (Strategy 1a). Dr. C imagined an object relation of a controlling, aggressive bully in relation to someone who is enraged, rebellious, and helpless, with the entire relationship colored by hostility and fear.

In her countertransference, Dr. C was aware of feeling controlled by Ms. M, at times victimized and at time helpless and afraid. In her behavior, Ms. M acted the bully; however, as Dr. C reflected on Ms. M's accusations and protestations, it seemed that the patient herself felt bullied and controlled by Dr. C, and it was not clear if Ms. M was aware of the impact of her own behavior. Thus, Dr. C formulated in her mind the dominant object relation of a helpless and rebellious patient-self, controlled by a bullying and aggressive therapist-other. Dr. C was also aware that this same pattern was being played out with Ms. M's mother, whom Ms. M experienced as bullying her to be in treatment while Ms. M felt controlled, enraged, and rebellious.

1b: Describing the Dominant Object Relations in Words

This process supports the patient's capacity for self-observation and provides containment of highly charged affect states.

In a particular session, Ms. M arrived 10 minutes late and then went on a rant about the inconvenience of the commute to Dr. C's office. She commented that Dr. C clearly didn't "give a shit" about Ms. M's time or convenience. Ms. M was quite agitated and was looking to Dr. C for a response. Dr. C used this opportunity to describe the dominant object relations in words (Strategy 1b), with the hope that this might provide some degree of affect containment and begin to stimulate a process of self-observation on Ms. M's part.

Dr. C attempted to put Ms. M's dominant conscious experience, as she understood it, into words: "I hear you. I am controlling and selfish, rigidly adhering to the treatment frame to meet my own needs, caring nothing about how difficult this is for you while you feel controlled, helpless, and frustrated; I can understand that this leaves you feeling very angry." Ms. M responded, "Yes, of course this is how I feel! How else *could* I feel?" At the same time, she seemed less agitated and afraid.

Comments: When working with BPO patients, the TFP-E therapist's first objective is to identify the salient idealized or persecutory object relation currently organizing the patient's experience in the session. Often this object relation will be affectively dominant in the transference. As a BPO patient's affects become more highly charged and are activated in the transference, the patient's nonverbal communication and the countertransference typically become the most useful channels of communication; verbal communications may at times be dissociated from what is affectively dominant in the session.

The therapist is called on first to tolerate her own confusion in what can be a potentially chaotic clinical situation, and to contain rather than act on her countertransference. Next, the therapist reflects on what she is feeling, what the patient is enacting, and what the patient is saying to construct a hypothesis about the object relations currently organizing the patient's experience. This internal process on the part of the therapist typically helps the therapist contain her own anxiety and confusion. Asking for additional clarification of the patient's experience, the therapist then works with the patient to put the *patient's perspective* on the relationship into words, creating a description of the representations involved and noting which side of the object relation the patient is consciously identified with.

Articulating and putting into words the dominant object relations can provide affective containment for the patient and reduce the overall level of confusion and anxiety for both patient and therapist in the session; identifying the dominant object relations introduces structure into what can feel like a chaotic clinical situation. Putting words to the patient's experience also allows the patient to feel understood and to see the therapist as trying to understand. Finally, defining the dominant object relations initiates a process of self-observation on the part of the BPO patient, a process on which the therapist builds in subsequent interventions.

Strategy 2: Calling Attention to the Repetitive, Rigid, and/or Contradictory Nature of the Patient's Experience and Behavior

The second TFP-E strategy in the treatment of BPO patients is conceptualized in terms of three generally sequential steps that build on one another:

- First, the therapist calls attention to repetition in the clinical process of a single dominant object relation that organizes the patient's experience and communications in session, and often across multiple sessions, inside and outside the transference.
- Next, the therapist focuses on role reversals within the previously defined object relation, highlighting how the patient is identified at different times with both sides of the object relation, or identified with one side while simultaneously enacting the other.
- Finally, the therapist invites the patient to attend to the dissociated quality of his experience across separate, idealized, and persecutory object relations and across time.

Each of these strategies calls on the patient to step out of his immediate affective experience—first, to become aware of the rigid, repetitive, and predictable nature of his experience (Strategy 2a); next, to see contradictions between his current experience and his current behavior (Strategy 2b); and finally, to note contradictions between his current dominant experience and experiences he has had at other times (Strategy 2c).[1]

> Over the next sessions, Dr. C called Ms. M's attention to how Ms. M frequently found herself feeling bullied, controlled, and angry (Strategy 2a). Ms. M agreed; she described feeling controlled and bullied in virtually all her encounters with others, but especially with her mother and with Dr. C. Ms. M said, "Of course I'm enraged. Who wouldn't feel this way if constantly treated as I am?"
>
> Dr. C and Ms. M began to identify the different ways in which Ms. M felt controlled, as well as the powerful negative emotions that accompanied seeing herself in that position. In relation to Dr. C, issues of control were organized around ongoing struggles in relation to the treatment frame: the inconvenience of transportation to Dr. C's office, the imposition of twice-weekly sessions, the request that sessions begin and end on time, and even the expectation that Ms. M speak in session all left Ms. M feeling bullied, controlled, hostile, and rebellious, with Dr. C cast as rigid, controlling, and self-serving. Similar difficulties emerged repeatedly in Ms. M's interactions with her mother as well.

---

[1]The exception to this general sequence of addressing role reversals before addressing splitting emerges in treatment of some high-BPO patients. With patients who are able to maintain relatively stable, defensive idealizations while splitting off the paranoid sector, the therapist begins by addressing splitting (Strategy 2c) before role reversals (Strategy 2b). For these patients, focusing on idealization will ultimately bring to light underlying paranoid object relations, along with identifiable role reversals. As a general rule, when both role reversals and splitting are in evidence, the therapist addresses role reversals first.

2a: Calling Attention to the Repetitive Nature of the Patient's Experience and Behavior as a Single Object Relation Predictably Organizes the Clinical Material Under the Impact of Splitting-Based Defenses

This process promotes self-observation and reflection.

Ms. M walked into a session 15 minutes late, ranting angrily about how she despised her mother. She went on to describe what she perceived as her mother's cruelty to her cat, whom her mother typically locked out of the living room before leaving for work; her mother didn't care about the cat, only about her own convenience. When Dr. C began to speak, Ms. M sat forward in her chair and glared at Dr. C in a threatening fashion, opening and closing her fists. Dr. C contained her own anxiety. She then shared with Ms. M that she had a thought and wondered if Ms. M would like her to share it. Ms. M considered and then acknowledged that she did.

Dr. C went on to say, "You know, this experience you describe of watching your mother control the cat, and her selfishly caring only about her living room and nothing about the cat's comfort, reminds me of how *you* feel in relation to your mother's insistence that you come to therapy when you don't want to, and when it's so difficult for you to be here" (Strategy 2a).

Ms. M did not acknowledge Dr. C's comment but instead complained about the traffic when coming to the office and the imposition of twice-weekly sessions. At this point, Dr. C went back to this pattern in the transference, commenting, "Your current complaints make me wonder if you're not having the same experience here with me now that you describe with your mother. This is a pattern we've observed many times between us; I seem controlling and selfish, and you are left feeling bullied and controlled" (Strategy 2a).

2b: Focusing on Role Reversals

This process introduces alternative perspectives, promoting reflection and self-awareness by focusing on the impact of projective identification on the patient's subjective experience and behavior.

In response to Dr. C's comment, Ms. M seemed calmer, more contained, and somewhat reflective. Dr. C felt that Ms. M might be at that moment in a frame of mind to be able to broaden her view to take into account her own behavior and her dissociated identification with the controlling bully that she had so frequently associated with Dr. C. At this point, Dr. C decided to attempt to call Ms. M's attention to the role reversal enacted in the clinical process. Accordingly, Dr. C said that while she understood

Ms. M's feeling of being controlled and bullied, she also wondered whether Ms. M could see the ways in which Ms. M herself was at times behaving in a controlling or bullying fashion in relation to Dr. C—for example, by cutting off Dr. C when she attempted to say something, or by sitting forward in her chair and glaring at Dr. C while opening and closing her fists. "At the same time that you feel I control you, you also are controlling me; and at the same time that you experience me as bullying you, in the same way, you can bully me" (Strategy 2c).

Over the ensuing months, Dr. C worked with Ms. M to identify the repetitive enactment of core dominant object relations in the transference, inviting Ms. M to join with her in noticing the impact of role reversals on the clinical process.

2c: Focusing on Dissociation of Idealized and Persecutory Object Relations

This process promotes reflection on internal states by highlighting the impact of splitting on the patient's subjective experience and behavior while inviting the patient to contextualize idealized and paranoid experiences across time.

Despite ongoing difficulty with the frame and intermittently stormy sessions characterized by Ms. M's hostile accusations and paranoia, Ms. M did stick with the treatment and started to make gains. Overall, she was less aggressive in sessions, and role reversals were less confusing and disruptive to the clinical process. She found steady employment, and things seemed to be less rocky at home. At the same time, she rarely let on that she was doing better and continued to complain (albeit not entirely enthusiastically) about Dr. C. Nevertheless, Ms. M would at times very tentatively acknowledge a positive view of the treatment or of her circumstances outside the treatment. She would then quickly return to her usual hostile, paranoid stance. These developments enabled Dr. C not only to articulate the familiar paranoid object relations that predictably organized the clinical process, but also to capture more hidden, idealized views of the relationship, in which Ms. M anticipated that Dr. C would solve all Ms. M's problems.

Having described and examined with Ms. M both the paranoid and newly evident idealized view of their relationship, Dr. C began to invite Ms. M to bridge contradictory and dissociated views of the relationship activated across time. For example, in a session 6 months into the treatment, in response to a return of Ms. M's paranoid agitation, Dr. C commented, "You feel angry and afraid that I am trying to control you and have no interest in helping you. This is different from what you were saying in our last session, when you acknowledged that you are doing better and that the treatment may have something to do with that" (Strategy 2c). Dr. C could see that Ms. M was listening and that she had experienced this intervention as a "bid for reflection."[2] Sensing curiosity on Ms. M's part in relation to the contradictions to which Dr. C had called her attention, Dr. C proceeded to move on to Strategy 3—that is, to offer a possible explanation of why Ms. M might shift between dissociated, persecutory, and idealized views of the relationship while focusing preferentially on the negative.

Comments: Over time, the TFP-E therapist helps the patient become familiar with the dominant object relations as they are enacted repeatedly and predictably, both in the transference and in the patient's relations with others (Strategy 2a). In calling attention to how a single dominant object relation repetitively organizes the patient's experience in different settings, the therapist is prompting the patient to observe his experience. This capacity is the first step in helping the patient create a psychological space for exploration, a space for "looking at," rather than simply "being in," a given moment or affective experience. Articulating these patterns and supporting the patient's capacity to observe his own experience in an area of conflict and in the setting of affect activation prepares the patient for addressing the impact of splitting-based defenses on his experience.

The therapist begins with projective identification, calling the patient's attention to role reversals (Strategy 2b). In addressing role reversals, the therapist first describes the dominant object relation from the patient's perspective (Ms. M feeling bullied by Dr. C), which the patient is consciously identified with and which he is attributing to the therapist or to an external object at the moment; once the patient has a clear view of this configuration, the therapist will tactfully call attention to the same object relation as it is enacted, but with roles reversed (Ms. M bullying Dr. C). This entails pointing out to the patient that at the same time that he is experiencing the therapist as abusive, for example, he is in fact behaving abusively toward the therapist. Alternatively, the therapist might point out one configuration early in a session, and then later in the session might point out to the patient that now the situation has become reversed, with the patient at this point in the role of abuser, formerly attributed to the therapist.

In contrast to Strategy 1, which approaches the clinical material entirely from the perspective of the patient, calling attention to role reversals (Strategy 2b) is a far more ambitious intervention. The therapist is inviting the patient to broaden his perspective to include aspects of experience that

---

[2]When a BPO patient is in a receptive frame of mind, interventions of this kind, classically described as *confrontations of defense*, can encourage the patient to step back to observe and reflect on her own internal experience.

are conflictual, expressed in behavior but defensively dissociated from his dominant experience. Focusing on role reversals invites the patient to entertain alternative perspectives ("You see me as bullying you, but if you step back and observe your behavior, can you see that you appear to be bullying me?"), while promoting self-observation and self-awareness in an area of conflict. To the degree that TFP-E supports these capacities in the BPO patient, the therapist is helping the patient move past a concrete, lost-in-the-moment experience, implicitly inviting him to step back, observe, and reflect.[3]

As clinical attention is focused on role reversals, associated affects tend to become better contained and less unstable. At the same time, working with role reversals calls on the patient to take at least partial responsibility for his aggression, rather than resorting entirely to projection and dissociation; attention to role reversals brings to the patient's awareness that he is inhabiting a largely paranoid universe, that it is not that the patient is "good," an innocent victim of a victimizing therapist, but rather that therapist and patient are both "bad," each both a victimizer and a hostile victim. This awareness on the part of the patient, of the split quality of his experience, creates a context for the next strategy of treatment, addressing splitting proper (Strategy 2c).

When the therapist moves on to address splitting, she focuses on shifts between idealized and persecutory object relations, mutually dissociated and enacted at different times in the session or across sessions. In this process, the therapist calls attention to the unstable and contradictory nature of the patient's experience across time, implicitly inviting him to cognitively "bridge the split" and to juxtapose differing, contradictory object relations that have been defensively dissociated from one another.

Making these links helps the patient begin to contextualize his current experience in relation to experiences he has had at other times. In this process, the patient develops a deeper appreciation of the degree to which neither side of the split is "real," but rather that both represent defensively distorted perspectives of his experience, aspects of his internal world rather than external reality. At the same time, the patient's developing awareness of the instability and potential distortions that characterize his

---

[3]This treatment goal of assisting the patient in observing and reflecting on repetitive interpersonal conflicts is similar to other treatment approaches, such as the goal of increasing mentalization in mentalization-based therapy (Bateman and Fonagy 2006) and the resolution of therapeutic ruptures (Safran and Muran 2000).

subjectivity help him shift from a singular focus on external events and material reality to exploration of his internal experience, and to a fuller appreciation of the extent to which his experience is subjective. (This is to say that after a time, the patient begins to appreciate that the gross inconsistencies he attributes to the therapist and to others in his life likely have something to do with his own internal experience.)

In sum, TFP-E Strategies 1 and 2 play a central and pivotal role in the treatment of BPO patients, particularly in the first half of the treatment. These strategies are responsible for the development of self-awareness and core psychological capacities, first for self-observation and affect containment, and next for reflection and entertaining alternative perspectives in the setting of psychological conflict. These capacities are the building blocks of identity consolidation, as the patient begins to contextualize his experience in the moment in relation to contradictory experiences he has had at other times.

Strategy 3: Exploring the Anxieties and Conflicts Motivating Splitting and Organizing the Dominant Object Relations, and Introducing Hypotheses About Underlying Wishes and Fears

This process promotes the capacity to tolerate awareness of anxieties driving the mutual dissociation of idealized and paranoid object relations, introducing greater flexibility into defensive functioning; this process also broadens the patient's perspective to appreciate the constructed, symbolic nature of subjectivity and, ultimately, the impact of psychological conflicts on his experience and behavior.

The impact of TFP-E Strategy 2 is that the patient has a developing awareness that the experiences he is exploring in treatment are reflections of his *internal* life, that his subjective experience is distinct from external reality—that is, the patient's perspective becomes less concrete and more flexible. This perspective is typically fleeting at first, but becomes more stable over time with ongoing clinical attention to role reversals and splitting. At those times that the BPO patient *does* have an awareness of the internal and subjective nature of his experience, the therapist can capitalize on moments of reflectiveness to initiate exploration of the anxieties and conflicts embedded in the dominant object relations. Here the therapist builds on earlier interventions, now focusing attention on the mutual dissociation of idealized and paranoid object relations to highlight how these defend against one another and to explore the anxieties motivating splitting.

> Dr. C sensed curiosity on Ms. M's part in relation to her previous intervention (Strategy 2c), in which Dr. C had called Ms. M's attention to the contradiction between her current and familiar, paranoid view of her relationship with Dr. C and the idealized version Ms. M had communicated in the previous session. With Ms. M seemingly attending closely, Dr. C proceeded to offer a possible explanation of why Ms. M might shift between dissociated, contradictory views of the relationship while focusing preferentially on the negative (Strategy 3).
>
> Dr. C suggested, "Perhaps you prefer to focus again on the negative relation between us because to do so feels familiar and safe. Experiencing the positive relation may feel good for a moment, but doing so is risky; the negative emotions are so overwhelming that all the good feelings could at any moment easily disappear. If you stick with the negative and keep the positive under wraps, it protects the good feelings in a secret place."

Comments: In Strategy 3, the therapist works with the patient to consider what might move him to organize his internal experience as he does. Building on earlier interventions, the therapist draws a relationship between idealized and persecutory object relations that have already been elaborated, now pointing out how each defends against the other and exploring anxieties motivating their mutual dissociation. Interventions of this kind provide support for the BPO patient's capacity to simultaneously hold in mind idealized and paranoid object relations while better containing anxieties motivating splitting.

At the same time, the interventions that make up the third strategy of TFP-E also have an explanatory quality, in that they offer possible explanations for what might motivate the patient to rely on splitting and to organize his experience as he does. Explanatory interventions of this kind focus on expanding not only self-awareness, as do earlier interventions, but also self-understanding. Interventions of this kind, introduced in the form of hypotheses about meanings and motivations driving defense, correspond with classical psychoanalytic conceptualizations of interpretation. (We discuss interpretation in detail in Chapter 10.) In the treatment of BPO patients, especially those in the low and middle range, interventions of this kind may not become effective until the more advanced phases of treatment, after the patient has benefited from more basic and concrete interventions (see Chapter 13 for discussion of treatment phases).

There is always a risk that the BPO patient will misinterpret and not understand explanatory interventions. The patient may interpret the therapist's intervention concretely and hear the therapist as saying, "Of course, you have to hide positive feelings or they will be destroyed." Alternatively, the patient may simply experience the therapist's communications as empty words.

Strategy 4: Working Through Identified Conflicts

4a: Working Through Identified Conflicts and Associated Anxieties as They Are Enacted in Different Contexts Across Time While Making Links to the Treatment Goals and the Patient's Interpersonal Relationships

This process enables the patient to contain anxieties associated with the expression of aggression and to relinquish splitting-based defenses, promoting integration of idealized and persecutory internal object relations and leading to a gradual process of identity consolidation while improving interpersonal functioning.

As part of the process of working through (Strategy 4a), during the middle phase of Ms. M's treatment, Dr. C made use several times of the strategies we have described. Working through allowed an exploration of the anxieties motivating Ms. M's use of splitting-based defenses and ultimately came to focus on Ms. M's fears of allowing Dr. C to be powerful: If the idealized version of Dr. C could help Ms. M, then Dr. C became very powerful. If Dr. C was powerful, then she was also dangerous; after all, she could at any moment turn on Ms. M and exploit or humiliate her, or she could decide to interrupt the treatment or to raise her fee to a rate Ms. M could not afford.

In subsequent interventions, Dr. C also suggested that just as Ms. M experienced her as an external enemy, she likewise struggled with an internal enemy: a powerful, controlling tyrant within that wanted to destroy the possibility of her making gains in life. Exploration of various anxieties underlying Ms. M's need to destroy her own possibilities included fear of attack from an envious, cruel, and aggressive parental figure and fear of her own intolerable disappointment and humiliation were she to allow herself to be duped into feeling falsely hopeful. Ultimately, the fear of losing a deeply held hope of attaining perfect love and care from a parental figure and the wish to hold on to the possibility of attaining such love and security from Dr. C were seen as motivations for maintaining a split view of the relationship.

As these anxieties were identified and explored, they became less concrete and less credible to Ms. M; they came to feel like fears and fantasies rather than actual dangers. In this setting, early depressive anxieties began to emerge, side by side with more familiar paranoid concerns. These anxieties revolved around Ms. M's sense that she was not deserving of Dr. C's help or of her mother's consideration, that she had been aggressive and had enjoyed bullying and frightening them and as a result did not deserve fair treatment from them.

In the later phases of treatment, Ms. M began to associate to early experiences with her father before he left the family, recalling that he would bully and frighten her, pulling out his belt and threatening to beat her if he thought she had not done as he asked. She reflected on how she had hated and feared him, and how as an adolescent she had been aware of her connection to him as she bullied her mother after her father left the family (Strategy 4b). Triangular and oedipal conflicts also emerged in later phases of treatment in terms of guilty wishes to triumph over and humiliate a highly successful younger brother whom their father manifestly preferred over the patient.

Toward the end of treatment, after Ms. M had begun working full-time and reconnecting with some of her high school friends, exercising at a gym, and helping out at home, she looked back on her earlier behavior, commenting on how angry and frightened she had been when she began therapy, and how challenging her behavior must have seemed. She commented that it had taken her a long time to be able to forgive herself. "I used to hate myself.... I used to hate everybody," she said, and she wondered how Dr. C had managed to put up with her. "A lot of other therapists would have run for the hills. But I can see now that somehow you always believed in the therapy, maybe even saw something in me...that I could do better. I no longer need you to be perfect. But you're okay. I guess I am, too."

Comments: The final strategy of TFP-E is to work through the conflicts elaborated in Strategy 3. With BPO patients, working through focuses on repeated identification, exploration, and interpretation of the anxieties, wishes, and fears associated with activation of splitting-based defenses and the mutual dissociation of idealized and paranoid object relations. Anxieties and defenses are explored from a variety of perspectives and in a variety of contexts, while at the same time the patient practices new ways of behaving, thinking, and feeling, both in the treatment and in daily life.

In the treatment of BPO patients, the process of working through begins with exploration of the paranoid anxieties motivating splitting; ultimately, depressive anxieties motivating splitting-based defenses are explored as well. As a result of working through the conflicts driving splitting-based defenses, the patient develops a greater capacity to contain the paranoid and depressive anxieties motivating defense; at those moments when anxieties are better contained, splitting becomes less extreme and rigid, leading to further containment of anxiety followed by further reduction in splitting. These dynamic shifts create a virtual cycle in which containment of anxiety promotes a (temporary) shift toward integration, and enhanced integration in the moment helps to temper aggression and reduces affective intensity, reducing the extremity of splitting and further promoting integration.

Over time, the process of working through leads to the gradual integration of persecutory and idealized internal object relations, with more realistic object relations and transferences being formed that are typical of patients organized at a neurotic level. As paranoid and depressive anxieties are worked through and object relations become progressively better integrated, links between the material explored in the session and the patient's developmental history tend to spontaneously emerge and can be fruitfully included in the exploratory and interpretive process. In the process of working through, the therapist focuses on the ways in which core conflicts relate to the treatment goals and to the difficulties that brought the patient to treatment, and on how changes in the patient translate into corresponding changes in his interpersonal relationships with important people in his life.

The successful integration of mutually dissociated idealized and persecutory internal object relations results in integration not only of corresponding self and object representations, but also of associated affect states. In this process, the patient develops a more complex and realistic experience of himself and others, and his emotional experience deepens as he relinquishes splitting-based defenses and as idealized and paranoid object relations coalesce. The patient's experience becomes better contextualized; he develops a core sense of self, corresponding with identity consolidation.

How does the therapist integrate material from the past into the treatment of the BPO patient?

When and how to make links between the BPO patient's current experience and difficulties and his developmental history is often a point of confusion. In TFP-E, it is only after the patient has attained some degree of identity consolidation that hypotheses of this kind should be introduced. Thus, although considered part of the fourth strategy of TFP-E with BPO patients, this strategy is typically not used until the later phases of treatment, as illustrated in the discussion of Strategy 4b.

4b: Linking Identified Conflicts to the Patient's Developmental History

This process deepens the patient's level of self-understanding while further promoting containment of anxieties motivating defense, supporting contextualization of experience across time and the process of identity consolidation.

In TFP-E, the focus is on object relations organizing the patient's experience in the here and now of the treatment setting, as enacted in the relationship with the therapist and in relationships with people in the patient's current life. As the therapist helps the patient elaborate the internal representations that emerge in the transference, her understanding of the patient's developmental history can inform her understanding of the patient's current experience. However, there are several important caveats here. Most important, the object relations that emerge in the transference and in the interpersonal relations of BPO patients are by definition contradictory, partial, and distorted representations of important figures from the patient's early life, as the patient's memories and accounts of his early history are similarly unreliable representations of actual events and people; although current representations may reflect aspects of early experience, they are organized through the lens of the patient's past and current wishes, fears, fantasies, and, of course, defenses.

With this in mind, when describing the transference, the therapist attempts to make reference not to actual past relationships but rather to prototypes, even when the transference seems to recapitulate the patient's relationship with a parent or sibling. For example, Dr. C would not say to Ms. M, "It is as if I am like your mother, who seems to care nothing for your feelings and controls you to meet her own needs." Instead, Dr. C would say, "It is as if I am a mother who cares nothing for your feelings and controls you to meet her own needs," appreciating that Ms. M will have many different and contradictory views of her mother, and of mothers in general, over the course of the treatment.

In later phases of treatment, as the BPO patient's experience becomes better integrated and more continuous across time, the therapist will notice that associations to and memories of early experiences and relationships with family members begin to emerge spontaneously and credibly in the patient's verbal communications. At this point, in the process of working through, making links between current conflicts and reconstructions of the patient's past can deepen the patient's sense of self-coherence as well as self-understanding and can promote further integrative processes as current experience is contextualized within a personal narrative.

For example, in the case of Ms. M, it was only in the later phases of treatment that the patient mentioned her early memories of and identifications with her father. By this time, Ms. M's identification with an abusive bully had been largely worked through in the transference, without the benefit of this historical reconstruction and, if anything, in the context of focusing on Ms. M's current struggles with her mother. However, introducing Ms. M's early experience with her father in the later phases of treatment shed light on how she came to be the person she was when she began treatment, and also deepened her forgiveness and appreciation of her mother, as well as ultimately of herself.

Patients Along the Neurotic Spectrum of Personality Organization

The overall psychotherapeutic strategy for the treatment of patients organized at a neurotic level can be conceptualized in terms of the four overall sequential tasks outlined at the beginning of this chapter, but with each task tailored to address the specific clinical challenges presented by the NPO patient, focusing on the impact of repression-based defenses on the patient's experience and behavior. The attentive reader will notice that for the most part, the overall strategies of treatment for NPO patients as described below are essentially the same as those outlined in the previous section on the treatment of BPO patients. Differences lie in the relative centrality of each of the strategies in the clinical process, as well as (to some extent) the functions that they serve.

Overall, in the treatment of NPO patients, there is much greater emphasis on the later strategies of treatment, Strategies 3 and 4, which can be effectively employed relatively early, whereas in the treatment of BPO patients, Strategies 1 and 2 play a more central role. These differences reflect the stability of repression-based defenses, coupled with the NPO patient's relatively well-developed capacities—conferred by identity consolidation—for self-observation, reflection, and consideration of alternative perspectives. As in the treatment of BPO patients, treatment strategies for NPO patients function to gradually broaden the patient's level of self-awareness and deepen his self-understanding. Table 6–3 outlines the strategies of TFP-E for NPO patients.

TABLE 6–3. Strategies of transference-focused psychotherapy—extended and their functions, modified for neurotic level of personality organization

Strategy 1. Defining the dominant object relations

    1a. Identifying the dominant object relations

        Function: Narrows the clinical focus to defensive object relations and an area of conflict

    1b. Describing the dominant object relations in words

        Function: Focuses exploration on the patient's internal experience in an area of conflict

Strategy 2. Calling attention to the repetitive, rigid, and/or contradictory nature of the patient's experience and behavior

    2a. Calling attention to the repetitive nature of the patient's experience and behavior as repetitive enactment of defensive object relations predictably organizes the clinical material

        Function: Promotes ego-dystonicity of defenses and promotes reflection in an area of conflict

    2b. Calling attention to inconsistencies, omissions, and systematic distortions in the patient's experience of self and other, reflecting the impact of repression-based defenses on the patient's subjective experience and behavior

        Function: Introduces alternative perspectives and reduces defensive rigidity while promoting reflection in an area of conflict

Strategy 3. Exploring the anxieties motivating repression and organizing the dominant object relations, and introducing hypotheses about underlying wishes, fears, and personal meanings

        Function: Supports the capacity to tolerate awareness of anxieties driving activation of defensive object relations by introducing hypotheses about underlying motivations and personal meanings; interpretation introduces greater flexibility into defensive functioning by supporting appreciation of the constructed and symbolic nature of subjective experience in an area of conflict

Strategy 4. Working through identified conflicts as they are activated in different contexts across time while making links to the treatment goals and the patient's developmental history

        Function: Enables the patient to tolerate awareness of anxieties associated with expression of conflictual motivations, to experience these anxieties as symbolic, and ultimately to contain conflictual motivations within dominant self experience; these integrative changes correspond with the patient's relinquishment of repression-based defenses in an area of conflict and with decreased personality rigidity

Clinical Illustration of Treatment Strategies in the Setting of NPO

Ms. S was 50 years old, married, and the mother of two successful adult children when she presented with problems of self-esteem, inability to assert herself, and social isolation. Though objectively extremely intelligent and quite engaging, she saw herself as inferior and unattractive, someone who had nothing of interest to offer. Socially isolated outside of her relationships with her husband and adult children, she seemed not to notice when others expressed interest in her ideas or in her as a person. Married right out of college, she had forfeited all professional and intellectual aspirations, and had devoted her adult life to raising children and supporting her husband's career. In recent years, she had taken on a series of volunteer positions.

Ms. S's manner was self-effacing but appealing, and in her interactions with Dr. C she was excessively accommodating and subtly submissive. After seeing the patient in consultation, Dr. C made the diagnosis of depressive personality disorder with dependent and hysterical features, organized at a neurotic level. Her STIPO-R profile was characterized by mild but global impairment across all STIPO-R domains.

Strategy 1: Defining the Dominant Object Relations

1a: Identifying the Dominant Object Relations

This process narrows the clinical focus to defensive object relations and an area of conflict.

Ms. S eagerly agreed to begin twice-weekly treatment and had no difficulty complying with the treatment frame and with the request that she speak openly and freely in session. In the early sessions, she spoke at great length about her current position as a volunteer research assistant to Dr. R, a highly regarded female scholar at a local university. Recently, Ms. S had begun to develop her own scholarly interests and to feel a glimmer of hope for herself in this setting. This, it seemed, had given her both courage and motivation to seek treatment for the first time in her life.

As Ms. S spoke about her experiences with Dr. R, it appeared to Dr. C that Dr. R both depreciated and took advantage of Ms. S, asking her to work long hours on a whim or to run personal errands, while excluding Ms. S from meetings in which her contributions to Dr. R's research were being discussed. When Dr. C inquired about whether Ms. S felt taken advantage of, Ms. S explained that she had lived her life "in the service of others"—in particular, her (now quite elderly) mother, her husband, and now Dr. R. All were people whom she viewed as vastly superior to herself.

Listening to Ms. S's descriptions of herself, as well as of her interactions with her husband and mother, and reflecting as well on Ms. S's attitude toward Dr. C herself, Dr. C developed an image in her mind of the dominant object relations (Strategy 1a). It seemed to Dr. C that the dyad dominating the clinical material was one of an inferior, inconsequential girl in relation to a superior maternal figure who was powerful, effective, and admired, reflecting feelings of inadequacy and wishes to please. This dyad colored Ms. S's self experience; her relationships with Dr. R, her husband, and her mother; her casual interactions with others; and her covert expectations of the therapist. Painful as it was, the patient's view of herself was *ego-syntonic*.

Habitual enactment of this dyad functioned as a character defense, organizing Ms. S's experience of herself in the world and her behavior in relation to others in all settings, leaving her meek, submissive, and easily pushed around; she seemed to never prioritize her own needs. At the same time, Dr. C sensed the object relations underlying this defensive dyad: a more autonomous and ambitious self in conflict with an exploitative and self-serving maternal figure, colored by feelings of self-assertion and resentment. Dr. C's hypothesis was that Ms. S's newfound scholarly interests and secret aspirations, perhaps in conjunction with her mother's progressive infirmity, had begun to shake what had been a long-standing, stable character defense. Her secret wishes to pursue long-suppressed professional aspirations were generating anxiety and were also bringing her to treatment. In relation to Dr. C, Ms. S was admiring, submissive, and girlish, although she also worked hard to understand herself in and between her sessions.

1b: Describing the Dominant Object Relations in Words

This process focuses exploration on the patient's internal experience in an area of conflict.

Dr. C listened to Ms. S's verbal communications and associations while paying attention to her behavior in session and to the countertransference. Ms. S began a session by apologetically explaining her need to cancel an appointment a few weeks hence; she explained that she was going on a business trip with her husband. Ms. S made no additional mention of her feelings about going. When Dr. C asked about Ms. S's attitude toward the trip, Ms. S explained that it required her to cancel other plans she had made, but it was "not a big deal." Her husband liked to have her travel with him when he was going to important meetings.

Ms. S then went on to speak about a new situation at the university: She was trying to find a place at the university to store her own papers but was finding this difficult. Dr. R had ignored—indeed, seemed not to register—Ms. S's subtle requests for help. Ms. S shared this anecdote in a matter-of-fact manner. She explained that Dr. R was working on an important deadline and had no time or attention for anything else.

Dr. C commented (Strategy 1b) that she was hearing a familiar and repeated pattern in Ms. S's description of her interactions with both her husband and her boss: "With both, it's as if you experience yourself as an inferior, inadequate girl in relation to a superior and powerful maternal figure on whom you are dependent. It's as if only their needs matter; yours are irrelevant."

Comments: In work with NPO patients, the TFP-E therapist's first objective is to identify the object relations organizing the patient's experience in session. What emerges are stable, ego-syntonic, relatively realistic views of self and others that appear and reappear throughout the clinical material. These object relations serve defensive functions, supporting repression of more conflictual object relations. In contrast to the setting with BPO patients, the NPO patient's verbal communications and associations tend to be the most useful indicators of the affectively charged object relations, supplemented by the patient's nonverbal communication and the countertransference. Also in contrast to the treatment of BPO patients, in the setting of neurotic pathology, early sessions are typically neither highly affectively charged nor confusing, and dominant object relations are not necessarily enacted in the transference.

The therapist listens for relationship patterns that tend to recur in the patient's descriptions of his interactions with others or in his descriptions of his internal experience. Often, these relationship patterns may be subtly mirrored in his interactions with the therapist, as they were in Ms. S's apologetic attitude toward Dr. C in relation to canceling a session. However, even when the therapist can identify the affectively dominant object relations enacted in the transference, these object relations are often less accessible to the patient in the transference than they are in other contexts and relationships. Once the therapist identifies the dominant object relations in his own mind, he will work with the patient to develop a description of that relational pattern. In contrast to the confusion of identifications introduced by role reversals in the treatment of BPO patients, the NPO patient will be stably identified with one side of the dominant object relationship, often putting himself in a childlike position.

As in treatment of BPO patients, the first strategy of treatment of NPO patients is to organize and put words to the patient's experience while communicating empathy. From the perspective of clinical process, identifying and then putting words to the dominant object relations focuses first the therapist's attention and then the patient's on an area of conflict, and on the patient's experience in that context. In work with an NPO patient, observing and describing dominant object relations calls on and supports capacities of self-observation and reflection that may be subtly compromised in the setting of conflict and defense, although these capacities are typically well developed and relatively stable in the NPO patient. Further, because the dominant object relations by definition serve defensive functions, focusing on the dominant object relations initiates a process of exploring the NPO patient's defenses.

Strategy 2: Calling Attention to the Repetitive, Rigid, and/or Contradictory Nature of the Patient's Experience and Behavior

The second strategy of treatment involves calling the patient's attention to the impact of enactment of defensive object relations on the patient's experience and behavior. The therapist will focus on rigidity, inconsistencies, and subtle but often systematic distortions introduced by repression-based defenses. In concert, Strategies 2a and 2b represent a process of "defense analysis" in the treatment of NPO patients. The ultimate outcome of the second strategy of TFP-E with NPO patients is that defenses gradually become ego-dystonic.

2a: Calling Attention to the Repetitive Nature of the Patient's Experience and Behavior as Repetitive Enactment of Defensive Object Relations Predictably Organizes the Clinical Material

This process promotes ego-dystonicity of defenses and promotes reflection in an area of conflict.

> Upon hearing Dr. C's description of the object relation organizing the clinical material (Strategy 1b)—that is, of Ms. S experiencing herself as an inferior, inadequate girl whose needs were irrelevant, living "in service" to a superior, powerful maternal figure—Ms. S immediately agreed, commenting that this was how she felt in most situations, and of course this was entirely warranted by her painful inferiority and inadequacy. From her perspective, there was nothing to notice or for Dr. C to comment on—the devalued view of herself that organized Ms. S's experience was entirely ego-syntonic. Dr. C responded that she was struck by how this pattern organized so many of Ms. S's relationships, and how rigid and fixed it seemed to be.

Dr. C worked with Ms. S to more specifically articulate the views of herself and others embedded in her notion of living "in service," and together they identified how Ms. S organized all her experiences according to this model—not only with her boss, her husband, and her mother, but also with her children, shopkeepers with whom she dealt, and even her housekeeper. Ms. S was an active and curious participant in a dialogue within which Dr. C highlighted both the rigidity and ubiquity of these patterns, along with how inappropriate they seemed in certain settings (Strategy 2a). For example, in one session, Ms. S blandly described organizing her daily schedule to accommodate her housekeeper, because the housekeeper juggled other jobs and personal commitments. Dr. C wondered out loud, "Who is working for whom?"

2b: Calling Attention to Inconsistencies, Omissions, and Systematic Distortions in the Patient's Experience of Self and Other, Reflecting the Impact of Repression-Based Defenses on the Patient's Subjective Experience and Behavior

This process introduces alternative perspectives and reduces defensive rigidity while promoting reflection in an area of conflict.

In another session, Ms. S arrived not only a few minutes late, but also dripping wet, explaining that Dr. R had asked her to serve as a courier to transport documents to another institution in the pouring rain. When Dr. C inquired whether there might have been other ways that she and Dr. R could have arranged for the documents to be transported, Ms. S responded that it hadn't crossed her mind to consider other options.

Dr. C responded, "It may well be that in the end there were no alternative solutions, but I am struck by how it did not even occur to you to consider if there were. As is your way, you automatically assumed that the obvious and perhaps only solution was that you be 'in service.'" As Dr. C listened to Ms. S speak about her day-to-day experiences and concerns, she called Ms. S's attention to the distortions resulting from her tightly held view of herself in the world: the extreme and profound devaluation of herself and of the value of her contributions, the minimization of her own needs, and the unquestioning elevation of the other embedded in this pattern (Strategy 2b; see also Comments below).

Comments: Focusing on the NPO patient's verbal communications, often mirrored in the transference-countertransference, the therapist helps the patient become aware of the repetitive and rigid nature of his experience in areas of conflict, as defensive object relations are repeatedly enacted. The therapist will also begin to call attention to subtle distortions and omissions introduced by the patient's need to sustain defensive views of self and others. These interventions introduce alternative perspectives—inviting the patient to step outside his customary, habitual, and defensive views of self and other—and lead the patient to become more reflective and curious about his experience in areas of conflict. The patient begins to call into question defensive views of self and others that he has for the most part accepted as "the way it is." For example, Ms. S began at times to wonder whether her view of herself was perhaps excessively self-denigrating rather than simply realistic, and she considered the possibility that there might be something a little off in her habitual and unreflective willingness to inconvenience herself to accommodate her housekeeper, or even perhaps Dr. R.

Overall, the impact of the interventions included in Strategy 2 with NPO patients is that defensive object relations become ego-dystonic; the patient is now aware of and curious, as he was not in the past, about the impact of his defenses on his subjectivity. This development represents a questioning of long-held, but subtly concretized and distorted, defensive views of self and others—and opens up the possibility of views of self and others in an area of conflict that are more complex and take into account more fully the constructed nature of subjectivity. To state it simply, Ms. S ultimately came to consider, "Maybe I am not entirely inconsequential; maybe I just think or feel I am." This shift represents a weakening of repressive defenses. As defenses become less effective, anxieties motivating defense become accessible, and underlying conflictual motivations are less stably repressed. In Strategy 3, the therapist's task is to help the patient tolerate awareness of these previously repressed aspects of his experience.

Strategy 3: Exploring the Anxieties Motivating Repression and Organizing the Dominant Object Relations, and Introducing Hypotheses About Underlying Wishes, Fears, and Personal Meanings

This process supports the capacity to tolerate awareness of anxieties driving activation of defensive object relations by introducing hypotheses about underlying motivations and personal meanings; interpretation in-

troduces greater flexibility into defensive functioning by supporting ap-
preciation of the constructed and symbolic nature of subjective experience
in an area of conflict.

As Dr. C continued to call Ms. S's attention to enactment of now-familiar defensive object relations, she began to notice a subtle shift in Ms. S's communications in session. What then became evident for the first time in therapy was the extent to which Ms. S denied that she indeed had her own quite well-developed and sophisticated intellectual interests. The extent to which Ms. S denied the positive attention that she received at work also became gradually more apparent; it seemed that others at the university library had noticed her talents, although Dr. R monopolized Ms. S's time with busywork and treated her dismissively.

Dr. C was aware that Ms. S's defenses were weakening, and other aspects of her behavior and aspirations were beginning to emerge in the treatment, despite her habit of hiding her assets and internally denying her successes. With the ongoing focus on Ms. S's out-of-session behavior and her tendency to minimize her successes and assets in session, Ms. S started at moments to be able to recognize and acknowledge, for a moment, an accomplishment or success. However, at these times, as soon as she became cognizant of feeling good about herself, she would immediately feel frightened and anxious, typically finding herself afraid of being in some way attacked—imagining a police officer yelling at her, or anticipating criticism from her boss, or worrying that perhaps Dr. C would not approve; shortly thereafter, Ms. S would find herself feeling even more inferior and inadequate than usual.

Dr. C began to call attention to the way in which Ms. S would vaguely allude in passing to a recent success (e.g., someone had commented on an essay she had written; someone else had sought her opinion about putting together a conference) and then quickly move on. Dr. C encouraged Ms. S to explore the anxieties and conflicts behind this behavior (Strategy 3). For example, Dr. C pointed out it was as if Ms. S *needed* to keep herself small, in her own eyes and in the eyes of Dr. C.

Ms. S responded that she was starting to have a different view of Dr. R, who now seemed in Ms. S's eyes less benign and more self-serving. Ms. S began to be more aware of and forthcoming about the ways in which Dr. R mistreated her and took advantage of her; at the same time, Ms. S persisted in feeling that she deserved to be treated badly and she continued to try to please Dr. R. Even so, Ms. S began tentatively to express criticism of Dr. R's treatment of her and at times demonstrated hints of resentment. As these feelings and the object relations embedded in them were explored, Dr. C and Ms. S were able to identify an object relation of a competitive, exploitative figure who grabs power and attention, in relation to someone who is weak, exploited, and resentful. To herself, Dr. C noted that this development represented the emergence of an underlying impulsive object relation, formerly repressed, corresponding perhaps more closely than the earlier defensive object relation with the reality of Dr. R, but more important, representing an expression of Ms. S's wishes to triumph and to gain attention, with the roles defensively reversed.

During this period, Ms. S published her first article, in a small journal run by the department at the university where she was a volunteer. She received positive feedback and was invited to give a lecture on her research in a graduate seminar. Ms. S reacted to the invitation with conviction that she would not be able to do it: she did not have the credentials or experience; this was a job for someone like Dr. R, not for her. As Dr. C pointed out to Ms. S that she had been invited on the basis of her article, and after all, the seminar instructor must feel that she had something to say, Ms. S became acutely anxious. She wondered aloud, "Perhaps I am a competitive exploiter? Maybe I want to show up Dr. R and make her feel small?"

This development led to exploration of Ms. S's anxieties about herself: If she is not inadequate, perhaps she wants to be the center of attention. Perhaps she is an exploiter, a user and a power-grabber, someone who wants only to succeed, to triumph over Dr. R, to triumph over her mother, defy her husband, and perhaps even defy Dr. C. These anxieties were linked to a deeply feared, formerly repressed object relation of a viciously competitive, exploitative self who wants to triumph over and diminish a despised and vulnerable maternal object. "Is this what I really am?" she asked. "If I no longer submit, is this what I become?"

Dr. C offered an explanatory hypothesis, a way to understand Ms. S's anxiety and self-effacement: "It sounds like, deep down, you believe that if you are not weak and submissive, you automatically become a monster. Perhaps you cling to the familiar view of being small, living in service, to protect yourself; at the moment when you begin to feel even the least bit competitive or to acknowledge even a small success, you immediately seem to see yourself as that feared monster, exploitative and cruel, taking advantage of those more vulnerable. It's as if in your mind there are only two, equally extreme ways that you can view yourself: either as entirely insignificant and submissive or powerful and cruel."

Comments: As the patient's defenses become less effective, anxieties motivating defense begin to emerge in the treatment, as underlying conflictual object relations and associated motivations become more accessible. (In our example, these anxieties were associated with Ms. S's wishes for autonomy, attention, and, ultimately, competitive triumph.) At this point, the therapist's task is to help the NPO patient explore his anxieties and elaborate underlying conflicts, with the objective of helping him tolerate awareness of repressed conflictual object relations. This process will involve identifying and exploring the functions of defensive object relations, linking their activation to the anxieties motivating defense and, ultimately, to underlying conflictual motivations. (This series of interventions corresponds with the interpretive process, discussed in detail in Chapter 10.) Often, the NPO patient is able to keep core conflicts largely outside the transference as they are collaboratively explored with the therapist, who is experienced as a relatively neutral and benign, helping presence.

Strategy 4: Working Through Identified Conflicts as They Are Activated in Different Contexts Across Time While Making Links to the Treatment Goals and the Patient's Developmental History

This process enables the patient to tolerate awareness of anxieties associated with expression of conflictual motivations, to experience these anxieties as symbolic, and ultimately to contain conflictual motivations within dominant self experience; these integrative changes correspond with the patient's relinquishment of repression-based defenses in an area of conflict and with decreased personality rigidity.

> Ms. S started to have more successes and to be more assertive, predictably stirring up anxiety at each step along the way, while providing ample opportunity in the therapy to work through the core conflicts that had been uncovered. With each success, Ms. S worried that she was exploitative, competitive, and rightfully hated by all; each time she put her own needs before her husband's, she wondered if she was cold and selfish, caring only for herself, staying with him only because he supported her financially. Dr. C repeatedly pointed out that in Ms. S's mind, it seemed she had only two choices—to be downtrodden and invisible or to be an exploitative, competitive user. Both choices left Ms. S filled with self-loathing; in her mind, there seemed to be no way to feel powerful without also feeling loathsome, and as a result it seemed she needed to see herself as powerless.
>
> In the process of exploring these anxieties, Dr. C and Ms. S made links to Ms. S's developmental history with a highly successful, competitive, but rather cold mother, and to the difficulties that had brought Ms. S to treatment. Dr. C and Ms. S repeatedly identified and explored Ms. S's depressive anxieties in relation to being powerful, competitive, or the center of attention ("I am a bad person, worse than those I despise." "Would I want to succeed at the cost of others? Would I enjoy that?" "Am I just like my mother?"), as well as her paranoid anxieties ("If I am successful, Dr. R will destroy me; the university will see me as an interloper and cast me out"; "My mother would have hated me"; "Would you still want to be my doctor?"). Over time, Ms. S became better able to tolerate awareness of her competitive aggression, ambition, and exhibitionism. These motivations came to seem less extreme, and she became increasingly confident in her ability to manage them internally, without having either to act on them or to repress or deny them.

As these conflicts were being worked through, Ms. S found herself looking back on how it had come about that she had dropped all her intellectual and professional aspirations at age 21. She revisited, now with horror, how her mother had pushed her to become a secretary, and contrasted this with how focused her mother had been on her own career. This led Ms. S to consider how many of her own life choices had represented efforts simultaneously to submit to her mother, who seemed not to want Ms. S to succeed or to get attention, and to ensure that she was different from her mother by entirely splitting off all competitive wishes of her own.

At the same time, it seemed that Ms. S had identified with and repressed a highly toxic view of her mother—and, she understood, a partially distorted one. This view was represented as an object relation of a sadistic, greedy, power- and attention-grabbing mother and a hateful, vengeful daughter, in which Ms. S was identified with both sides of this object relation. During this period, Ms. S's father emerged in the treatment as a more central figure; Ms. S looked back on how attached she had been to him. She remembered, with feelings of longing, the happy times they had spent alone together reading books. Ms. S recalled childhood fantasies that her father must prefer her, love her more. Perhaps, Ms. S reflected, she had wanted to triumph over her mother even then. But she now understood how devoted her father had been to her mother, and also understood that despite her mother's failings as a mother, she was in many ways admirable and desirable.

Toward the end of the treatment, Ms. S had begun in earnest to do independent research in an area of her interest and had started working on an invited article for publication in a scholarly journal. She also had become more active socially and more assertive at work, making contacts and appropriately developing collegial relationships.

Ms. S arrived at therapy one day and announced, very uncharacteristically, that her paper was "going great." And she had decided to color her hair. She was feeling "very positive." She told about a dream the previous night: She was carrying a white bag. She realized that one side was dirty, but rather than panicking and feeling she had to run home, as would be her typical reaction, she felt relaxed. She could just turn the bag around and the dirt wouldn't really show. And even if it did, it was okay; she could clean it when she got home.

In the same session, Ms. S uncharacteristically voiced criticism of Dr. C, albeit indirectly. She told Dr. C she had read a newspaper story about a doctor who had skied to the hospital in a recent blizzard, but Dr. C had canceled patient appointments because of the bad weather. Later in the session, Ms. S said she thought the bag dream was very positive; it was about her secrets, such as her published paper and all the positive things she had been afraid to talk about in the past. Dr. C suggested it was also about her angry and critical feelings toward Dr. C. These feelings now seemed less frightening and more acceptable; she no longer needed so desperately to hide them. Ms. S concurred; she never would have articulated her thoughts about the cancellation in the past. She commented that maybe Dr. C would hate her now—but then added that she knew this wasn't true.

Comments: In the treatment of NPO patients, Strategy 4 makes up the vast majority of psychotherapeutic work; the bulk of clinical time and attention from relatively early in treatment is focused on the working through of conflicts underlying defensive object relations. This strategy entails working through the depressive and also paranoid anxieties linked to the conflicts that have been elaborated in Strategy 3 and that motivate the activation of defensive object relations. In this process, the patient will work through the fear, guilt, and regret associated with tolerating awareness of and ultimately taking responsibility for formerly unconscious motivations, needs, wishes, and fears, represented as affectively charged internal object relations. He will also at some point in this process become aware of his unconscious identification with both halves of defensive and impulsive object relation dyads.

In the process of working through, as the therapist deepens the patient's self-understanding and self-acceptance, the therapist facilitates integrative processes by making links between core conflicts and the patient's developmental experience. The therapist also returns to mutually agreed-upon treatment goals, focusing on how the patient can now understand the difficulties that brought him to treatment and directing therapeutic efforts to the patient's relinquishing maladaptive patterns linked to presenting complaints. Finally, as part of the process of working through, it is often possible to relate conflicts that have been explored and elaborated outside the transference to subtle transference manifestations that color the therapeutic relationship, even for those NPO patients who tend to avoid working with transferences. As conflicts are worked through and the patient is better able to tolerate awareness of conflictual object relations, he may become more able to be conscious of the ways in which his conflicts have been played out in relation to the therapist.

The outcome of the process of uncovering, understanding, and taking responsibility for conflictual needs, wishes, and fears is that object relations associated with expression of these motivations become less threatening and extreme; as previously repressed aspects of self experience are consciously tolerated and explored, they come to be viewed less concretely. Thus, rather than experiencing conflictual motivations and the fears associated with their expression as concrete realities ("My being competitive is the equivalent of my being a monster"), the patient can experience conflictual motivations as internal wishes, needs, and fears.

For example, Ms. S came to feel that her competitive wishes did not concretely turn her into a monster, but rather that she *feared* they would—that is, she came to understand her fears in symbolic terms, as fearful fantasies about what it means to be aggressively competitive, rather than as damning, concrete realities. Thus, as conflictual object relations become less concrete and less extreme, the patient is able to incorporate them into and contain them within his dominant sense of self, in the process deepening and enriching his experience of self and others.

What role did exploration of transference play in Ms. S's therapy?

For the most part, Ms. S maintained a relatively neutral, positive (quietly idealizing) relationship with Dr. C. Early in the treatment, Ms. S described worrying that Dr. C might not see her as deserving of the therapist's time and attention; later on, she at times feared that Dr. C would be critical and rejecting were Ms. S's aspirations to be too great or were she to be too aggressive. At these times, the transference briefly assumed affective dominance. However, as Dr. C helped Ms. S to articulate and reflect on the object relations being enacted, Ms. S quickly came to see them as mirror images of the object relations explored in relation to the important figures in her life, and also as expressions of her own anxieties (this is in marked contrast with Ms. M, presented earlier in this chapter, who for extended periods of time experienced her transferential anxieties as concrete realities). Ms. S would explain that she was not really worried about her relationship with Dr. C; her feelings and fears were far more intense in relation to Dr. R, her husband, her mother, and even at times her housekeeper.

Dr. C, for her part, was well aware of how often the object relations, in particular those involved in defensive idealization, were more or less chronically enacted in the transference. However, efforts to make these transferences the focus of exploration typically fell flat, leaving Ms. S feeling that Dr. C's interventions, though not necessarily wrong, were off target. Thus, although it was clear that the same dominant object relations were simultaneously activated in relation to Dr. C and in relation to the important figures in Ms. S's external and internal life, often these transferences remained largely unconscious, and even when conscious, they rarely assumed affective dominance; in Ms. S's treatment, references to transferential phenomena were most effective when Dr. C presented them in the form of "and so it must be here with me as well."

How does the therapist integrate material from the past into the treatment of the NPO patient?

NPO patients, in contrast to those who begin treatment organized at a borderline level, provide a coherent history and a vivid description of important early relationships from the earliest sessions. However, even though NPO patients' descriptions of early childhood experiences and important relationships, past and present, tend to be realistic and credible, especially when compared with the unstable and partial representations presented by BPO patients, these descriptions remain constructions. During the course of treatment, the therapist can expect patients' descriptions and memories of early objects to evolve, as the therapist can expect patients' descriptions of current objects to evolve. These changes reflect shifting defenses and processes of integration as conflicts are worked through.

For example, Ms. S initially presented with a benign and superficial view of her mother, then later entertained a highly negative but equally superficial view, and ended up with a more complex view that included both positive and negative elements. Her image of Dr. R at the university evolved as well, becoming more complex, more realistic, and predominantly but not entirely negative. As a result, and as discussed in relation to the BPO patient Ms. M earlier in this chapter, when the therapist refers to parental or other important figures in the process of describing the dominant object relations in the here and now, the therapist tends to speak in terms of prototypes, rather than in terms of individuals—for example, a submissive, girlish self in relation to *a domineering mother* or a *maternal figure*, rather than in relation to "your mother."

Because NPO patients are typically able to provide a coherent life narrative, it can be tempting to engage with them in generating hypotheses about the impact of early developmental experiences on their current psychological situation and difficulties. However, although entertaining such hypotheses is perhaps at some level satisfying to both patient and therapist, this approach is generally ill advised insofar as it tends to result in intellectualized discussions that are to some degree removed from the immediacy of the patient's current affective experience and his current life, and therefore of limited therapeutic benefit. In fact, early in treatment, NPO patients tend to make efforts to engage in theories about the impact of the past on their difficulties to avoid experiencing conflicts in a more immediate fashion, and these theories can be seen to interfere with deepening of the clinical process.

In contrast, further along in treatment, when it comes to the process of working through, generally it is helpful to make links between the anxieties and conflicts being worked through in the here and now and important figures and experiences from the patient's developmental history. These links tend to present themselves organically in the clinical process, emerging in the form of spontaneous associations and memories on the part of the patient, and function to deepen his level of self-understanding and self-acceptance, promoting integrative processes.

Key Clinical Concepts

- The strategies of treatment organize the TFP-E therapist's overall approach, in each session and throughout the treatment, to promote treatment goals.

- The strategies of treatment are closely tied to our model of change.

- TFP-E can be described in terms of four overarching strategies, each of which fills specific functions in supporting the development and stabilization of core capacities within the patient.

- Each of the overall TFP-E strategies is tailored to meet the needs of the patient, based on the patient's level of personality organization and dominant defensive style. The different TFP-E strategies serve different functions and vary in their relative centrality in the clinical process, depending on severity of personality pathology and phase of treatment.

References

Bateman A, Fonagy P: Mentalization-Based Treatment for Borderline Personality Disorder. New York, Oxford University Press, 2006

Clarkin JF, Caligor E, Stern BL, Kernberg OF: Structured Interview of Personality Organization—Revised (STIPO-R), 2016. Available at: www.borderlinedisorders.com. Accessed September 20, 2017.

Joseph B: Psychic Equilibrium and Psychic Change: Selected Papers of Betty Joseph. Edited by Feldman M, Spillius EB. London, Tavistock/Routledge, 1989

Safran JD, Muran JC: Negotiating the Therapeutic Alliance. New York, Guilford, 2000

Section III

The Skillful Consultation

EVERY TREATMENT BEGINS WITH CAREFUL
assessment, followed by discussion of the patient's treatment goals and
therapeutic options. A consultation that is completed skillfully and in
depth, and with the patient's active participation, sets the stage for recommendations and any treatment to follow.

The consultation begins with a comprehensive assessment, focusing
on the patient's presenting problems, symptoms, and maladaptive personality traits; current functioning in work; relationships and leisure time;
and level of personality organization. In evaluating personality functioning and level of personality organization, we draw upon the model of personality disorders and classification described in Chapter 2. We also fill
in that discussion by further considering factors within and across each
level of severity likely to impact clinical course and outcome.

Assessment provides both therapist and patient with a clear understanding of the nature and severity of the patient's difficulties. After completing the assessment, the consultant shares diagnostic impressions with
the patient and works with the patient to define treatment goals. The consultant outlines treatment options and their relative risks and benefits, and
helps the patient come to an informed decision regarding how to proceed—
a decision that reflects the patient's personal goals and needs and that draws
upon the consultant's expertise. By the end of the consultation, the patient
will have an understanding of the diagnosis and how this interferes with
functioning, will have identified specific and realistic treatment goals, will
have a general understanding of what transference-focused psychotherapy—extended entails, and will have expressed interest (or lack of it) in
initiating treatment.

Patient Assessment and Treatment Planning

WHEN FIRST MEETING WITH A PATIENT, WE
always begin with comprehensive assessment. Described further in Part 1 of this chapter, assessment entails characterizing the patient's presenting symptoms and pathological personality traits, general personality functioning, level of personality organization, and DSM-5 (American Psychiatric Association 2013) diagnoses, if applicable. The clinical diagnostic interview can be complemented by introduction of structured questionnaires inquiring about symptoms and maladaptive personality traits. In addition, the Structured Interview of Personality Organization—Revised (STIPO-R; Clarkin et al. 2016) can be integrated into clinical assessment to enhance evaluation of personality organization. A comprehensive assessment, including DSM-5 and structural diagnoses, paves the way for treatment planning.

As detailed in Part 2 of this chapter, the second half of the consultation entails sharing diagnostic impressions with the patient, defining treatment goals, describing treatment options and their relative risks and benefits, and helping the patient come to an informed decision with regard to how to proceed—a decision that reflects the patient's personal goals and needs and draws on the therapist's expertise as consultant.

It is the assessment of personality organization, leading to a structural diagnosis, that informs the clinician's understanding of prognosis, treatment options, and contracting needs, while the assessment of symptoms, traits, and functional deficits informs the clinician's understanding of issues likely to be a focus of intervention during the course of treatment. The transference-focused psychotherapy—extended (TFP-E) model of assessment is both clinically focused and embedded in the object relations model of personality pathology and classification presented in Section I of this book. Assessment focuses on domains most relevant to treatment planning and enables the clinician to tailor treatment to the needs of the individual patient based on the level of severity of structural pathology, along with presenting symptoms and personality traits. In sum, in the TFP-E model, thorough assessment guides the selection of treatment structure, focus, and level of care.

The Therapeutic Consultation

The psychotherapeutic consultation is more than simply a clinician-guided battery of self-report questions or a rundown of evidence-based treatment options; the consultation is a clinical interaction between two people (Figure 7–1). The interviewer conducts the evaluation and consultation with two main objectives: 1) to gain a complete understanding of the patient's difficulties, strengths, and personality functioning; and 2) to lay the groundwork for the development of a relationship in which the patient views the interviewer as interested, knowledgeable, and able to understand her and the nature of her difficulties. The manner in which the clinician organizes and conducts the consultation process can lay the groundwork for developing a therapeutic alliance and help the patient engage in the treatment process (Bachelor 1995; Hilsenroth and Cromer 2007).

   This overall approach to the consultation is consistent with the findings of Hilsenroth and Cromer (2007), who identified features of the consultation that promote the development of an alliance and engagement in therapy. They found that a longer, collaborative, and in-depth assessment, one that allows ample opportunity for the patient to voice concerns and discuss them with the interviewer, is of significant value. Detailed exploration of the patient's immediate concerns fosters the alliance and helps the patient commit to therapy, as does seeking feedback from the patient about how she thinks the assessment is going and how she feels while discussing her problems with the interviewer. Hilsenroth and Cromer recommend that the evaluator use jargon-free, experience-near language when discussing the patient's difficulties and sharing impressions—in the process helping the patient develop new ways to think about her presenting problems and making use of psychoeducation.

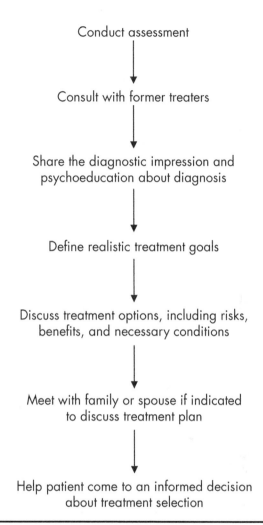

Conduct assessment

↓

Consult with former treaters

↓

Share the diagnostic impression and
psychoeducation about diagnosis

↓

Define realistic treatment goals

↓

Discuss treatment options, including risks,
benefits, and necessary conditions

↓

Meet with family or spouse if indicated
to discuss treatment plan

↓

Help patient come to an informed decision
about treatment selection

FIGURE 7–1. The therapeutic consultation.

Structure of the Consultation

Allocating 90 minutes for the initial consultation is recommended. A viable
alternative is to arrange two shorter appointments; however, the relatively
leisurely feeling of a 90-minute initial meeting is desirable as long as scheduling allows. It is often useful after the initial meeting to have the patient
return for a 45-minute session to complete discussion of the diagnostic impression and treatment planning. A second meeting with the patient in consultation has the advantage of allowing patient and therapist time to reflect

on the initial interview, and then the therapist can use the second meeting to address aspects of the patient's internal and external situation that may have been omitted or inadequately explored in the initial meeting. In addition, a second meeting provides an opportunity for the therapist to explore the patient's reactions to the initial interview and to completely answer the patient's questions and address her concerns. Some patients, especially those with more complex problems or for whom there is diagnostic uncertainty, may require two or even three follow-up sessions in the form of an extended consultation, in order for a treatment plan to be determined.

Part 1
Diagnostic Assessment

PATIENTS WITH PERSONALITY PATHOLOGY seek treatment for a wide variety of reasons. Many present seeking relief from symptoms such as depression, anxiety, or disturbing thoughts; others complain of difficulty regulating their emotions, or managing anger or fluctuations in self-esteem; still others present with maladaptive behaviors that may be impulsive, compulsive, or self-destructive, including substance misuse and eating disorders. Many patients with personality disorders present with difficulty functioning in certain domains of their lives—for example, getting along with others or maintaining relationships, establishing or maintaining intimate relationships, or functioning or succeeding in work. Still others seek treatment complaining of painful or dysphoric subjective states linked to personality pathology, such as constant self-criticism, feelings of emptiness, chronic boredom, a global lack of satisfaction, or an inability to identify meaningful goals.

Within the framework of object relations theory, many of the complaints that bring patients with personality pathology to clinical attention are understood as direct expressions of personality pathology—for example, self-destructive behavior, feelings of emptiness, or chronic dysphoria. Other complaints are best conceptualized as co-occurring disorders embedded in the patient's personality—for example, substance misuse or major depression.

At times, it can be difficult to distinguish between direct expressions of personality pathology and symptoms of co-occurring disorders. For example, the therapist may ask himself questions such as these: Are these complaints best understood as part of a mood disorder or as the dysphoria associated with poorly consolidated identity? Does this patient suffer from a primary anxiety disorder or from free-floating anxiety associated with personality pathology? In longitudinal studies of individuals with and without personality disorders, the interaction of symptoms, such as anxiety and episodic personality dysfunction, raises questions about the boundaries between personality pathology and symptom expression (Hallquist and Lenzenweger 2013), at least in some cases.

Because the presence of a personality disorder adversely affects the prognosis for treatment of co-occurring disorders (Grilo et al. 2004) and because some symptoms—such as feelings of emptiness and, in some cases, depressive symptoms—are likely to improve only with treatment of underlying personality pathology (Gunderson et al. 2004; Skodol et al. 2011; Zanarini et al. 2006), it is of value to do the complete assessment outlined in this chapter with *all* patients presenting for *any kind* of treatment, not only with those presenting for treatment of a personality disorder or those who on presentation clearly have significant personality pathology.[1]

In sum, in the TFP-E approach to the general psychiatric consultation, presenting difficulties, symptoms, pathological personality traits, and functional difficulties are always conceptualized as embedded in a particular personality organization. When the clinician first meets with a patient, she begins with comprehensive assessment, regardless of the setting or the nature of the problems that bring the patient to clinical attention:

- Presenting symptoms and pathological personality traits are clearly characterized, leading to a descriptive diagnosis (e.g., DSM-5 [ICD-10-CM] or ICD-10 diagnosis).
- Personality functioning is evaluated, leading to an assessment of the patient's overall level of functioning (e.g., Global Assessment of Functioning Scale).
- Personality organization is explored in depth, leading to a structural diagnosis (e.g., level of personality organization [see Table 7–2 later in this chapter] or dimensional rating on the STIPO-R).

---

[1]For example, even for patients with a high borderline level of personality organization who may appear superficially "normal" (e.g., some individuals with narcissistic personality disorder), the personality disorder diagnosis will complicate treatment and adversely affect the prognosis for treatment of co-occurring disorders.

The Clinical Diagnostic Interview

The TFP-E approach to assessment rests primarily on the clinical diagnostic interview, which continues to have advantages over other, more structured approaches (Clarkin and Livesley 2016). In particular, the clinical diagnostic interview allows the clinician to elicit information in ways that foster the alliance and engage the patient in treatment, while also providing opportunity to attend to and explore the patient-interviewer interaction as part of the assessment process. The role of the interviewer is to be directive, asking specific questions of the patient and ensuring coverage of presenting difficulties, symptoms, maladaptive traits and behaviors, personality functioning, and whatever additional information is needed to characterize the patient's level of personality organization. The interview focuses on the here and now—both the patient's current life situation and her current interactions with the interviewer, in contrast to the developmental past. During the course of the interview, the interviewer relies on clarification of—and, to some degree, confrontation of—the patient's communications, while attending to the relationship emerging between patient and interviewer.

The clinical diagnostic interview can be complemented and is often enhanced by the introduction of structured assessment instruments in the form of self-report questionnaires inquiring about symptoms and maladaptive traits (see Clarkin et al. 2018). Integrating the STIPO-R, a semistructured interview, facilitates the clinical assessment of personality organization. This hour-long interview focuses on the domains of identity formation, defenses, object relations, aggression, and moral values. The STIPO-R may be particularly helpful for relatively inexperienced clinicians, as well as for more seasoned clinicians who are less familiar with our model of pathology and assessment, and of course is useful in research settings.

The 55-item STIPO-R interview provides specific examples of questions that can be used in the clinical diagnostic interview to evaluate personality organization, as well as follow-up probes. The STIPO-R example questions contain tactful phrasing that can help the reader more concretely appreciate the nature of the content in each domain, as well as the TFP-E approach to the evaluation of domains. In addition, the STIPO-R includes helpful anchors that can guide the clinician in assessing identity formation and locating severity of pathology on a scale of 1–5. The STIPO-R is discussed further in Part 1 of this chapter in the later subsection, "Structured Assessment and the STIPO-R." The complete STIPO-R interview, with questions and probes, along with the accompanying score sheet, are available at www.borderlinedisorders.com.

For convenient clinical reference, a version of the STIPO-R anchors developed for clinicians ("STIPO-R Clinical Anchors for Personality Organization: Identity, Object Relations, Defenses, Aggression, and Moral Values Across the Range of Severity") is available in the appendix of helpful resources at the back of this book. As illustrated in Chapter 2, these STIPO-R anchors provide a summary of the contents of each domain of functioning assessed in the diagnostic interview. In essence, these anchors offer a clinical scale for classification of identity, object relations, defenses, aggression, and moral values based on the STIPO-R ratings. We suggest that as readers move through this chapter, they refer to these clinical anchors that accompany each domain of functioning in our discussion.

For purposes of clarity and economy, our discussion of the clinical diagnostic interview proceeds in three parts, as follows: First, we outline the conceptual flow of the interview and the data that the interview is designed to provide, describing the information that the clinician should have in order to make a diagnosis (Table 7–1). Second, we outline methods and procedures whereby data are collected, which is derived from the Structural Interview of Kernberg (1984) and the STIPO-R. Third, we discuss personality types and diagnosis that result from the clinical diagnostic interview.

Conceptual Flow and Data Collection

The conceptual flow of the clinical diagnostic interview and the resulting data collected comprise the following aspects of personality assessment: descriptive features of personality functioning and pathology; structural features of personality, including dimensional assessment of personality organization and structural diagnosis; and domains of functioning central to personality functioning and pathology.

Descriptive Features of Personality Functioning and Pathology

Presenting Symptoms, Pathological Personality Traits, and Psychiatric History

Patient assessment begins with identification and characterization of the symptoms and pathological personality traits that brought the patient to treatment, followed by a thorough and systematic evaluation of all symptoms and difficulties, beginning with current areas of difficulty and incorporating a review of the past psychiatric history. This portion of the

TABLE 7–1. Content domains of clinical diagnostic interview

Presenting symptoms, pathological personality traits, and psychiatric history

Symptoms and pathological personality traits that brought the patient to treatment

Thorough and systematic evaluation of all symptoms and difficulties, beginning with current areas of difficulty and also reviewing past history

History of prior psychiatric treatment, medication, and/or hospitalization

Medical history; history of substance misuse; family history of psychiatric illness; history of trauma, physical or sexual abuse, or neglect

Complete psychiatric review of symptoms, including symptoms of affective, anxiety, psychotic, eating, and learning disorders; substance misuse; self-destructive behaviors; history of violence or illegal activity

Review of previous treatments, including difficulties that emerged in the course of treatment, how the treatment ended, and the patient's view of each previous treatment experience

Personality functioning in relationships, work, and leisure time

Degree to which symptoms and pathological personality traits interfere with personality functioning

Interpersonal functioning, including intimate relations and sexual functioning

Work functioning, current and past

Personal interests and use of free time

Structural features of personality: dimensional assessment of personality organization and structural diagnosis

Identity formation—sense of self, sense of others, and capacity to invest in and pursue longer-term goals

Quality of object relations—interpersonal functioning, understanding of relationships in terms of mutuality vs. need fulfillment

Defensive style—predominantly flexible-adaptive, repression-based, or splitting-based

Management of aggression—well-modulated adaptive expression of aggression vs. inhibited expression or maladaptive aggressive behavior directed toward self and/or others

Moral functioning—internalized values and ideals that guide behavior vs. failure of internal values and ideals with unethical or antisocial behavior

Complete dimensional appraisals of health vs. severity of pathology covering each of the five domains listed above

Personal/developmental history[a]

Developmental history—history of trauma, antisocial behavior, positive relationships

[a]For further discussion, see the subsection "Phase IV: Past History" in Part 1 of this chapter.

consultation involves data collection that would be part of any general psychiatric assessment. If the patient has a history of prior psychiatric treatment, medication, and/or hospitalization, this information is reviewed in depth, as are the patient's medical history and history of substance misuse, as well as family history of psychiatric illness and substance use. In addition, the interviewer inquires specifically about any history of trauma, physical or sexual abuse, or neglect.

A thorough review of previous treatments, including any difficulties that emerged in the course of treatment, how the treatment ended, and the patient's view of each previous treatment experience (i.e., what felt helpful and what did not), is especially helpful when it comes to treatment planning. Such a review aids in anticipating difficulties likely to emerge during the consultation as well as during any treatment that may follow. Although it may be tempting to anticipate that difficulties that emerged in past treatments will not reemerge with a different treater, clinical experience suggests the opposite; in short, careful review of prior treatment experiences, both positive and negative, can provide invaluable information. The interviewer follows up on this line of inquiry by contacting previous treaters to obtain a complete history of past treatments.

Personality Functioning in Relationships, Work, and Leisure Time

Having characterized the patient's difficulties, the consultant turns to the next phase of the assessment: exploring the patient's personality, focusing on the degree to which symptoms and maladaptive personality traits interfere with personality functioning. The interviewer prompts the patient to describe her interpersonal functioning, intimate relations, current functioning at work and work history, and use of leisure time.

In evaluating interpersonal functioning, the consultant addresses the extent to which the individual has relationships and the duration and stability of those relationships. Does she have friends? How many and of what duration? Does she trust her closest friends, is she able to depend on them, and does she derive satisfaction from these relationships?

When evaluating interpersonal functioning, the consultant also inquires specifically about intimate relations. Does the individual currently have a partner? If so, what is the nature of that relationship? If not, has she been able to establish and sustain intimate relations in the past? Has she ever been in love? Does she have enjoyable sexual relations? Have her intimate relations been stable, stormy, satisfying, or ultimately boring? If she has children, what is the nature of her relationships with them?

The consultant also inquires in detail about current and past work functioning. Is the individual engaged in full-time employment or academic studies? Is her level of employment consistent with her level of education and her abilities? In the workplace, does she get along well with peers, bosses, and subordinates, or does she have a tendency to develop interpersonal problems? Does she derive satisfaction from her work and/or studies? What are her long-term goals in this regard? Are they realistic goals, and is she taking practical steps to attain them? Does the individual have a history of significant failures or disappointments at work? If so, what happened? If the individual is not engaged in full-time employment, why not, and how is she supporting herself?

Finally, the consultant asks about personal interests and what the patient does with her free time. Does she have activities that she is invested in or has stayed with over time? Does she derive pleasure from her leisure time, or does she find herself feeling aimless and bored when her time is her own?

By the time this phase of the clinical interview is complete, the consultant will have obtained an in-depth view of the patient's functioning and pathology, including present and past symptoms and difficulties, maladaptive personality traits, and personality functioning. This information should be sufficient to diagnose or rule out affective or anxiety disorders, eating disorders, or substance abuse disorders, and to make a DSM-5 Section II personality disorder diagnosis, if one is present.

Structural Features of Personality: Dimensional Assessment of Personality Organization and Structural Diagnosis

As described in Chapter 2 and listed in Table 7–1, structural assessment focuses on the following domains:

- Identity formation—sense of self, sense of others, and capacity to invest in and pursue longer-term goals
- Quality of object relations—interpersonal functioning, capacity for intimacy, and the individual's internal working models of relationships
- Defensive style—predominantly flexible-adaptive, repression-based, or splitting-based
- Management of aggression—well-modulated adaptive expression of aggression versus inhibited expression or maladaptive aggressive behavior directed toward self and/or others

- Moral functioning—internalized values and ideals that guide behavior versus a failure of internal values and ideals; unethical or antisocial behavior

Structural assessment results in dimensional appraisals of health versus pathology, as well as severity of pathology, for each of the five domains listed above. This assessment informs the clinician's understanding of prognosis and guides treatment planning.

Level of Personality Organization, Severity of Pathology, and Prognosis

Dimensional assessment across the five domains of identity formation, quality of object relations, defensive style, management of aggression, and moral functioning can be combined to determine the patient's *level of personality organization*—normal, neurotic personality organization (NPO), high borderline personality organization (BPO), middle BPO, or low BPO (see Figure 2–1 in Chapter 2)—representing increasing degrees of severity. The various levels of personality organization are not hard-and-fast categories but rather represent common presentations of personality pathology across the dimension of severity, with important implications for prognosis and treatment planning. Alternatively, dimensional assessment across the five domains can be combined to construct an individualized dimensional profile of personality organization by making use of the STIPO-R anchors to rate the clinical interview. Both these approaches and the relationship between them are illustrated in Chapter 2.

Structural assessment of personality organization complements and deepens the DSM-5 personality disorder diagnosis and/or assessment of personality traits by focusing on those dimensions that within the TFP-E model of personality functioning and disorder are most relevant to long-term prognosis and treatment planning. A fair amount of variability exists within any DSM-5 diagnostic category regarding severity of pathology (e.g., some patients with histrionic personality disorder have only mild pathology of identity and object relations and function quite well, whereas others have more severe pathology that is disruptive of functioning). Variability also occurs in relation to combinations of traits, some of which may be more or less problematic in terms of prognosis and treatment (e.g., borderline personality disorder may be manifest either with or without recklessness and stimulus-seeking or impulsive aggression).

Similarly, although dimensional assessments of traits can provide clinically useful information about treatment goals and clinical focus, they fail to adequately address the issue of severity or to provide information needed for treatment planning. In sum, neither DSM-5 personality disorder diagnoses nor dimensional description of traits specifically reflect the severity or prognosis of personality pathology, and neither is linked to specific models of treatment as is a dimensional assessment of personality organization (Meehan and Clarkin 2015).

In contrast, the TFP-E model of *levels of personality organization* is specifically organized to provide information about a patient's "treatability" and overall prognosis (Table 7–2). The diagnosis of a particular level of personality organization provides an assessment of severity of personality pathology, in which severity is understood as related to prognosis (i.e., "this patient is likely to do better in life and in treatment than a patient organized at a lower or higher level of personality organization") regardless of presenting complaints. At lower levels of personality organization, any form of treatment carries greater risk, and the treatment frame will require a more extensive contracting process and a higher level of structure; also, the treatment itself becomes more challenging, both at the level of clinical technique and in terms of management of countertransference.

Domains of Functioning Central to Personality Functioning and Pathology

Identity Formation: Sense of Self, Sense of Others, and Capacity to Invest in and Pursue Longer-Term Goals

Evaluating identity formation is a cornerstone of structural assessment. In assessing identity, the consultant evaluates the extent to which the individual has 1) the capacity to establish and pursue long-term goals and to invest in work/studies and personal interests; 2) an integrated, well-differentiated, realistic, and stable experience of herself; and 3) a similarly integrated, well-differentiated, realistic, and stable sense of her significant others. Throughout the clinical interview, the consultant makes an ongoing assessment of the degree to which the patient has a consolidated identity versus evidence of pathology of identity formation.

Overall Presentation.   At the most broad-stroke, subjective level, the consultant will have a variable experience of the patient and of the interview depending on the patient's level of personality organization in general and her identity formation in particular.

TABLE 7–2. Severity, prognosis, and clinical course of personality pathology at different levels of personality organization

---

Patients with NPO	Have mild pathology; excellent overall prognosis.
	Treatment need not be highly structured.
	Do well in variety of treatments, particularly in transference-focused psychotherapy—extended (TFP-E) for neurotic pathology (see Caligor et al. 2007).
	Pathology best characterized as "maladaptive personality rigidity" rather than "personality disorder," given relatively mild severity of impairment and typically high level of functioning.
	More focal pathology (i.e., limited predominantly to a particular domain of functioning rather than globally affecting all domains of function) and less severe rigidity have better prognosis.
	Often present with obsessive-compulsive, depressive, and hysterical personalities.[a]
Patients with high BPO	Have least severe personality disorders within BPO spectrum; positive prognosis, but less consistently so than NPO group.
	Do poorly in unstructured treatments.
	Do well in structured forms of therapy and generally do extremely well in TFP-E.
	Relative absence of significant pathology of moral functioning and presence of capacity to form dependent relationships characterize this group and are positive prognostic features for TFP-E.
	Often diagnosed with histrionic, dependent, and avoidant personality disorders and may present with healthier narcissistic traits.
Patients with middle BPO[b]	Despite severity of symptoms, have relatively positive prognosis and benefit from a variety of specialized treatments.
	Require highly structured frame and contract, and early phases of treatment often characterized by acting out.
	Can do well in TFP-E.
	More severe impairment of moral functioning and object relations brings more guarded prognosis.
	Often diagnosed with borderline, paranoid, and schizoid personality disorders.

TABLE 7–2.   Severity, prognosis, and clinical course of personality pathology at different levels of personality organization (continued)

Patients with low BPO	Have extremely guarded prognosis; treatments carry a high risk of destructive acting out.
	Contracting must be extensive and involve participation of third parties.
	Commonly diagnosed with narcissistic personality disorder with significant antisocial features (often comorbid with borderline personality disorder), malignant narcissistic personality disorder, and antisocial personality disorder.
	Antisocial personality disorder is a contraindication to outpatient psychotherapy.

Note.   BPO=borderline level of personality organization; NPO=neurotic level of personality organization.

aSome patients fall on the border between NPO and high BPO; these patients present with more global and severe pathology than do NPO patients, with mild instability in the sense of self and/or other, reflecting a combination of repression- and splitting-based defenses, in the setting of a generally consolidated identity. The healthiest avoidant, histrionic, and narcissistic patients may fall into this group. The term *higher level personality pathology* describes this group, along with the familiar neurotic personality types.

bMiddle-level and low-level BPO groups together are referred to as the *severe personality disorders*. Patients in these groups have more pathology of aggression than do patients in the high-BPO group. The low-level BPO group is distinguished from the middle-level BPO group by more severe pathology of moral functioning and object relations; both are primary indicators of poor prognosis in the BPO spectrum.

When seen in consultation, patients with consolidated identity are able to provide information about themselves and their difficulties in an organized fashion. During the course of a 90-minute consultation, the interviewer will easily develop a progressively clear and detailed impression of the patient's internal experience and external functioning, including both strengths and weaknesses. In the patient with consolidated identity, apparent distortions in self-perception or self-presentation and poorly integrated aspects of self experience will be limited to specific areas of conflict; for example, a successful professional may not appreciate that he is valued by his employers. Similarly, as the patient describes her relationships with others, the important people in the patient's life will emerge as three-dimensional, realistic, understandable, and complex individuals.

In contrast, the clinical interview with the patient with poorly consolidated identity is likely to leave the interviewer with a vague, incomplete, or confused understanding of the complaints and motivations for the patient's coming to treatment. The patient's presentation of her history may be nonlinear or chaotic, or may focus on some events or areas of difficulty while omitting other important information, requiring the interviewer to actively and frequently guide and redirect the patient. Even so, not infrequently, the interviewer will be left unclear as to what the patient hopes to gain from treatment.

In the setting of poorly consolidated identity, the information that the patient provides about herself will typically be vague and lacking in detail, superficial, and often internally inconsistent. For example, a patient may describe herself as chronically suicidal and overwhelmed by anxiety, and in the next sentence maintain that she has a highly successful professional life, or she may describe herself as "very outgoing and social," even though she has no friends in the city in which she lives. Similarly, in the setting of identity pathology, the patient's descriptions of the people in her world tend to be superficial and poorly differentiated, "black and white" or caricature-like, and internally inconsistent, making it difficult for the interviewer to develop a complete or coherent sense of others in the patient's life. For example, a patient may describe his girlfriend as "the best thing that ever happened to me" in one moment, but as a bore and a burden in the next, so that it is difficult for the interviewer to develop a clear impression of the patient's internal experience or external functioning.

Goal-Directedness. In the evaluation of identity formation, the interviewer explores the individual's capacity to organize and pursue long-term goals and to invest over time in work/studies and personal interests—that is, capacities conferred by normal identity formation. This information typically emerges over the course of the clinical interview as the therapist evaluates the patient's presenting difficulties, personality functioning, and personal history. Individuals with poorly consolidated identity typically demonstrate a lack of investment in work/studies and a work/educational history that is unstable or lacking in direction or foresight. In some cases, the complete absence of any long-term goals, associated with low motivation and a pervasive sense of passivity, may be striking. In milder cases, the patient may set goals but have difficulty sustaining the necessary effort to achieve longer-term objectives. Low self-directedness, low self-efficacy, and lack of purpose often become especially evident in evaluating the patient's work functioning or in taking the personal history. To clarify, the interviewer might inquire, "Do you feel as though you are not in control of your life, or that there is nothing you can do to change the things you are describing?"

Sense of Self and Sense of Significant Others. To evaluate the patient's sense of self in a focused fashion, the interviewer can follow up on material that emerges organically in the patient's description of presenting problems. For example, if the patient presents with "depression" but then describes his mood as unstable rather than consistently depressed, the interviewer might ask for clarification in the following way:

> Perhaps in addition to your mood, the feelings you describe have something to do with your sense of self or your self-esteem. Would you say that your view of yourself seems to shift so that at times you see yourself in very positive terms—for example, as special and unique—while at other times you see yourself in negative terms—for example, as small or defective?

If the patient's answer is yes, the interviewer might ask, "Does your mood tend to fluctuate with your view of yourself?"

Or with a patient who complains of chronic dysphoria, the interviewer might ask, "Do you feel as if you are empty or hollow inside, or that life has no meaning?"

Or with a patient who presents with marital problems, describing mutual resentment and enmeshment between himself and his wife, the interviewer might ask questions like these:

> In the course of your marriage, has it been difficult for you to maintain your own sense of self? Has it been hard to maintain your own interests, attitudes, or tastes, and do you find yourself taking on your wife's tastes, interests, and preferences?
>
> Would you say that this experience extends beyond your marriage— that in general you look to others to see what views and opinions they hold, and adopt them as your own because you don't really know your own mind? Do you do this in regard to how you feel about a new friend, for example, or a job opportunity, or even something trivial such as style of dress or taste in music?

The patient's sense of significant others can be explored in similar fashion. For example, if a patient presents with stormy, short-lived romantic relationships, the interviewer might seek more information:

> When you're in a relationship, do you find that your image of your girlfriend can shift when she disappoints you or when you get angry at her? At those times, is it as though you see her as simply awful—that you can't stand her or are disgusted by her, or that you can't remember what you ever saw in her? Or is it more like "Okay, I'm really angry, but she is still someone I'm very close to," where you can hang on to being angry and being close at the same time?

We encourage the reader to review the STIPO-R Identity section, which provides ready-formed questions similar to those included above, along with the follow-up probes that can aid assessment. For more comprehensive examples of useful questions pertaining to identity formation, the reader can consult the original 87-item STIPO (both the STIPO-R and the original STIPO are available at www.borderlinedisorders.com.

In the structural assessment, the clinician completes the evaluation of identity formation by asking the patient to describe herself and a significant other. Asking for a description of someone outside the patient's family of origin is recommended, as descriptions of parents and siblings may not be representative of the individual's overall experience of others. These questions and requests consistently prove to be the most sensitive and the most efficient clinical probes in the evaluation of personality pathology, quickly shedding light on the degree of integration and differentiation of the patient's sense of self and her sense of significant others. This line of inquiry comes toward the latter part of the interview (see "The Structural Interview" later in chapter) and often serves to confirm hypotheses about personality organization already formulated on the basis of the patient's presenting problems and current functioning.

Asking the patient to provide a self-description calls on her to self-reflect as well as to present an integrated view of her internal experience and her external functioning. Patients with consolidated identity may require some prompting but are able to provide a three-dimensional and complex description of themselves, focusing on core values and personality traits. For example, a patient might say,

> That's a difficult question.... Let's see. I'm intelligent, a bit of a nerd—a workaholic, actually. I like to keep busy, love a good project. I'm not a very emotionally expressive person.... I like my job, I'm a lawyer.... I'm devoted to my family, take pride in providing for them, though sometimes I get cranky with the kids at the end of a hard day, you know how it is.... I try to be a devoted son, my parents are aging.... I guess you could say I'm someone who always tries to do the best I can and to make the best of things. Is this the kind of thing you had in mind?

In contrast, patients with identity pathology will have much greater difficulty responding. Some patients may openly struggle with the task and comment about being unsure of who they are, whereas others may provide a brief, superficial description consisting of a few nonspecific or concrete attributes. For example, a patient might say, "I am not sure what to say. I'm tall, have brown hair.... I'm not very smart, I don't earn much money so I live with my mom.... Is that what you're asking?"

Patients with milder identity disturbance can, with help, provide a general self-description, typically characterized by concrete qualities and a string of adjectives, or by a description of things they do rather than who they are. The interviewer might follow up along these lines: "You've used several adjectives to describe yourself. I'm wondering if you could fill in your description a bit, perhaps bringing it to life with an example or story that illustrates some of those qualities."

In contrast, with severe identity disturbance, the sense of self may be so vague, confused, and impoverished that it becomes difficult for the patient to identify anything but the most basic, often physical attributes, as illustrated by the patient with brown hair, above. Or the patient may be simply nonplussed and say, "Can you tell me again what you're asking?" or "My feelings about myself change all the time, so I can't really say."

When patients have difficulty, the interviewer can prompt the patient to provide additional information: "Is there anything else you can tell me so that I get a full picture of your personality, of what you're like as a person?" "I notice you describe largely negative attributes. Are there positive qualities that you can tell me about briefly?" "You have highlighted the things you are good at. Are there areas in which you face greater difficulty?" Or perhaps the interviewer may point out that the patient has done a good job of describing how others see her but has said little about how she feels about herself inside.

Having explored the degree of integration of the patient's sense of self, the interviewer can revisit the patient's experience of the important people in her world. In this phase of the interview, the clinician focuses on the most intimate relationships, because in patients with severe personality disorders—who lack a stable and integrated picture of the people in their lives—deficits in sense of others are typically most pronounced with the people who are important to a patient. In addition, better-integrated narcissistic patients who have a relatively stable sense of self can be clearly identified at this point in the interview by virtue of the absence of subtlety and depth in their descriptions of others—findings that are most dramatic when the patient is describing the people with whom she is most closely involved.

The interviewer asks the patient to provide a description of an important person in her current life. If the patient has difficulty, the interviewer can prompt her by specifically asking the patient to identify the person to whom she is closest, and then inviting the patient to describe the person as if she were writing a paragraph about him in a story.

As with self-description, with prompting, individuals with consolidated identity are able to provide a three-dimensional description of significant others, characterized by subtlety and depth, making it easy for the interviewer to imagine the person described. The following is an example:

Patient: Well, the person I'm closest to is definitely my wife. We've been together since our freshman year of college. Let's see.... She's caring, organized, forthright, and reliable. She's home with the kids these days and is a great mom, very patient, much more than I am. She also has a part-time job at an art gallery. The job doesn't pay much but is enough to cover the nanny, and she says it lets her engage her creative side. She majored in art history in college so she knows a lot about art, and she really loves it. Also she's good at tuning in to people, to what they're thinking or what they might be looking for, which helps a lot with making sales at the gallery.

Interviewer: That's a pretty glowing description. Any shortcomings?

Patient: She does need time to herself or she gets kind of overwhelmed and, to be honest, kind of irritable—not so much with the kids, but with me. I try to give her a break these days, maybe take the kids for a morning or afternoon on a weekend. She tells me how much she appreciates my making the effort; it seems to mean a lot to her.

In contrast, patients with identity pathology often describe others using a string of adjectives: "She's nice, pretty…. What else do you want me to say?" Also, descriptions are often self-referential: "She's good to me, always knows how I'm feeling and is willing to help me out," or "She's smarter than I am. Not as pretty as me."

Sometimes the patient may provide a highly polarized view—"She's wonderful, the best wife a guy could have, pretty, smart"—or entirely negative—"A disaster of a person, clingy, demanding. I can't understand how I ended up with such a wife." When a patient gives a polarized description, it is helpful to point out the one-sidedness to the patient and to inquire whether he can provide additional qualities: "You've described your wife in entirely positive terms. Does she have any shortcomings as a person?" "You've presented a string of adjectives to describe your best friend. I'm wondering if you can fill in your description a bit, perhaps bringing it to life with an example or a story that illustrates these qualities." With prompting, patients with less severe identity pathology can introduce more specific and less polarized elements into their descriptions. In contrast, for a patient with more severe pathology, the patient's experience of the significant other is too rigidly polarized and/or superficial to leave room for introduction of any complexity or subtlety.

As described in Chapter 2, identity consolidation differentiates normal personality and higher level personality pathology (i.e., NPO) from failure of identity consolidation in the more severe personality disorders (i.e., BPO spectrum). Identity pathology can be characterized across a spectrum of severity, from mild to most severe. With increasing severity, there is an increasing distortion of and instability in the experience of self and others, and an increasing impairment in the capacity to establish and pursue goals and to invest in work/studies and personal interests.[2]

Quality of Object Relations: Interpersonal Functioning, Capacity for Intimacy, and Internal Working Models of Relationships

When evaluating the quality of object relations, the clinician is interested in 1) the patient's interpersonal functioning, 2) his capacity for intimacy, and 3) his internal investment in others—that is, his basic understanding of the nature of close relationships, along with his capacity to appreciate and care about the needs and feelings of others (empathy).

When evaluating capacity for intimacy, the clinician considers whether the patient has been able to establish intimate relationships, whether he has been able to sustain them over time, and whether he can integrate gratifying sexual experiences into intimate and tender relations. When evaluating the patient's internal investments in others, the clinician considers whether the patient sees relationships in terms of need fulfillment or in terms of who gets what from the relationship and which person gets more, or whether he has a sense of mutual give and take. Does he have a capacity for empathy—can he accurately perceive and care about the needs and feelings of others? Is he exploitative in his relationships, or does he take satisfaction in giving to and caring for others? Does he have the capacity to allow himself to be cared for?

As described in Chapter 2, interpersonal relationships in the normal personality and in NPO are stable in quality and sustained over time, marked by trust and respect for the other as an individual. There is a fully developed capacity for intimacy, though there may be difficulty in fully integrating intimacy and tenderness with sexuality in the setting of NPO;

---

[2]Of note, patients with narcissistic personality disorder can pose a particular challenge to assessment of identity formation. Diagnostic confusion reflects the specific presentation of identity pathology in narcissistic personality disorder; identity pathology may be less evident on initial assessment than it is, for example, in borderline or even histrionic personality disorder. Identity pathology in narcissistic personality disorder is characterized by a superficially integrated sense of self, albeit one that lacks depth and is often fragile, which may be coupled with the ability to pursue professional and personal goals. This constellation can lead to underestimation of the extent and severity of identity pathology. However, when the interviewer remembers that assessment of identity formation focuses on the sense of others as well as sense of self, the diagnosis of identity pathology in narcissistic personality disorder becomes difficult to miss; in narcissistic personality disorder, a seemingly relatively well-integrated self experience is coupled with an experience of others that is markedly superficial, often strikingly so—vague, shadowy, and lacking in specificity.

to the degree that disruption of interpersonal functioning occurs in NPO, it is limited to specific areas of conflict. Object relations in the normal personality and in NPO are characterized by concern for the needs of others independent of the needs of the self; a fully developed capacity to empathize with the feelings of others; the capacity for mutual give and take; and the capacity to depend on others, as well as to be depended on.

In patients with severe personality disorders, interpersonal relationships are often stormy, unstable, and chaotic, colored by mistrust and hostility and lacking in intimacy; in some patients, there may be an extreme paucity of relationships or even a complete absence. Object relations are characterized by a need-fulfilling view of relationships—for example, they are organized in relation to a search for caretaking, managing fears of being alone, wishes to attach to someone of status or wealth, fears of being exploited, or, at the most extreme end of the spectrum, ego-syntonic exploitation of others for personal or financial gain. In the latter case, there is limited capacity to focus on or care about the needs of others independent of the needs of the self—with, for example, resentment at having to cancel personal plans because a loved one or family member is ill. Thus, in the severe personality disorders, the capacity for empathy is compromised or may be entirely lacking.

In the high-BPO group, milder pathology of object relations is seen, often characterized by the capacity to sustain mutually dependent and caring—albeit often stormy—relationships, but with less stability and depth than is characteristic of the NPO group. Patients in the high-BPO group are heterogeneous with regard to the capacity for empathy, which is often in conflict with concerns about the needs and wishes of the self.

As is the case with evaluation of identity formation, much information regarding the patient's quality of object relations will emerge spontaneously during the description of presenting problems and evaluation of current functioning. This information can be supplemented by interjecting focused questions designed to more specifically flesh out the quality of the patient's interpersonal functioning and internal investments. For example, when a patient tells the interviewer that he has been married for 5 years, the interviewer might follow up with these questions:

Would you say that your relationship with your wife is characterized by intimacy and trust? Can you share things openly with her?

When you have sex, does it make you feel closer to her?

In your relationship, are you dependable?

Or in response to a patient reporting difficulties in his friendships, the interviewer might ask these questions:

> In those relationships, do you find yourself "keeping score"—thinking about who is getting more out of the relationship—or do you frequently have the experience of feeling taken advantage of?
>
> Do you tend to drop people to whom you were once close?
>
> Are your close relationships characterized by trust, openness, and disclosure, or would you say that you are cautious and guarded, even with those closest to you?

The quality of object relations can be characterized across the dimension of severity, from normal through the most severe level of pathology. As illustrated in Chapter 2, Figure 2–1 and Table 2–1, severe pathology of object relations (i.e., STIPO-R Levels 4 and 5), along with pathology of moral functioning, distinguishes low BPO from middle and high BPO, and bodes poorly for prognosis.

Defenses and Personality Rigidity: Predominant Defensive Style

When assessing defensive operations, the clinician evaluates 1) the degree to which the individual relies predominantly on a) healthy, adaptive defenses, b) repression-based defenses, or c) splitting-based defenses; and 2) the degree to which defenses are maladaptive, introducing rigidity and interfering with personality functioning.

In the severe personality disorders, lower-level, or splitting-based, defenses are highly maladaptive, affecting the patient's behavior and grossly distorting her subjectivity; as discussed in Chapter 2, many of the core features of severe personality pathology reflect the impact of splitting-based defensive operations on the patient's internal experience and external functioning. As a result, the predominance of splitting-based defenses characteristic of the patient with severe personality pathology are typically relatively easy to diagnose during the course of a clinical diagnostic interview, and will invariably prove to be adversely affecting the patient's functioning. The patient's descriptions of her relationships and personality functioning, along with presenting difficulties, will typically quickly highlight the black-or-white, hot-or-cold, and unstable and contradictory quality of experience introduced by splitting-based defenses.

The impact of lower-level defenses will also often emerge during the interview as the patient describes contradictory personality traits—for example, a demure elementary school teacher may earn extra cash by working as an escort. In addition, during history taking, the patient will often show striking evidence of denial of important aspects of reality; for example, a patient on academic probation may describe himself as an excellent student, and when asked in follow-up about the apparent contradiction, he responds that probation merely reflects his grades, which are not a good measure of academic ability or success.

To further clarify the patient's reliance on splitting-based defenses, the interviewer can follow up with specific questions. For example, with the student with chronic academic difficulties, the interviewer might ask these questions:

> Do you tend to deny painful or disturbing realities, to put them "out of mind"? Do you do that to the extent that it gets you into trouble—for example, not leaving you with enough time to write a paper or study for an exam?

Or with the patient who describes his experience in a superficial and polarized fashion, the interviewer might inquire as follows:

> Do you tend to see yourself, others, or situations in black-and-white, all-or-nothing terms?

> Does it happen that you idealize people, expecting a lot from them or even putting them up on a pedestal, only to realize after a while that they weren't all you thought they were? Do you then feel very disappointed in them and find fault with them?

In interactions with the interviewer during the consultation, the patient who relies predominantly on splitting-based defenses will often employ defenses that involve controlling the interviewer in one way or another; in particular, projective identification, omnipotent control, and idealization/devaluation can be diagnosed in the countertransference during the clinical assessment of the patient with severe personality pathology. For example, the interviewer may become aware that he has sidestepped certain central issues for fear of angering the patient; or that he has been uncharacteristically "gentle and encouraging," fearing that the patient is "fragile" and "needs to be handled with special care"; or perhaps that his interactions with the patient are leaving him feeling uncharacteristically devalued and irritated.

Moving from the severe personality disorders toward the healthier end of the BPO spectrum, the interviewer continues to see the impact of splitting and dissociative defenses but typically in more subtle forms and in a manner that is less pervasive, interfering less dramatically or more focally with functioning, and combined with an admixture of higher-level defenses. For example, a young woman, happily married, noted that she would periodically find her opinion of her husband abruptly shifting—from seeing him as an ideal partner to considering him irritating and boring. The patient described doing her best not to act on the coldness she felt at the latter times, aware that her feelings were inconsistent with her usual, somewhat idealized feelings toward her husband.

In contrast to splitting-based defenses, repression-based defenses can be more difficult to identify in a diagnostic interview because they are less likely to affect the patient's behavior or the interviewer's experience. As a result, the interviewer tends to infer rather than observe the predominance of repression-based defenses when he sees personality rigidity in conjunction with a consolidated stable, integrated, and realistic sense of self and others. Repression-based defenses will be reflected primarily in rigidity of functioning; difficulty coping with stress and change; and/or a history of repetitive, maladaptive behavior patterns that the patient is either unaware of or unable to change—in contrast to the flexible and adaptive coping mechanisms characteristic of the normal personality. In the diagnostic interview, maladaptive personality traits reflecting activation of repression-based defenses, such as an excessive need to please or to feel in control, may be enacted in the patient's interactions with the interviewer.

Healthy defenses are more or less conscious coping mechanisms, as expressed, for example, in the patient's use of humor to deal with a painful situation, or in her planning ahead to manage anxiety associated with a stressful event. As is the case with splitting-based defenses, healthy defenses can be assessed directly through focal inquiry:

> When you anticipate stressful events or periods of time in your life, do you take time in advance to plan how you will handle the stress?

> When plans that you are counting on fall through, are you the kind of person who can easily adapt, roll with the punches, and make a new plan, or do you tend to get stuck when this happens?

Management of Aggression: Internally and Externally Directed

Assessment of the individual's capacity to manage aggression plays a central role in evaluation of personality disorders. As personality pathology becomes more severe, maladaptive expressions of poorly integrated forms of aggression tend to play an increasingly central role in pathological personality functioning. Aggression is often expressed in behavior, either toward others or toward the self, and as a result assessment of aggression tends to be largely behaviorally focused.

If management of aggression is a central problem, this will most often become evident during the clinical interview when discussion focuses on the history of presenting problems and current personality functioning. Specific questions pertaining to aggression included in the psychiatric review of systems—including questions about a history of self-destructive or destructive behavior, aggressive outbursts, and verbal or physical threats or assault—should not be overlooked in assessment of personality pathology. Self-directed aggression can be as severe and disruptive as aggression directed toward others. Milder forms of self-directed aggression may manifest as chronic suicidal ideation or self-destructive fantasy, self-neglect, skin picking, or risk-taking behaviors. As severity increases, the therapist sees purposeful self-harm—for example, cutting, burning, or sublethal suicide attempts—and at the most severe end of the spectrum, there may be chronic engagement in severe or potentially lethal self-harming or parasuicidal behavior.

Specific inquiry in relation to expression of aggression, initiated in a systematic fashion by the interviewer, is essential in the evaluation of personality disorders. Patients may actively conceal a history of aggressive behavior or, under the impact of dissociation or denial, may not think to mention it during the initial interview unless explicitly asked.

Here are some questions that the interviewer might ask:

Do you sometimes neglect your physical health? For example, do you go to the doctor when you are ill? Do you take care of injuries? Have there been serious consequences to your neglect?

Do you sometimes do things that seem unwise and potentially dangerous, such as having unprotected sex, engaging in heavy drinking or drug use, or getting yourself into situations in which you could be in physical danger?

Do you hurt, cut, or cause physical pain to yourself—for example, by scratching, cutting, or picking your skin; picking at pimples; binge eating or purging food; or doing other things?

Have you made a suicide attempt in the past 5 years?

Do you tend to lose your temper with others? Can you give me an example of when this happened recently?

In the past 5 years, have you at any time intentionally harmed someone physically? If yes, please tell me what happened.

In addition to inquiring about behavioral expression of aggression, the interviewer also evaluates internal, subjective expressions of aggression, such as overwhelming feelings of envy, intense hatred, or recurrent, often pleasurable fantasies of revenge. The following are examples of questions:

> Do you enjoy causing or witnessing the pain or suffering of others, emotional or physical?

> If someone has hurt you or you feel slighted or mistreated, do you find yourself responding with a wish to seek revenge on that person? Do you play out scenes of revenge in your head? Have you actually set those scenes in motion, enacting scenarios involving revenge?

Moral Functioning

As with the evaluation of aggression, evaluation of moral functioning is less central when evaluating patients along the NPO spectrum. In patients with higher level personality pathology, there are relatively well-integrated and stable internalized value systems and moral functioning. To the extent that pathology of ethical functioning interferes with other functioning, these patients may demonstrate inflexibility, often characterized by a tendency toward excessive self-criticism and unduly high internal standards. As the clinician moves into and through the BPO spectrum of personality organization, evaluation of moral values becomes an increasingly central, and ultimately critical, aspect of assessment. As with assessment of aggression, assessment of moral functioning is largely behavioral, combined with evaluation of the patient's experience (or lack) of an internal moral compass and capacity for experiencing guilt.

Within the spectrum of patients presenting with identity pathology, moral functioning can be quite variable (see Figure 2–1 and Table 2–1 in Chapter 2). Individuals with milder forms of identity pathology, typically falling into the high-BPO group, often present with value systems that are not fully internalized or are inconsistent. A patient's moral values can be seen to guide behavior in some areas, even rigidly so, but may coexist with "lacunae" (e.g., a scientist dedicated to the ethics of his field falsifies data; a nurse, highly conscientious about patient care and excessively self-critical in relation to any self-perceived shortcomings in her work, forges prescriptions). Alternatively, moral functioning may be more consistently organized, but largely in relation to fears of getting caught rather than internalized values; in other cases, excessively harsh or rigid moral functioning is colored by aggressive and painful self-attack for even minor transgressions (e.g., a young man viciously berates and attacks himself for days after a minor oversight at work, becoming anxious and somewhat paranoid in relation to his superiors).

More severe pathology of moral functioning involves lying, cheating, and stealing. Some individuals may chronically use deception (e.g., a respected member of the clergy is found to have pilfered from his church's coffers for years; after many years of marriage, a wife discovers that her loving husband and the father of her children, often traveling for work, has long concealed that he has a second family in another city). Further along the spectrum of pathology of moral functioning are manifestations in the form of frankly aggressive antisocial behavior—for example, blackmail, embezzlement, robbery, or assault. At the most severe end of the spectrum, beyond the presence of antisocial behavior or traits, is the total breakdown of all moral functioning and standards, which characterizes antisocial personality disorder. There is evidence that standard psychological interventions for antisocial and psychopathic individuals is ineffective, and multifaceted treatment programs may provide the best hope for some success (Patrick 2007).

In evaluations of patients with severe personality disorders, assessment of moral functioning becomes a critical—perhaps the *most* critical—consideration, guiding differential treatment planning and greatly (adversely) impacting prognosis. As a result, specific questions designed to facilitate a complete review of systems of moral functioning and antisocial behavior are essential in assessment of patients with personality disorders, especially those with more severe pathology. These questions might include the following:

> Are there times when you deliberately deceive others—for example, stretching the truth on a résumé or job application, or plagiarizing someone else's work? Do you tell outright lies? Have you been deceptive or untruthful in answering questions in this interview?

> In the past 5 years, have you done anything illegal? Do you have a criminal record?

> Have you ever engaged in shoplifting or stealing, or in illicit drug use or drug trafficking? Have you had sex in exchange for money or drugs?

> Have you ever embezzled money, written checks that you knew were not good, or failed to pay your taxes?

In contexts in which significant pathology of moral functioning is diagnosed or suspected, it becomes necessary to involve third parties (significant others, parents, siblings, or guardians) in the evaluation process, in order to obtain an accurate history and to complete the assessment of the patient who cannot be relied on to provide honest information about herself. Patients in this group—even those who do not meet criteria for antisocial personality disorder proper—carry a poor prognosis and present significant treatment challenges. Individuals with extremely poor moral functioning (STIPO-R Levels 4–5) fall in the low-BPO group (see Table 2–1 in Chapter 2). Any form of treatment of patients in this group will require special conditions, including a highly structured treatment frame and ongoing involvement of third parties, to manage antisocial features and accurately inform the therapist of the patient's behavior outside sessions. In the high-BPO group, the presence versus absence, as well as the extent, of significant pathology of moral functioning is an especially helpful predictor of treatment course and prognosis.

Methods and Procedures

Thus far, we have focused predominantly on the flow of the interview and the data collected during the assessment phase that enable the interviewer to make a complete diagnostic evaluation of the patient, her difficulties, and her personality, and that are used to guide treatment planning. We turn now to a consideration of the process by which these data are acquired.

There are different ways to collect the data needed for assessment of patients with personality pathology. In research settings, self-report questionnaires and structured interviews are favored insofar as they enhance reliability and ensure even coverage of core domains across raters. However, in clinical settings, most practitioners prefer the clinical diagnostic interview, often complemented by self-report questionnaires, and this is our preference as well (Clarkin et al. 2018). Although structured assessments may improve reliability, the clinical diagnostic interview enables the interviewer to attend not only to the contents of the patient's verbal communication of her difficulties and her responses to the evaluator's questions, but also to the patient's behavior during the consultation, her interactions with the interviewer, and the interviewer's countertransference (i.e., the clinical interview can make use of the *three channels of communication*, as discussed in Chapter 4).

Although different clinicians favor different approaches to the clinical interview, what matters is that at the end of the process, the data and domains of functioning outlined in Table 7–1 (earlier in this chapter) have been clearly elaborated. The TFP-E approach to the clinical interview 1) evaluates descriptive features of personality functioning and pathology while 2) inquiring about the patient's understanding of and attitudes toward her problems and 3) attending to her experience in the interview and of the interviewer. This multipronged approach, derived from the Structural Interview (Kernberg 1984), enables the interviewer to evaluate defensive functioning and reflective capacities in real time, while at the same time obtaining a psychiatric history. Discussed further in the next section of this chapter, the Structural Interview is designed to distinguish BPO from NPO; it focuses on assessing identity formation and defenses, as well as reality testing and subtle forms of psychosis. At the same time, descriptive information about symptoms and personality traits typically gathered in a general psychiatric interview is obtained.

The overall structure of the content domains explored in the Structural Interview follows the flow outlined in Table 7–1 earlier in this chapter. Within this overall linear structure, however, the interviewer has a great deal of flexibility. As he moves through the interview, he will toggle back and forth between taking the history and attending to the patient's behavior and experience in the interview. Also, during the course of the interview, the interviewer will return—repeatedly, if need be—to material that was initially unclear or is contradictory with material emerging later. This recursive process is especially helpful with BPO patients, whose communications about themselves and their difficulties are often vague, incomplete, and/or contradictory and confusing, and who often rapidly develop transferences to the assessor in the initial meetings.

This overall framework for the clinical interview—moving through content domains while toggling between history and experience in the interview, and returning in a cyclical fashion throughout the interview to material that is unclear or contradictory—will bring to light the nature of the patient's defenses as they impact her communications in the interview and her experience of the interviewer. At each level of inquiry, information is acquired and used to generate hypotheses that will guide and focus the clinician's approach at the next level of inquiry. As the interviewer moves through the interview, he assimilates a progressively more fully developed understanding of the patient's personality functioning and organization, circling back to a previous level of inquiry to clarify any areas that emerge as contradictory or that remain unclear.

The Structural Interview

The TFP-E approach to the clinical interview is derived from Kernberg's (1984) Structural Interview. The Structural Interview is a loosely structured clinical interview that can be administered by an experienced clinician in approximately 90 minutes, making use of the interviewer's clinical judgment and skill. The interview focuses on the patient's symptoms and pathological personality traits, as well as the functional difficulties associated with them; on the patient's capacity to reflect on her difficulties; and on the particular ways in which her problems are manifested in her interactions with the interviewer.

In the Structural Interview, the consultant will periodically diverge from exploring the patient's difficulties and level of functioning in order to make use of clarification and confrontation, employed to highlight and explore the defensive operations and conflictual issues activated in the patient-interviewer interaction. This process provides the interviewer with additional data that complement what the patient provides in her narrative; ultimately, this process enables the clinician to rule out psychotic illness and to pursue the differential diagnosis of neurotic versus borderline level of personality organization.

During the course of the Structural Interview, the interviewer will ask for *clarification* of the patient's subjective experience whenever information is vague, is unclear, or contains gaps. In addition, the interviewer will use *confrontation* to gently point out omissions or contradictions in the patient's narrative, or inconsistencies between verbal and nonverbal communications. The interviewer will go on to ask how the patient understands these contradictions or inconsistencies, and will encourage the patient to provide additional information that might clarify what has been occurring. For example, the interviewer might say, "I notice that you are describing your wife in quite negative terms. Earlier you told me that she was the best partner you could imagine. How does this fit together?"

The interviewer will pay close attention to how the patient responds to these interventions; this sequence challenges the patient to reflect on and explore defensively organized behaviors and communications, and provides the interviewer with the opportunity to evaluate the patient's capacity to do so. In the end, the consultant will combine the clinical history with what he hears about the patient's subjective experience and what he observes in the patient's behavior and interactions with him during the interview, in order to make inferences about the patient's level of personality organization.

The Structural Interview is divided into four phases and a final phase that provide an overall structure to the interviewer's approach and that correspond quite closely with the outline provided in Table 7–1. The phases are as follows:

- Phase I: Presenting complaints and symptoms and general psychiatric data

- Phase II: Personality functioning
- Phase III: Identity formation
- Phase IV: Past history
- Final phase: Outstanding issues and questions

Phase I: Presenting Complaints and Symptoms and General Psychiatric Data

The clinical diagnostic interview begins with inquiries about the patient's presenting difficulties. The interviewer begins with a request for information, saying something like "Please tell me what brought you to this interview. What is the nature of your difficulties, and what are your expectations as to how treatment might be of help to you?" This opening provides the patient with the opportunity to discuss her symptoms, her chief reasons for coming to treatment, and any other difficulties she is experiencing in her present life.

In listening to the patient, the interviewer can assess the patient's awareness of her pathology, her appreciation of the need for treatment, and the degree to which her expectations of treatment are realistic or unrealistic. Failures of reality testing and thought disorders typically become apparent quickly as the patient struggles (or fails to struggle) to answer this complex, abstract, and unstructured request for information. Further, patients with poorly consolidated identity often identify themselves by responding to the initial inquiry with apparently thoughtless and chaotic presentation of their difficulties, life situation, and expectations for treatment.

If the patient responds to the initial request for information in a fashion that is easy to follow and understand, clearly describing her symptoms and presenting problems and responding appropriately to the interviewer's request for clarification, the first part of the interview closely resembles a general psychiatric interview. The interviewer proceeds through the history of present illness, past psychiatric history, treatment history, and psychiatric and medical review of systems. In contrast, if the patient's responses to these early inquiries and/or her behavior in the interview are poorly organized, peculiar, or confusing, the interviewer focuses attention in this area, or makes a note to return to it later. The interviewer begins by pointing out areas of vagueness or contradiction, asking for clarification, and inquiring as to whether the patient can understand the interviewer's confusion. Patients with psychotic disorders have difficulty following this line of inquiry and understanding the interviewer's confusion, while becoming increasingly disorganized.

Clinical Illustration 1:
Structural Interview of Ms. A,[3] Phase I

Ms. A, a 30-year-old single woman, was referred for treatment by her general practitioner. She arrived at the interview with Dr. U casually but stylishly dressed, wearing makeup and having well-coiffed hair. The interviewer began with the standard opening to the Structural Interview, made up of a series of open-ended questions:

Dr. U: What are the problems that bring you here? Are there other difficulties in your life? What do you hope to get out of treatment? [*The complex and relatively unstructured nature of these questions requires that the patient have a clear sensorium and is an initial screen for psychotic illness.*]
Ms. A: I'm depressed. It's gotten so bad that I've spent the past 2 weeks in bed. I can't stop crying. I feel paralyzed—literally can't move. I can't go on. I wake up, can't face it, and go back to sleep—cannot leave my bed.
Dr. U: What is it you cannot face?
Ms. A: My life—it's a disaster. Nobody cares about me. There's no point.... I just can't face my life. I just lie there.

At this point, Dr. U inquired about neurovegetative symptoms of depression, which were negative. Ms. A denied suicidal ideation but endorsed a feeling of "not wanting to go on." Dr. U decided to learn more about Ms. A's present difficulties and why she was staying in bed.

Dr. U: How long have you been depressed like this?
Ms. A: A month now. I can't get out of it—I can't move.
Dr. U: Has this happened to you before?

Ms. A gave a history of several similar episodes, of variable duration, over the past 10 years. She had been treated with various antidepressants, with minimal benefit.

Dr. U: When you became depressed a month ago, how were things going? Were you aware of anything that triggered the depression?
Ms. A: My boyfriend, Mike, broke up with me. Well, he wasn't my boyfriend *really.* I knew him through work for many years; we were best friends and then we got involved. But he said he didn't believe in monogamy. He never lied—and

---

[3]This case illustration is of an interview with a BPO patient. For a detailed illustration of an interview with an NPO patient, we refer the reader to Caligor et al. (2007), Chapter 9, "Patient Assessment and Differential Treatment Planning," pp. 175–201.

honesty is really important to me, so I'm glad he was honest. But he would never go out with me or meet my family. It was all on his terms; he'd call me to come over at night. I was in love with him and thought he was in love with me. He was so patient with me, so kind. But then about a month ago, out of the blue, he told me he wanted to be on his own.

Dr. U: Did it bother you that he saw other women?

Ms. A: Of course it did! It drove me crazy. We fought all the time about it.

Dr. U: So is that why you two broke up?

Ms. A: No—like I said, it was out of the blue. I have no clue what happened. He said he'd given me plenty of warning, had been suggesting I move on for a long time, but that I wouldn't hear it. But I don't think that's really true. And now he won't talk to me, won't answer my texts.

Dr. U was struck by Ms. A's rather chaotic and seemingly contradictory description of Mike and of their relationship. Dr. U planned to return to this issue in later phases of the interview. Before doing so, Dr. U decided to ask Ms. A about other symptoms, inquiring about anxiety disorders, eating disorders, bipolar or psychotic illness, attentional disorders, learning disabilities, and substance abuse. Ms. A endorsed a lifelong history of intermittent "panic attacks," typically lasting hours to days, treated with clonazepam. She carried a diagnosis of attention-deficit/hyperactivity disorder, also treated with medication in the past. She denied a history of self-destructive, dishonest, or illegal behavior. She had never been hospitalized.

Phase II: Personality Functioning

The second phase of the interview involves inquiring about the patient's personality. The interviewer begins by following up on aspects of the patient's personality functioning that have emerged in earlier parts of the interview, filling in whatever was unclear and revisiting areas of confusion. In this portion of the interview, the evaluator prompts the patient to describe her interpersonal functioning, her current functioning at work and her work history, and her use of leisure time. The possibility of a diagnosis of clinically significant identity pathology is raised if, in the course of presenting further data about herself, the patient conveys information that the interviewer cannot put together in his mind—particularly contradictory data that do not fit with the internal image of the patient and her life that the interviewer is building (e.g., a patient's chief complaint was that he was excessively anxious, passive, and timid, yet later in the interview, when describing his work history, he told the interviewer that he had recently been fired after an employee under his supervision complained that the patient had bullied him and other coworkers).

This is a juncture in the interview at which tactful probing of potential or apparent contradictions may be indicated in order to evaluate the extent to which contradictory self-images are present or the extent to which the patient presents a solid, well-integrated conception of herself, if this is unclear. The goal is to distinguish higher level personality pathology, in which conflictual aspects of functioning are split off from a consolidated, central self experience, from identity diffusion, in which there is a lack of central sense of self and instead a globally dissociated quality of self experience. In practice, this distinction is generally made quite easily; by exploring areas of apparent contradiction in the communications from patients with significant identity pathology, the interviewer can identify multiple contradictory aspects of functioning and self experience in the absence of an underlying or central sense of self. (For example, upon further probing, the anxious, passive patient fired for being a bully described shifting self states: at times feeling superior to everyone else, which was seen as justification for bullying those beneath him, and at other times feeling that he was inferior and that those same employees beneath him were contemptuous of him.)

Clinical Illustration 1 (continued): Structural Interview of Ms. A, Phase II

Dr. U began to systematically evaluate Ms. A's present life situation and functioning. He introduced this line of inquiry: "I have gotten a pretty clear sense of the symptoms and difficulties that bring you to treatment. Can you tell me now about how you function in your daily life, and about the ways in which your difficulties have or have not interfered with your functioning?" In this way, Dr. U examined both Ms. A's current functioning and her longer-term functioning in order to differentiate between a present disorder (e.g., a depressive episode) and more chronic impairment (e.g., long-term low functioning due to a personality disorder). This is accomplished by referring to different time frames and modes of functioning, as well as frequency, pervasiveness, and severity of the behavior under investigation (e.g., "Is this how you typically deal with work problems?").

Dr. U inquired in detail about Ms. A's vocational functioning, relationships, romantic life, and use of free time, as well as what impact, if any, her symptoms had on her functioning in these areas. With some effort by making extensive use of clarification to organize Ms. A's communications in her own mind, Dr. U ascertained that Ms. A had held several entry-level jobs since graduating from college but lacked professional direction, skills, or interests. The patient reported that she had most recently been working on and off as an assistant to the brother of Mike, the man who had recently broken up with her. When her relationship with Mike ended, Ms. A precipitously left her job with his brother. She was currently unemployed and looking into collecting unemployment benefits.

Ms. A had a circle of women friends, several dating back to middle school. She described these relationships as stormy and for the most part unsatisfactory, with several more positive connections with friends currently living in other cities. She had had a series of long-term romantic relationships with men, all ending in her being rejected. She lived alone and spent her days watching television, going to the gym, and meeting up with friends. She described wanting a career but had no specific professional goals and no personal interests.

Dr. U noted to herself that Ms. A's functioning was consistent with BPO; she lacked professional or personal goals, she described significant pathology in her interpersonal and romantic life, she felt directionless and empty, and she had no developed interests. The absence of antisocial features, the presence of a capacity to sustain long-term relationships with men (albeit unsatisfactory ones) and to maintain a circle of friends, and the absence of highly aggressive behavior suggested high BPO.

Phase III: Identity Formation

The next step in the Structural Interview is to focus explicitly on identity formation by asking the patient to provide a description of herself and of a significant other, and then targeting any remaining lack of clarity in the quality of object relations, moral functioning, or aggression in order to evaluate the level of personality organization and to guide treatment planning. This is another juncture in the interview that provides an opportunity for tactful confrontation of vagueness and contradictions.

As illustrated by the vignette of Ms. A, much of the data needed to evaluate personality organization will have already emerged spontaneously and in the answers to follow-up questions in earlier portions of the diagnostic interview, in the course of evaluating maladaptive personality traits and overall personality functioning. By the time these initial portions of the clinical interview have been completed, the experienced interviewer will typically already have a fairly clear understanding of the patient's level of personality organization on the basis of what she has communicated about her personality functioning and how she has communicated it, as well as her interactions with the interviewer.[4]

In the TFP-E approach, the therapist concludes the personality assessment by evaluating the patient's sense of self and others with open-ended questions that invite the patient to provide a self-description and to describe a significant other. In clinically evaluating the patient's response, the therapist attends not only to the content of what the patient says but also to the process of thinking and articulation in which the patient engages. For example, is she coherent and specific or is she vague and disorganized? Is she thoughtful or is she glib? Is she able to be reflective? The interviewer follows up on the patient's responses by tactfully pointing out discrepancies, contradictions, omissions, and/or notable patterns that have emerged during the course of the interview.

The extent to which the patient can engage in a lucid, detailed, and multilayered construction of a description of herself and of her significant others is an indication of identity integration versus pathology and helps the interviewer determine the level of personality organization. In addition, these questions allow the interviewer to learn more about the patient's inner experience and to identify more subtle forms of identity pathology, as well as better-integrated narcissistic pathology, which may present with a relatively stable sense of self but can be clearly identified at this point in the interview by virtue of the often dramatic vagueness and superficiality in descriptions of significant others.

The following two video clips illustrate the impact of a severe identity disturbance (Video 1) in contrast to normally consolidated identity (Video 2) on a patient's capacity to provide a coherent self-description.

In Video 1, "Assessment of Identity Integration: Borderline Level of Personality Organization," Dr. Caligor is evaluating a man who presented with suicidal ideation after the breakup of a relationship. The patient initially responds with confusion to Dr. Caligor's request that he describe himself, and the description he ultimately provides is superficial, sparse, and polarized, all reflective of severe identity pathology. Later in the interview, Dr. Caligor completes her evaluation of the patient's identity formation by asking him to provide a description of a significant other. Consistent with the patient's self-description, his description of his former girlfriend is vague, superficial, and highly idealized. This video clip illustrates the impact of identity disturbance on the capacity to organize a coherent description of self or other. Specifically, we see the impact of splitting, idealization, and lower level denial on the patient's experience of himself and of his girlfriend.

---

[4]For example, in describing many brief, chaotic, and failed romantic relationships or recurrent problems with employers, a patient will provide the interviewer with information about the patient's experience of others and the quality of his object relations. Similarly, the interviewer will gather information about moral functioning by listening to a patient describe his marriage in terms of financial exploitation, or his interruptions in his work history in terms of recurrent episodes of petty theft in the workplace, and by exploring the patient's attitude toward his own behavior. In the TFP-E approach, the interviewer uses these moments to ask specific questions that target and elaborate expressions of pathology, as outlined in earlier sections of this chapter.

Video Illustration 1
Assessment of Identity Integration:
Borderline Level of Personality Organization (8:33)

In Video 2, "Assessment of Identity Integration: Self Description; Normal Identity Formation," Dr. Caligor evaluates a young woman who presented with anxiety and problems with self-esteem. As in Video 1, Dr. Caligor asks the patient to describe herself. In contrast to the patient in Video 1, this patient is able to provide a clear, specific, and nuanced description of her personality, consistent with normal identity formation. Also consistent with a fully consolidated identity, in response to Dr. Caligor's pointing out a potential contradiction in her narrative, the patient demonstrates a high level of self-awareness and reflectiveness.

Video Illustration 2
Assessment of Identity Integration: Self Description;
Normal Identity Formation (3:36)

Clinical Illustration 1 *(continued)*: Structural Interview of Ms. A, Phase III

Dr. U began by asking Ms. A to provide an in-depth description of herself.

> Dr. U: You have told me about your symptoms and your difficulties. I'd like now to shift gears a bit, to hear more about you as a person. Could you describe yourself, your personality, what you think is important for me to know about you, the way you perceive yourself, the way you feel others perceive you, anything you think might be helpful for me to get a real feeling for you as a person.
>
> Ms. A [*appearing confused*]: What do you mean? What do you want to know? I've been depressed—is that what you mean?
>
> Dr. U: You've told me about your depression. I'd like now to hear more about you as a person—what you're like. For example, if you were to write a paragraph about yourself, what would you include so that I could get to know who you are as a person and what your personality is like?
>
> Ms. A: Well, I guess I'd say I'm stupid. And I can't get anything right. And my family always picks on me. Is that what you mean?

> Dr. U: Well, are there other things about you as a person, things that would be important to know about you?
>
> Ms. A: Other than that I'm stupid and unemployed and don't have a boyfriend?
>
> Dr. U: Are there positive things you would say about yourself?
>
> Ms. A: Well, I think I'm a nice person. In fact, I'm too nice. Everyone takes advantage of me. I always do what other people want.

Dr. U viewed the impoverished and inconsistent quality of Ms. A's sense of herself, along with the marked difficulty she had in approaching his questioning, as supporting the impression of identity pathology. Consistent with this, Dr. U noted that Ms. A's description of herself as "too nice" and excessively accommodating was frankly discrepant with her behavior with Dr. U early in the interview, when she had seemed at times petulant and quietly oppositional.

Dr. U moved on to ask Ms. A for a description of a significant other.

> Dr. U: I would now like to ask you about the people who are most important to you in your current life. For example, who is the person who is most important to you right now?
>
> Ms. A: The most important person to me is Mike. Even though we've broken up, I still think about him all the time, and he is the most important person to me. Even now I love him and cannot live without him.

Dr. U noted the self-referential quality of Ms. A's description of Mike, and her lack of information about Mike as an individual.

> Dr. U: Can you tell me more about Mike so that I might form a real, live impression of him? What is he like as a person—how would you describe his personality?
>
> Ms. A: He is the only person who has ever understood me. He was so kind and patient with me. No one has ever treated me so well. He made me feel so safe. He was my best friend. He was always supportive.

Dr. U was again struck by the superficial, idealized, and self-referential description that Ms. A provided, confirming his impression of Ms. A's identity pathology. He decided to complete the assessment of identity pathology by offering a tactful confrontation of Ms. A's contradictory description of Mike, to see if the patient could be reflective and possibly integrate Dr. U's comments, to some degree.

> Dr. U: You are telling me now that Mike is the only person who has understood you, that he was kind and patient and he made you feel safe. I remember that earlier in the interview, you painted a different picture: you told me that he wasn't faithful to you,

> which was very upsetting to you and became the cause of arguments. What do you make of that seeming contradiction?
>
> Ms. A: He was just wonderful, that's what I'm telling you. You really don't understand—the other stuff is meaningless, and he never lied to me.

Thus, Ms. A responded to Dr. U's confrontation by maintaining a highly idealized view of Mike, denying the impact of the negative history she had described and demonstrating a lack of concern or reflectiveness in response to Dr. U's intervention. This response to confrontation was further evidence of identity disturbance and reliance on the defenses of splitting, idealization, and lower-level denial. Dr. U followed up to see whether, with prompting, Ms. A might be able to empathize with his confusion, a final check on her reality testing.

> Dr. U: What is it that I do not understand? Can you see why I might be confused by what you are telling me?
>
> Ms. A [*now somewhat more reflective*]: I get it—why this is all confusing. I know this may sound crazy, but without personally knowing Mike and how special he is, you wouldn't be able to get the picture.

At this point, the diagnosis of high BPO, as opposed to NPO or more severe personality disorder or psychosis, seemed clear to Dr. U—as manifested by identity pathology and use of lower-level defenses and intact reality testing, in the presence of relatively intact moral functioning, the capacity to establish and maintain long-term friendships and romantic relations, and the absence of a significant history of overtly aggressive behavior, either inwardly or outwardly directed.

Phase IV: Past History

Once the interviewer has a clear picture of the patient's presenting difficulties, personality functioning, and level of personality organization, he briefly inquires about the patient's past as it relates to her current difficulties. In Phase IV, the interviewer obtains information about the patient's developmental history and her current and past relationships with parents and siblings. When a patient has higher level personality pathology, information regarding the patient's past follows naturally from exploration of her present personality. The patient's description of her history and her family of origin deepens the interviewer's understanding of the patient and typically enables the interviewer to develop preliminary hypotheses about the nature and origins of the patient's conflicts.

In contrast, when a patient has identity pathology, information about the past is generally sufficiently contaminated by the patient's present personality difficulties that it becomes difficult to know how to make use of the information the patient provides. The patient's descriptions of her past will be as confusing, chaotic, and internally contradictory as her descriptions of her current life. As a result, interviewing a patient with severe personality pathology requires careful assessment of her present life, identity consolidation, and quality of object relations in order to obtain the data necessary for assessment of personality pathology; at this point, it is preferable to explore the past only along general lines, without trying to clarify or confront the patient's characterizations of her past experiences. The interviewer focuses on obtaining a general history, including information about the patient's family members and about her important, meaningful, positive relationships while growing up (a positive prognostic sign), as well as any history of antisocial behavior (a negative prognostic sign).

Clinical Illustration 1 (continued): Structural Interview of Ms. A, Phase IV

In response to Dr. U's queries, Ms. A described her family members in highly polarized terms. She described her mother and siblings entirely negatively, in words colored by hostility and resentment, but presented a more idealized, though somewhat contradictory, picture of her father. Ms. A's descriptions of her early life, adolescence, and post-college years were vague and superficial. She had graduated from both high school and college in specialized programs for students with attention-deficit/hyperactivity disorder and learning disorders. Her academic history was marked by multiple failures, leaves of absence, and changes of schools.

Ms. A's description of the details of her rather lengthy history with Mike, her boyfriend, spanned much of her adult life and was vague, confusing, and extremely inconsistent. Friends were poorly differentiated from one another, and apart from her relationship with Mike, no single past relationship emerged as especially important or meaningful.

Final Phase: Outstanding Issues and Questions

The final phase of the interview begins with the interviewer acknowledging to the patient that he has completed his task. At this point, the patient is invited to raise any additional issues that she considers important to discuss before moving on to a discussion of diagnosis and recommendations for treatment.

Structured Assessment and the STIPO-R

For assessment of patients in a clinical setting, the clinical interview can be complemented and enriched by a more structured approach. In research settings, structured assessment is required to ensure that patients are evaluated in a uniform fashion and that diagnostic assessments are reliable across different raters and different sites. Both to meet clinical demands and to facilitate the evaluation of personality organization in clinical research trials, we developed the STIPO-R, which is available on our Web site (www.borderlinedisorders.com). The semistructured interview format of the STIPO-R provides a standardized way in which to gather information about personality organization and to score it objectively. **In contrast to the clinical diagnostic interview, the STIPO-R does not inquire about symptoms, past treatment, or personal history.**

Although the STIPO-R was originally developed for research purposes, it can easily be integrated into clinical settings. It serves as a useful educational tool as well; experience with the STIPO-R greatly enhances the skill with which trainees can clinically assess general personality functioning and pathology in their practices. For the clinician who is relatively new to structural assessment and psychodynamic interviewing, the STIPO-R offers a series of specific questions and follow-up probes used to evaluate the dimensions of personality relevant to assessing the level of personality organization.

Within the semistructured format of the STIPO-R, the interviewer has the freedom to follow clinical inference when selecting follow-up probes, and also when selecting from among anchors for scoring, both at the item level and at the domain level. Thus, the STIPO-R represents a semistructured interview format that is flexible, leaving room for clinical judgment while reducing variability across interviewers. Because the flow of the STIPO-R is similar to that of a clinical evaluation, the STIPO-R can be easily introduced into a clinical assessment; patients typically value the experience, learning about themselves in the process and appreciating the clinician's taking the time to be thorough.

The STIPO-R interview takes about 60 minutes to administer. It assesses the same domains of personality functioning as does the clinical assessment of personality organization, while providing clearly formulated questions and anchors to aid the scoring process and the classification of personality organization. The STIPO-R consists of 55 questions assessing six domains: 1) identity, 2) object relations, 3) lower-level (primitive) defenses, 4) higher-level defenses, 5) aggression, and 6) moral values (see also Chapter 2 for a discussion of the STIPO-R and its role in classification of personality disorders).

Scores are obtained on the item level, following probes and using individual anchors for the item-by-item rating process (e.g., "Do people tell you that you behave in contradictory ways, or would you say that people pretty much know what to expect from you in terms of your behavior?"); scores are also obtained through the consultant's assignment of overall clinical ratings per domain and subdomain (e.g., the patient's sense of self and sense of others). Finally, an overall level of personality organization is assigned clinically, ranging from normal to neurotic to borderline levels of personality organization.

Other instruments have been developed for the systematic assessment of patients who present with personality pathology. The Quality of Object Relations Scale (Piper and Duncan 1999) has been found to predict patients' responses to different forms of brief psychotherapy. The Shedler-Westen Assessment Procedure (SWAP; Westen and Shedler 1999a, 1999b) uses Q-sort methodology to reliably assess personality and personality pathology. The SWAP is scored on the basis of patients' descriptions of themselves and others, captured in interpersonal narratives in clinical interviews or therapy sessions. The Level of Personality Functioning Scale—Brief Form (Hutsebaut et al. 2016) is a user-friendly self-report instrument that is in development as a quick screener for severity of personality pathology. The Structured Clinical Interview for the DSM-5 Alternative Model of Personality Disorders (SCID-5-AMPD; First et al. 2018) is a newer instrument developed to accompany and enhance research and clinical use of the DSM-5 Section III Alternative Model for Personality Disorders. The interview has three separate modules that respectively assess level of personality functioning, personality traits, and categorical personality disorders.

Personality Types and Diagnosis

In addition to assessing personality organization, the clinical interview will enable the assessor to diagnose one of the following:

- One or more of the 10 personality disorders in DSM-5 Section II, on the basis of the patient meeting those specific diagnostic criteria as emerges during the course of the clinical interview
- DSM-5 other specified personality disorder or DSM-5 unspecified personality disorder, when the patient meets general criteria for a personality disorder but fails to meet full criteria for any one disorder
- No personality disorder (many if not most NPO patients fall into this category), with traits specified

Most of the time, whether the patient meets DSM-5 personality disorder criteria and has dominant maladaptive traits will emerge clearly in the course of the interview, reflected both in the clinical history and in the patient's behavior and interactions with the consultant in the interview. In cases in which DSM-5 diagnostic criteria remain in question after the clinical interview, the interviewer can explicitly evaluate the patient in regard to these criteria to clarify issues of differential diagnosis. For a complete evaluation of traits, when needed, it may be helpful for the interviewer to ask the patient to fill out one or more self-report questionnaires prior to the clinical interview. These could include the carefully developed Schedule for Nonadaptive and Adaptive Personality (SNAP; Clark 1993) or the Personality Inventory for DSM-5 (PID-5; Krueger et al. 2012), which was constructed to accompany the alternative model for personality disorders that appears in DSM-5 Section III.

Figures 7–2, 7–3, and 7–4 summarize the familiar personality disorder types, many of which are included in DSM-5 Section II (see also Chapter 2, Figure 2–2, for the relationship between levels of personality organization and DSM-5 Section II). The framework outlined in these figures provides an extremely useful approach to conceptualizing and classifying familiar personality types. The assessor focuses on the patient's identity integration, affective tone, cognitive style, interpersonal style, and attitude toward self to characterize the patient's personality and then adds to that picture common symptoms associated with the various personality disorders. This information enables the assessor to describe the patient's personality type, while also making inferences about the core dynamics likely underlying the patient's difficulties, and to anticipate initial transferences and dominant object relations likely to emerge early in treatment.

For a comprehensive discussion of the descriptive, psychodynamic, and clinical features of the different types of personality disorders, the following two volumes are especially helpful: *Psychoanalytic Diagnosis: Understanding Personality Structure in the Clinical Process* (McWilliams 1994) and *Psychodynamic Diagnostic Manual*, 2nd Edition (Lingiardi and McWilliams 2017).

	Obsessive-compulsive	Depressive	Hysterical
Identity	Consolidated	Consolidated	Consolidated
Affective tone	Emotionally constricted	Somber Serious	Emotional
Cognitive style	Focused on detail	Thoughtful, thorough	Impressionistic
Interpersonal style	Controlling, stubborn, judgmental	Seeking love Sensitive to loss	Attention seeking Seductive
Attitude toward self	Morally superior Perfectionistic	Perfectionistic Self-critical	Childlike and inadequate, restricted to sexually meaningful settings
Common symptoms	Anxiety, anxious ruminations	Depression, guilty ruminations	Sexual inhibitions
Core dynamics	Compromise formations around oedipal aggression and dependency with defensive retreat to struggles over control of self and others	Intolerance of aggression, which is turned against the self; conflicts around being cared for defend against oedipal conflicts	Oedipal conflicts around sexuality and dependency
Initial transferences/ Dominant object relations	Dutiful but covertly critical, rebellious self and judgmental parent	Pleasing, ingratiating, inferior self and admired caretaker	Engaging, childlike self and admiring, responsive other

FIGURE 7–2. Core descriptive features of personality disorders organized at a neurotic level.

| | INTROVERTED → | | EXTRAVERTED | |
	Avoidant	Dependent	Narcissistic	Histrionic
Identity pathology	Mild failure of consolidation	Mild failure of consolidation	Pathological consolidation ("grandiose self")	Mild failure of consolidation
Affective tone	Anxious and fearful Shameful Depressive	Anxious, needy	Cold	Hyperemotional Superficial
Cognitive style	Vigilant	Variable	Variable, superficial use of detail or vague and exaggerated	Lacking in detail Superficial
Interpersonal style	Shy Hypersensitive to slights or criticism	Ingratiating Submissive Clinging	Seeking attention and admiration Self-focused and unrelated	Demanding of attention Aggressively seductive
Attitude toward self	Inferior Undesirable	Ineffectual Needy	Idealized and grandiose and/or devalued	Infantile, grandiose, eroticized
Common symptoms	Social anxiety, social isolation Imagined derision from others	Fears of abandonment Sadness and fear when relationships end	Failure of intimacy Unstable self-esteem Constant need for attention	Sexual promiscuity Affective lability Temper tantrums
Core dynamics	Conflicts around dependency with projection of aggressive self-criticism and wishes to devalue vulnerable objects	Conflicts around dependency and trust defended against via idealization of powerful significant others and devaluation of self	Split between idealized and devalued images of self interferes with integration; projection of devalued self onto others	Conflicts around dependency with defensive use of sexuality to gratify dependent and aggressive needs
Initial transferences/ Dominant object relations	Inferior, defective, undesirable self and superior, rejecting other	Well-taken-care-of self and idealized caretaker	Detached, therapist as sounding board Superior, grandiose self and inferior, devalued other	Sexually desired and stimulated self and responsive other

FIGURE 7–3. Core descriptive features of personality disorders organized at a high borderline level.

INTROVERTED ⟷ EXTRAVERTED

	Paranoid	Schizoid	Borderline personality disorder	Narcissistic	Antisocial
Identity consolidation	Moderate to severe failure	Moderate to severe failure	Moderate to severe failure	Moderate to severe failure with "grandiose self"	Moderate to severe failure
Affective tone	Hostile, irritable, resentful, fearful	Affectless Flat Absence of anger	Charged, unstable Predominance of negative affect	Cold, hostile	Malevolent
Cognitive style	Hypervigilant Extremely rigid Concrete	Intellectualized Ruminative Internally directed	Vague, extreme Contradictory	Hyperbolic and vague or excessive superficial detail Blurring of fact and convenient fiction	Glib
Interpersonal style	Suspicious Resentful Vindictive Grandiose	Aloof, cold, passive detached, wooden	Dependent, demanding, controlling	Attention-seeking, seductive vs. devaluing, exploitative	Exploitative Sadistic Controlling Contemptuous
Attitude toward self	Under threat Humiliated Despised vs. omnipotent Vindicated, triumphant	Superior Apart Hyperattuned and self-protective	Confusion about identity Self-loathing	Grandiose, may alternate with devalued self states	Superior
Common symptoms	Irritability Suspiciousness Paranoid thoughts	Isolation Apathy Lack of pleasure Lack of interest in sexual relations	Stormy relationships Affective instability Destructive behavior	Unstable self-esteem Need for constant attention Depression, emptiness, boredom	Amorality Lack of empathy Recklessness Somatization

FIGURE 7–4. Core descriptive features of personality disorders organized at middle and low borderline levels.

	Paranoid	Schizoid	Borderline personality disorder	Narcissistic	Antisocial
Core dynamics	Projection of hatred and envy creates world of hostile, devaluing enemies. Projective identification leads to hostile provocation of others	Core conflict between wish for closeness and fear of engulfment met with defensive isolation and withdrawal	Splitting to defend against excess of poorly integrated aggression leads to instability and wish for perfect caretaker	Idealization of the self and projection of devalued aspects of self; need for chronic admiration to sustain grandiose defensive self-structure	Projection of hatred creates world of hostile enemies; failure of idealization leaves only amoral "dog-eat-dog" world
Initial transferences/ Dominant object relations	Persecuted, hateful self and critical, devaluing, superior other	Emotionally distant, grandiose self and intrusive, omnipotent other	Paranoid, enraged victim-self and victimizer-other; or perfectly gratified self and idealized caretakerg	Dismissive, superior, ideal self and inferior, devalued other	Dishonest, manipulative self and threatening, manipulative, and deceitful other

FIGURE 7–4. Core descriptive features of personality disorders organized at middle and low borderline levels. (*continued*)

Part 2

Sharing the Diagnostic Impression and Differential Treatment Planning

THE FIRST HALF OF THE CONSULTATION, discussed in Part 1, is organized around acquiring the information needed to make DSM-5 and structural diagnoses. The second half of the consultation involves 1) sharing the diagnostic impression with the patient, 2) determining treatment goals, and 3) reviewing the available treatment options and helping the patient make an informed choice regarding the kind of treatment(s) to pursue.

Sharing the Diagnostic Impression and Psychoeducation

The second half of the consultation begins with the interviewer sharing his diagnostic impressions with the patient. It is important that the consultant, in sharing his impressions, review both symptomatic disorders *and* personality pathology. It is not uncommon that a patient with a personality disorder will never have been told of the diagnosis, despite a long and complex history of treatment. The consultant's description of the patient's difficulties and discussion of diagnostic issues should be clear, neutral, and as specific as possible, linking discussion of diagnosis to the patient's presenting problems. Throughout this process, the consultant should avoid using technical terms or jargon. After completing the task of sharing the diagnosis, the consultant will educate the patient about the implications of the diagnosis, including course, etiology, and associated symptoms, as well as expected outcome if the patient does not pursue treatment.

In the TFP-E approach, when discussing diagnostic issues, the consultant first offers a summary of the patient's symptoms, presenting difficulties and maladaptive personality traits, and then asks the patient if the formulation seems accurate and if there is anything the patient would like to add or modify. At this point, the diagnosis of any symptomatic disorders (anxiety, affective, or eating disorders; substance misuse; or psychosis) should be shared with the patient.

Next, the consultant discusses personality functioning and pathology with the patient. Before addressing DSM-5 diagnoses or personality disorder types, the consultant discusses personality pathology by focusing on the issue of identity formation and personality rigidity, two central aspects of self functioning and functioning with others. This approach serves multiple functions in that it 1) provides the patient with an experience-near description of his difficulties; 2) introduces a way to relate the patient's seemingly disparate presenting complaints; 3) begins the process of educating the patient about personality functioning and disorder; and 4) introduces self and interpersonal functioning as potential organizers of the patient's difficulties and targets of treatment.

When discussing neurotic-level personality pathology with patients, the consultant begins by addressing personality *rigidity*. She highlights whatever maladaptive patterns have emerged in the consultation, framing them as reflective of familiar, self-protective ways of viewing the self and others, and as an inability to fully, comfortably experience certain aspects of self experience that are out of awareness but somehow threatening.

When discussing personality disorder with BPO patients, the consultant organizes discussion around the construct of identity, helping the patient to conceptualize his problems from the perspective of his having an incompletely consolidated or unstable sense of self that makes it difficult for him to feel at ease, interferes with his ability to function to the best of his ability in relationships and work/studies, and makes it difficult to organize and pursue long-term goals.

In discussions with NPO patients, it is generally neither helpful nor necessarily accurate to use the term *personality disorder*.[5] To describe higher level personality pathology in terms of a personality disorder can be confusing to patients and is to some degree misleading. Instead, the consultant explains the constructs of personality and personality rigidity and dis-

---

[5]In the TFP-E approach, neurotic-level pathology is most accurately described as clinically significant but *subthreshold* or *subsyndromal* with regard to the diagnosis of a personality disorder. This practice is consistent with the general consensus that "moderate impairment" is required for diagnosis of a personality disorder (see the Alternative Model for Personality Disorders in DSM-5 Section III, Criterion A).

cusses how they relate to the patient's presenting problems and maladaptive personality traits, perhaps adding comments about personality "style" (e.g., obsessive-compulsive, histrionic, avoidant, narcissistic).

In discussions with BPO patients, it is useful—and also necessary from the perspective of informed consent—to move from discussion of identity to discussion of how identity relates to personality and personality disorder. As to the question of whether to go into specifics of the *type* of disorder during the consultation, the current literature recommends sharing the borderline personality disorder diagnosis (Yeomans et al. 2015), and increasingly the narcissistic personality disorder diagnosis as well (Caligor and Petrini 2016); these diagnoses are increasingly attached to an empirical literature on psychopathology, prognosis, and treatment.

Many if not most BPO patients will not fit clearly into a DSM-5 personality disorder category or will fit into many. Attempting to share a DSM-5 diagnosis may be less helpful for these patients, especially if limited literature is available on a given disorder. Frequently, however, BPO patients express interest in what kind of personality disorder the consultant is diagnosing, in which case sharing impressions openly and tactfully is recommended. In our experience, discussion of the severity of personality disorder, especially as it links to prognosis, is consistently useful. In sum, in the consultant's discussion of the diagnostic impression, the overall goal is to share with the patient how the consultant thinks about the patient's difficulties and his personality, providing him with a way to think about himself that may be new to him, while also creating a context for the discussion of treatment options.

To illustrate the process of sharing the diagnostic impression with patients of different levels of personality organization, we return to the patients introduced in Clinical Illustrations 1–3 in Chapter 2.

Clinical Illustration 2: Sharing the Diagnostic Impression With an NPO Patient

Ms. N, the 28-year-old teacher with a neurotic level of personality organization who sought help for "problems with men," was introduced in Clinical Illustration 1 in Chapter 2.

> Interviewer: You describe yourself as someone who in many ways is living a full life, with social connections and a profession that you enjoy and value. At the same time, there are certain areas in which you seem to have gotten "stuck" and with which you are not completely satisfied. It seems the central issue on your mind is your romantic

life; you would like a partner but have not been able to find an appropriate one, and you describe feeling less attractive than your friends and not worthy of male attention and admiration. In addition, though seemingly of less concern to you, you describe some difficulty appropriately asserting yourself at times—as you put it, "pushing back"—which can leave you excessively accommodating of others. And finally, you have described a tendency to become overly self-critical when you do not live up to your own relatively high expectations, and a recent lowering of your mood. Would you say this is an accurate summary of the difficulties that you have described?

Ms. N: Yes, it is.

Interviewer: Shall I share with you my understanding of what you have told me, how I put it together in my mind?

Ms. N: Yes, please.

Interviewer: Well, let me say first that different people might have different perspectives on the situation; some might focus first and foremost on your mood, and others perhaps on negative thoughts or on interpersonal skills. But I see the picture in terms of your personality and what I would call rigidity in your personality. When I say *rigidity*, I mean, for example, that in theory you would like to be more flirtatious, but you cannot get yourself to do it, and instead feel shy in social situations where you might meet a man, in your mind automatically ceding to your girlfriends. Similarly, you would like to be more assertive; maybe you even go into certain situations with a plan to stand up for yourself and push back, but then you end up feeling uncomfortable and are unable to follow through. These are behaviors that you would like to change, and you understand you would feel better and be better off if you were able to do so. But it's as though you're stuck in some way; you haven't been able to change these behaviors despite your best efforts. That is what I mean by *rigidity*. Does what I'm saying make sense to you? Shall I go on?

Ms. N: Please do.

Interviewer: It seems to me that perhaps out of your awareness, it is as if you are wedded to a somewhat narrowly defined view of who you are or are supposed to be. You see yourself as a caring and nurturing person who always does her best—something of a "good girl," if you will. While this is perfectly fine, the problem with this view is that it is inflexible; it is as if at some level you believe that you must be *only* this way. If you were to want things for yourself that could involve doing things that in your mind are incompatible with this self-image, you would find it difficult to pursue them; to do so, you would have to broaden your view of yourself, and that's something you've not been able to do. If you try to step out of the box, as it were, and deviate from this rigidly held self-image, you get anxious, you retreat…and we see what I referred to before as *rigidity*. And even more striking, it's as if you're so invested in maintaining this view of yourself that you even fail to see, or neglect feedback that contradicts, this image of yourself. We see this, for example, when you describe feeling surprised at getting attention at a party, even though it has happened many times. Because it's discrepant with your strongly held view of yourself, you can't see it or take it in; you don't fully appreciate how others see you.

Ms. N: I have to admit, I've never really thought about this, even though I guess it's true.... It just feels so wrong to get attention and so surprising whenever it happens. I do understand what you're saying about me.... It seems accurate, but it also makes no sense.

Interviewer: Well, yes and no. Typically, personality rigidity and the kind of difficulties you describe are driven by psychological forces outside our awareness, so on the surface it may not make sense, but from a psychological perspective it does. [*Pause.*] I have said a lot. What are your thoughts about my comments? What are your questions?

As illustrated in the above case, at various points in sharing impressions, the interviewer will leave time for the patient to ask for clarification or to express disagreement; in addition, the interviewer will attend to and explore any nonverbal communication on the part of the patient that reflects her attitude toward what the interviewer is saying—for example, any silent expression of doubt, disagreement, confusion, shame, mistrust, or hostility.

Clinical Illustration 3: Sharing the Diagnostic Impression With a BPO Patient

Ms. B, the 28-year-old patient with a borderline level of personality organization who sought help for "problems with men," was introduced in Clinical Illustration 2 in Chapter 2.

Interviewer: You describe a number of areas of difficulty, but it sounds like the primary one that troubles you and brings you here today is the stormy and unsatisfactory nature of your relationships with men. Is this correct? [*The patient nods in agreement.*] It sounds like these relationships start off well but end badly; you suggested that part of the problem may be your temper—you are vulnerable to lashing out when a man disappoints you or doesn't meet your expectations. It also sounds to me as though there may be similar problems with girlfriends, but this is less troubling to you. Would you say that what I have described thus far is accurate? Shall I go on?

Ms. B: Sure.

Interviewer: In addition, I hear that you have been unable to identify or pursue a satisfying career path, or to develop interests that might help you feel more engaged in the world, more alive. It seems to me that you have not been able to achieve the milestones you might have hoped for at this age: a stable relationship with a man, some kind of career path or stable job, perhaps an active social life. These disappointments make it difficult to feel good about yourself and tend to leave you feeling resentful of others who seem to have more, and you find yourself increasingly unhappy and angry.

Ms. B: That really is true. I've been feeling lousy…angry all the time.

Interviewer: I understand that, and that it's become painful. In my mind, I see the various difficulties you describe as related to one another. Would you like me to explain? [*The patient nods.*] I understand your difficulties as expressions of an underlying problem having to do with your personality. For starters, what do I mean by *personality*? Everyone has a personality; our personality organizes how we feel about ourselves and others and how we function in the world. A particularly important part of personality functioning is our identity or sense of self, and also our sense of others. It seems to me that a big part of your problem is that you don't have a stable, coherent, organized sense of yourself or of the people important to you. It's as if your views can shift—one moment, your boyfriend seems like a wonderful guy and a solution to your unhappiness, and you feel great about him, and then in a flash he can become an enemy and you attack him. This kind of instability makes it difficult to sustain relationships or to pursue goals, and it tends to leave people with a kind of empty, meaningless feeling, a feeling that can be very painful. Does what I'm saying ring true?

Ms. B: I guess so…. Yeah, it does.

Interviewer: Are you saying yes just to agree with me, or does what I'm saying really make sense to you?

Ms. B: No, I know that what you're saying applies to me. I just don't like it.

Interviewer: Okay, I can understand that, and down the road we'll have the opportunity to discuss further what it is you don't like. But for now, let me continue…. The kinds of problems we're talking about—given your sense of yourself and your problems in relationships—are described in terms of a personality disorder. Have people spoken with you before about this, or has anyone suggested that you suffer from a personality disorder?

Ms. B: Yes, a couple of therapists have said I have borderline personality disorder. One person told me I'm narcissistic and histrionic.

Interviewer: Good, so you are likely to be already pretty well informed. We've learned a lot about personality disorders in recent years and have come to feel that they are far less static and far more treatable than was thought in the past. This applies to borderline personality disorder in particular and to personality disorders in general. One advantage of a DSM diagnosis is that it can provide you with information about the disorder and relevant treatments. I'd say you likely do have borderline personality disorder, though often the specific DSM-5 personality disorder labels don't tell us that much;

there are lots of different ways that someone can have borderline personality disorder. Having said that, I do think it's important that we share a clear understanding of your problems before talking about treatment goals and possible treatment approaches. What questions do you have for me?

Clinical Illustration 4: Sharing the Diagnostic Impression With a High BPO Patient

Mr. H, the 38-year-old lawyer seeking help for anxiety, was introduced in Clinical Illustration 3 in Chapter 2.

> Interviewer: As I hear it, you complain primarily of anxiety, and while you may be a generally anxious person, most of your anxiety is organized in relation to concerns about work and is experienced while you are at work. Is this correct?
>
> Mr. H: It is.
>
> Interviewer: The other major area of difficulty you describe has to do with your self-esteem: it seems you feel overall inadequate and inferior. In fact, if you think about it, much of your anxiety at work has to do with fears of not measuring up or worrying that your colleagues are looking down on you or deriding you behind your back. So it seems likely to me that these two areas of difficulty are connected; from what you describe, much of the anxiety you feel is linked not only to work, but also to these feelings of inferiority.... They leave you always looking around anxiously and comparing yourself to others, feeling you come up short, or fearful that others are looking down on you. Does what I am saying sound accurate?
>
> Mr. H: Yes, it is very accurate.
>
> Interviewer: Outside of problems with your work and self-esteem, you describe yourself as happy in your marriage, and clearly you think the world of your wife. At the same time, from your description, it sounds as though in some ways she kind of supports your view of yourself as inadequate. I'm glad to see you nodding, because I was somewhat hesitant to say anything about this; it isn't clear to me that you see this as a problem.
>
> Mr. H: I really don't.
>
> Interviewer: Okay, so we agree that how things are between you and your wife is okay with you, at least for now—not something you'd necessarily want to change.
>
> Mr. H: Exactly.
>
> Interviewer: So it sounds like we agree on the major issues: anxiety, insecurity at work, and problems with self-esteem, or at least particular aspects of your self-esteem. So how can we understand all of this? Well, it does seem to me that you likely suffer from a clinical anxiety disorder, and we will talk about possible medications or targeted psychotherapies that might help you with your anxiety. But before

jumping ahead to that, I want to consider how the various difficulties you face may be connected; this may sound strange to you, but I see them all as connected to an underlying problem with your personality. Shall I go on?

Mr. H: Sure.

Interviewer: Everyone has a personality; our personality organizes how we view and feel about ourselves and others and how we function in the world. A particularly important part of personality functioning is our identity, or sense of self. It seems to me that a big part of your problem is that you have a fixed view of yourself as inferior, inadequate, and lesser than, and a corresponding view of others—most pointedly your wife, and also the guys at work—as superior to you, better in a variety of ways. In the ideal situation, it's not that way; a person has a more complex view of himself and also of his significant others, one that incorporates both good and bad qualities. But for you, it's as if you have only bad qualities and others have only good qualities—like your wife: entirely strong, admirable, effective. Your views seem kind of polarized, and as if there's something kind of flat, or somewhat two-dimensional, about them. Does that make sense to you? Do you follow what I am saying? [*The patient nods.*] Well, I think that this way of experiencing things makes the world somewhat confusing—and is certainly demoralizing; it leaves you feeling anxious and fearful of criticism. [*Pause.*] The kinds of problems we're talking about—your rigid and negative sense of yourself and your tendency to see others as better than you, and the impact this way of seeing things has on your relationships—are usually described in terms of a personality disorder. Have people spoken with you before about this, or has anyone suggested that you may suffer from a personality disorder?

Mr. H: No, never. I've been treated for anxiety, but no one ever discussed a personality disorder with me. That sounds scary—does it mean I'm dangerous?

Interviewer: Absolutely not. Personality disorders are not at all scary, and it is clear that you are not dangerous—except perhaps to yourself, to the degree that you sometimes neglect your health. Personality disorders can be relatively mild or relatively severe. You are correct that more severe disorders can be associated with violence or antisocial features, but in your case, violence is not an issue. I want to emphasize that you have a relatively mild personality disorder, with many personality strengths: you are honest; you have a stable relationship with your wife; and you have a career, even if there are problems there. We've learned a lot about personality disorders in recent years and have come to feel that they are far more common, less static, and far more treatable than was thought in the past, especially the milder personality disorders such as the one that I think you have.

Mr. H: Do I have a particular kind of personality disorder? I know my uncle was diagnosed with narcissistic personality disorder.

Interviewer: Many people have a disorder that doesn't fit into the category of a particular personality disorder, but rather have a combination of features. If anything, I'd say your difficulties come closest to the description of avoidant personality disorder as described in the literature or in DSM-5. You might want to read up on this online and see what you think. Narcissistic personality disorder is a lot about problems with self-esteem, so you might have some narcissistic traits, and also perhaps some dependent traits, based on your description of your relationship with your wife. [*Pause.*] Well, we have covered a lot of ground. What questions do you have for me?

Determining Treatment Goals

The consultation in TFP-E emphasizes helping the patient identify explicit goals for treatment. Different forms of treatment have different objectives; the therapist cannot select a form of treatment without first identifying what he hopes to accomplish in the treatment. Further, once a treatment is selected, the possibility of success for that treatment rests on identified goals that are realistic, given the patient's pathology and motivation for treatment and the form of treatment selected. Identified goals orient the therapist during the course of treatment, focusing his thinking and interventions, and goals make it possible for therapist and patient to assess progress in treatment over time. It is the task of the therapist to ensure that both patient and therapist agree on suitable goals before starting treatment.

In the broadest sense, the goals of TFP-E are *to improve self and interpersonal functioning*—changes that are understood as reflections of identity consolidation and/or integration of conflictual aspects of functioning into dominant self experience. In terms of the more specific goals of a particular therapy, when the therapist is discussing goals with the patient, it can be helpful to distinguish between *personal goals* and *treatment goals*. A patient's personal goal may be to get married; to hold down a job; or to be a better spouse, parent, or friend. The corresponding, respective treatment goals would be to address those aspects of the patient's internal experience and behavior that interfere with finding a partner and falling in love; with working more consistently and conscientiously; or with being more agreeable, realistic, and flexible in relationships.

Frank discussion of treatment goals makes clear that different forms of treatment are designed to facilitate different kinds of changes, and that part of the patient's job is to identify what it is that she hopes to accomplish and to understand what that requires in terms of necessary conditions for treatment. This process also underscores that the patient is to be an active participant in the treatment to follow, something that may not always be apparent to the patient with a personality disorder, who may expect to "receive" rather than to participate in treatment; in addition, the process sets the stage for the contracting phase to follow (discussed in Chapter 8).

Determining treatment goals is not always a straightforward process, especially when treating patients with identity pathology. It is not uncommon for patients with personality disorders to be seen in consultation while in the midst of some sort of crisis; the patient may be feeling overwhelmed, desperate, or confused—as in the case of Ms. A (Clinical Illustration 1 in this chapter), who had been flattened by her breakup with Mike. In the setting of a crisis, the patient's goals for treatment may well be limited to obtaining relief from acute distress, and she may be unable or unwilling to think beyond the current moment. Even when not in crisis, many patients with identity pathology present without specific goals beyond "to feel better," "to be happy," or "to understand myself." Other patients present their chief complaints in ways that are so poorly formed or so vague as to leave the therapist struggling to understand what the patient is looking for and whether the therapist can help.

In contrast, some patients with personality disorders present with very specific—and in some cases, relatively limited—treatment goals, despite descriptions of broad areas of difficulty during the assessment. For example, a therapist might have a patient like Mr. H, who wants treatment for anxiety and has no interest in addressing underlying personality pathology; or a patient with global and severe personality pathology like Ms. B, whose goal is to better regulate her temper, with no interest in changing her sense of self or the instability in her experience of others; or a patient like Ms. N, who appears to have the goal of addressing her romantic difficulties but who might eventually request specific treatment for sexual inhibitions, or for a mild depressive episode.

It is the responsibility of the consultant to help the patient to determine exactly what he is seeking treatment for—that is, what he hopes will be ameliorated by the time treatment ends—and to think about whether his motivation for treatment is compatible with his goals. The consultant should not agree to treatment goals that are frankly unrealistic; for example, if Mr. H anticipated becoming "a powerful personality and an extravert," this would not be considered practical to achieve. The consultant should educate the patient about what kinds of changes are realistic to work toward. The consultant should also avoid pushing the patient to adopt goals that are overly ambitious; for example, with Mr. H, the consultant's job was to accept that after explaining his assessment of Mr. H's difficulties and his recommendation for psychotherapeutic treatment of his personality disorder, Mr. H might want treatment simply for anxiety, even while understanding that his personality disorder could compromise the outcome of that treatment.

In sum, the consultant's task is to share with the patient his understanding of the total picture, including the patient's presenting complaints and additional areas of difficulty, and then help the patient decide on his goals, weighing relative risks and benefits of different treatment options, including the possibility of no treatment.

Differential Therapeutics and Discussing Treatment Options

The nature of the patient's goals and motivation, combined with her structural and DSM-5 diagnoses, determines treatment options. The consultant will present the options and then help the patient make an informed and autonomous decision in relation to selecting a treatment. Treatment planning will be guided by the consultant's expertise and recommendations, but ultimately determined by the needs and wishes of the patient, as reflected in her personal goals and level of motivation for treatment. As he reviews treatment options and recommends a particular form of treatment—psychotherapeutic and/or psychopharmacological—the clinician initiates a process of obtaining informed consent (Beahrs and Gutheil 2001). It is incumbent upon the clinician to disclose enough information for the patient to make a reasoned decision about whether to undertake the treatment.

For patients who are financially supported by someone else, such as a family member or significant other, and particularly if someone other than the patient will be paying for the treatment, discussing treatment options with the relevant third party as well as with the patient is recommended. This can best be accomplished in a family meeting with the patient and her significant others in which the consultant shares the treatment plan, including risks and benefits and expected outcomes. During the process of discussing treatment options and selecting a treatment, meeting with family members or significant others of any patient who is at high risk for destructive or self-destructive behavior is also highly recommended. We address this topic in greater depth in the discussion of contracting in Chapter 8.

Informed Consent for Psychodynamic Therapy

The goal of the process of informed consent is to facilitate autonomous decision making. Informed consent entails the following:

- Discussion of the diagnosis and formulation of the patient's difficulties
- Discussion of the course, etiology, and associated symptoms of the patient's presenting complaints
- Discussion of expected outcome if the patient does not pursue treatment
- Description of TFP-E and its associated risks and benefits, including the expected duration of treatment and possible side effects (e.g., a temporary increase in anxiety or other symptoms)
- Discussion of significant alternative treatments, including their attendant risks and benefits

Informed decision making begins with the process described in earlier sections, in which the consultant shares his impressions and diagnostic assessment with the patient, and then helps the patient clarify his goals. The next step is for the therapist to review possible treatment options, along with potential benefits, costs, and risks of each treatment approach. With patients with personality disorders, it is important to outline the treatment frame and necessary conditions of each treatment discussed. The consultant will also cover potential risks and benefits of not pursuing treatment at the current time.

For patients who present with mild or subsyndromal personality pathology—for example, Ms. N, who functions at a neurotic level and who exhibits relatively focused personality rigidity—there are many possible treatment options, including brief dynamic, supportive, and cognitive-behavioral therapies (CBTs), as well as TFP-E. The consultant will describe each of these various options, explaining that brief dynamic, supportive, or CBT would likely be less time intensive, less expensive, and perhaps less stressful options than TFP-E; on the other hand, the other treatments have less ambitious goals than TFP-E, and only TFP-E would specifically target her conflicts in relation to getting attention from men, with the goal of resolving her romantic inhibitions. The consultant would help Ms. N weigh the costs and benefits of each approach, and would also make a personal recommendation that Ms. N would be free to accept or reject.

For patients like Ms. B who present with significant identity pathology, supportive psychotherapy is widely accessible, and increasingly Good Psychiatric Management (GPM; Gunderson 2014) also is. However, more specialized treatments—notably, cognitive-behavioral treatments, including dialectical behavior therapy (DBT; Linehan 1993); mentalization-based therapy (MBT; Bateman and Fonagy 2006); schema-focused therapy

(SFT; Young et al. 2003); and TFP-E—may be best suited to specific aspects of pathology or to the patient's preferred approaches to change. Furthermore, the specialized treatments may have more to offer in relation to different presenting problems in the patient with identity pathology: DBT targets behavioral and emotional dysregulation; MBT aims to improve the ability to accurately identify mental states in self and others; SFT is intended to modify maladaptive schemas; and TFP-E has the explicit goal of improving self and interpersonal functioning and promoting identity consolidation.

Because patients with personality disorders often present with co-occurring disorders—most often affective, anxiety, eating, or substance misuse disorders—the clinician faces the task of helping the patient decide whether to focus on treating underlying personality pathology or to first attempt to treat presenting symptoms. Some patients want to address only the presenting symptoms or co-occurring disorders, whereas others want to address only the personality pathology. When a patient wants to focus exclusively on the treatment of presenting complaints or a co-occurring disorder to the exclusion of personality pathology, the consultant can help the patient 1) develop a suitable treatment plan and 2) appreciate that the presence of a co-occurring personality disorder (especially if it is in the BPO range) complicates treatment and the prognosis of other psychiatric syndromes.

Patients who prefer to be treated only for personality pathology, to the neglect of co-occurring disorders, often need help understanding that 1) TFP-E is not a treatment for co-occurring disorders, including major affective, anxiety, eating, and substance misuse disorders; and 2) treatment of co-occurring psychiatric disorders, either before or concurrent with treatment for personality pathology, is necessary if the latter is to be effective.

In many cases, medication management or a specific symptom-focused treatment (e.g., for substance misuse or eating disorder symptoms) can be introduced with another provider, a self-help group, or 12-step program while the patient begins TFP-E. With patients who are more symptomatic (e.g., those with major depression, severe panic disorder, or obsessive-compulsive disorder, or those whose substance use or eating disorder symptoms would complicate a course of TFP-E), a sequential treatment model is recommended before TFP-E begins, in which treatment of these disorders is initiated first, with the therapist either seeing the patient in a more supportive treatment or referring him for specialized treatment. For patients with a history of significant substance abuse or substance dependence, at least 6 months of stable sobriety is recommend before TFP-E can be considered.

When co-occurring disorders are incompatible with beginning TFP-E, the consultant should share his assessment with the patient and agree upon a plan. He should explain that the patient's current symptoms preclude beginning TFP-E at the moment; that the recommendation is to focus first on symptom-focused and behaviorally aimed treatment using evidence-based modalities; that this treatment may include medication, focal forms of psychotherapy, and substance abuse or eating disorder treatment; and that when co-occurring disorders are stabilized, beginning TFP-E can be revisited as a treatment option.

Patients who present with severe active symptoms or in crisis often benefit from either an extended consultation or a brief course of supportive therapy that targets symptom relief or resolution of the crisis, before beginning TFP-E. For example, Ms. A, introduced earlier in this chapter to illustrate the Structural Interview, began a brief, supportive treatment with the goal of transitioning to TFP-E as her current crisis resolved; in the supportive treatment, the therapist assumed a pragmatic approach, providing structure combined with limit setting, and reevaluated her medications. These interventions helped Ms. A get out of bed and return to her baseline, rather low level of functioning. At that point, the therapist helped Ms. A transition from supportive therapy to TFP-E, making clear that the nature of the treatment was changing, as were the goals and the manner in which therapist and patient would be working together, all of which would now be focused on helping her improve her self and interpersonal functioning. Before making the transition, Dr. U helped Ms. A establish specific goals for treatment, and they negotiated a TFP-E treatment contract.

In the case of Ms. B, the consultant made use of an extended consultation, focusing on psychoeducation and enabling Ms. B to elaborate the unhappiness that was often hidden by her hostility, and helping her share her underlying feelings of isolation and emptiness. This process, extending over a number of weeks, helped Ms. B develop confidence in the consultant and consolidate her motivation to initiate treatment of her personality disorder. During the consultation, it also emerged that she was using alcohol more extensively than she had originally acknowledged, and she agreed to begin attending Alcoholics Anonymous as a precondition for treatment.

In contrast to Ms. B, during the course of an extended consultation, Mr. H remained uninterested in treatment of his personality pathology. The consultant referred him for a course of CBT in conjunction with medication for treatment of his anxiety. Over time, this evolved into longer-term, supportive treatment with the CBT therapist, focusing on helping Mr. H manage his anxiety and question his constant negative thoughts about himself.

In sum, it is the role of the consultant to honestly share with the patient his assessment of which treatments will address which aspects of the patient's pathology, as well as the costs in terms of time, money, and any potential side effects. To our knowledge, TFP-E is the only available treatment for personality disorders that specifically targets self and interpersonal functioning while remaining embedded in a comprehensive model of personality functioning. When recommending TFP-E, the consultant should describe the potential benefits of the treatment, as well as the costs and potential risks, along with information about the expected course.

To describe TFP-E for patients with higher level personality pathology (see Caligor et al. 2007), the consultant might say something like this:

> TFP-E is a treatment designed to help us learn more about aspects of your internal experience connected to the problems that brought you to treatment—to help you become more self-aware and better understand yourself. The treatment involves your speaking openly and honestly about what is on your mind while you are in sessions. My role is to help identify the patterns of behavior, emotion, and thinking that underlie your difficulties. The general idea is that as you become more aware of some of the things you do, think, and feel, and as you come to better understand what drives them, you will be able to manage your internal experience and your external behavior in a more flexible and adaptive fashion.

In addition, the consultant should explain that TFP-E is a twice-weekly treatment that lasts at least 1 year and typically from 2 to 4 years. There are few serious risks associated with the treatment, although it can stir up strong feelings, and the patient may experience heightened anxiety or other symptoms as transient "side effects" at various points during the treatment. With patients with more severe personality pathology, the consultant might add that emotions stirred up by the treatment can lead to impulses to act out, and that the therapy includes a treatment contract designed to help the patient control such impulses. The patient should understand that although the consultant recommends TFP-E for treatment of personality pathology, other treatment options exist, each with its own rationale and risk-benefit profile.

Key Clinical Concepts

- The therapeutic consultation comprises assessment, sharing of the diagnostic impression, determination of treatment goals, discussion of treatment options, and helping the patient make an informed treatment selection.
- Diagnostic assessment includes thorough evaluation of personality functioning and personality organization, as well as of the domains covered in a standard psychiatric interview.
- The determination of personality organization, along with the presence or absence of co-occurring disorders, guides treatment planning.
- Assessment of personality organization focuses on the domains of identity, defenses, object relations, aggression, and moral functioning.
- Personality organization can be assessed in the clinical interview or by using the Structured Interview of Personality Organization—Revised.
- Sharing the diagnostic impression and providing psychoeducation about the patient's diagnosis are important components of the consultative process.
- In discussing treatment options, the consultant describes potential benefits and risks of available treatments.

References

American Psychiatric Association: Diagnostic and Statistical Manual of Mental Disorders, 5th Edition. Arlington, VA, American Psychiatric Association, 2013

Bachelor A: Clients' perception of the therapeutic alliance: a qualitative analysis. J Couns Psychol 42:323–337, 1995

Bateman A, Fonagy P: Mentalization-Based Treatment for Borderline Personality Disorder. New York, Oxford University Press, 2006

Beahrs JO, Gutheil TG: Informed consent in psychotherapy. Am J Psychiatry 158(1):4–10, 2001 11136625

Caligor E, Petrini MJ: Treatment of narcissistic personality disorder, in UpToDate. Available at: http://www.uptodate.com. Accessed December 9, 2016.

Caligor E, Kernberg OF, Clarkin JF: Handbook of Dynamic Psychotherapy for Higher Level Personality Pathology. Washington, DC, American Psychiatric Publishing, 2007

Clark LA: Manual for the Schedule for Non-adaptive and Adaptive Personality (SNAP). Minneapolis, University of Minnesota Press, 1993

Clarkin JF, Livesley WJ: Formulation and treatment planning, in Integrated Treatment for Personality Disorder: A Modular Approach. Edited by Livesley WJ, Dimaggio G, Clarkin JF. New York, Guilford, 2016, pp 80–100

Clarkin JF, Caligor E, Stern BL, Kernberg OF: Structured Interview of Personality Organization—Revised (STIPO-R), 2016. Available at: www.borderlinedisorders.com. Accessed September 20, 2017.

Clarkin JF, Livesley WJ, Meehan KB: Clinical assessment, in Handbook of Personality Disorders: Theory, Research, and Treatment, 2nd Edition. Edited by Livesley WJ, Larstone R. New York, Guilford, 2018, pp. 367–393

First MB, Skodol AE, Bender DS, Oldham JM: Structured Clinical Interview for the DSM-5 Alternative Model for Personality Disorders (SCID-5-AMPD). Arlington, VA, American Psychiatric Association Publishing, 2018

Grilo CM, Sanislow CA, Gunderson JG, et al: Two-year stability and change of schizotypal, borderline, avoidant, and obsessive-compulsive personality disorders. J Consult Clin Psychol 72(5):767–775, 2004 15482035

Gunderson JG: Handbook of Good Psychiatric Management for Borderline Personality Disorder. Washington, DC, American Psychiatric Publishing, 2014

Gunderson JG, Morey LC, Stout RL, et al: Major depressive disorder and borderline personality disorder revisited: longitudinal interactions. J Clin Psychiatry 65(8):1049–1056, 2004 15323588

Hallquist MN, Lenzenweger MF: Identifying latent trajectories of personality disorder symptom change: growth mixture modeling in the longitudinal study of personality disorders. J Abnorm Psychol 122(1):138–155, 2013 23231459

Hilsenroth MJ, Cromer TD: Clinician interventions related to alliance during the initial interview and psychological assessment. Psychotherapy (Chic) 44(2):205–218, 2007 22122211

Hutsebaut J, Feenstra DJ, Kamphuis JH: Development and preliminary psychometric evaluation of a brief self-report questionnaire for the assessment of the DSM-5 level of Personality Functioning Scale: the LPFS Brief Form (LPFS-BF). Personal Disord 7(2):192–197, 2016 26595344

Kernberg OF: Structural diagnosis, in Severe Personality Disorders: Psychotherapeutic Strategies. New Haven, CT, Yale University Press, 1984, pp 3–26

Krueger RF, Derringer J, Markon KE, et al: Initial construction of a maladaptive personality trait model and inventory for DSM-5. Psychol Med 42(9):1879–1890, 2012 22153017

Linehan MM: Cognitive-Behavioral Treatment of Borderline Personality Disorder. New York, Guilford, 1993

Lingiardi V, McWilliams N (eds): Psychodynamic Diagnostic Manual, 2nd Edition. New York, Guilford, 2017

McWilliams N: Psychoanalytic Diagnosis: Understanding Personality Structure in the Clinical Process. New York, Guilford, 1994, pp 168–188

Meehan KB, Clarkin JF: A critical evaluation of moving toward a trait system for personality disorder assessment, in Personality Disorders: Toward Theoretical and Empirical Integration in Diagnosis and Assessment. Edited by Huprich SK. Washington, DC, American Psychological Association, 2015, pp 85–106

Patrick C: Antisocial personality disorder and psychopathy, in Personality Disorders: Toward the DSM-V. Edited by O'Donohue W, Fowler K, Lilienfeld S. Thousand Oaks, CA, Sage, 2007, pp 109–166

Piper WE, Duncan SC: Object relations theory and short-term dynamic psychotherapy: findings from the Quality of Object Relations Scale. Clin Psychol Rev 19(6):669–685, 1999 10421951

Skodol AE, Grilo CM, Keyes KM, et al: Relationship of personality disorders to the course of major depressive disorder in a nationally representative sample. Am J Psychiatry 168(3):257–264, 2011 21245088

Westen D, Shedler J: Revising and assessing Axis II, part I: developing a clinically and empirically valid assessment method. Am J Psychiatry 156(2):258–272, 1999a 9989563

Westen D, Shedler J: Revising and assessing Axis II, part II: toward an empirically based and clinically useful classification of personality disorders. Am J Psychiatry 156(2):273–285, 1999b 9989564

Yeomans F, Clarkin JF, Kernberg OF: Transference-Focused Psychotherapy for Borderline Personality Disorder: A Clinical Guide. Washington, DC, American Psychiatric Publishing, 2015

Young JE, Klosko J, Weishaar ME: Schema Therapy: A Practitioner's Guide. New York, Guilford, 2003

Zanarini MC, Frankenburg FR, Hennen J, et al: Prediction of the 10-year course of borderline personality disorder. Am J Psychiatry 163(5):827–832, 2006 16648323

Section IV

Establishing the Treatment Frame

IN TRANSFERENCE-FOCUSED PSYCHOTHER-apy—extended (TFP-E), the treatment frame is established in the form of a treatment contract, which is agreed upon by patient and therapist before treatment begins. Negotiating a treatment contract and establishing the treatment frame—a process referred to as *contracting*—bridge the consultation and the formal beginning of the therapy.

The treatment contract defines the necessary conditions for treatment, those under which patient and therapist can successfully work together. The tasks of the contracting phase are to introduce the patient to the general frame of the treatment, the respective tasks of patient and therapist in the treatment, and any specific modifications to the frame necessitated by the patient's personality pathology, treatment history, or current life circumstances. Therapist and patient discuss these arrangements until they are able to reach a mutual agreement about how they will work together. This process begins with revisiting the goals discussed in the assessment phase—ensuring that patient and therapist share an understanding of problem(s) to be addressed in treatment—and ends with mutual agreement on how the two will work together to achieve these goals.

Essential Treatment Contracting

Behaviors, Adjunctive Treatments, and Medication

THE TREATMENT CONTRACT IN TRANSFER-ence-focused psychotherapy—extended (TFP-E) establishes the treatment frame and ensures that the patient understands and agrees upon the *necessary conditions for treatment*. The process of contracting picks up where the consultation leaves off, further developing a working relationship between patient and therapist by specifically defining the role of each party in the treatment to follow. The treatment contract grounds the treatment in reality and recognizes the limitations of both patient and therapist. As the severity of personality pathology increases, threats to the contract also increase (Links et al. 2016).

This chapter provides a comprehensive discussion of contracting in TFP-E, beginning with Part 1, which provides an overview of the treatment frame and contract, including topics and roles addressed during contracting. Part 2 discusses universal elements of any TFP-E treatment contract, and Part 3 provides discussion of the individualized elements of the TFP-E contract tailored to the specific patient regarding destructive or treatment-interfering behaviors, co-occurring disorders, medication management, and other special topics.

Part 1

Overview of the Treatment Frame and Contract

THE TREATMENT FRAME DEFINES AND OR-
ganizes the treatment and the relationship between patient and therapist
(Table 8–1). Without a treatment frame, there is no treatment, and when
the treatment frame is not maintained, the treatment is destined to founder.
In TFP-E, the treatment frame provides a contained setting within which
the patient's conflictual object relations can unfold and be explored; the
treatment frame establishes the *necessary conditions for exploration* and
helps protect the therapist's neutrality. Thorough discussion of the treatment contract ensures that the patient understands the terms upon which
both beginning and continuing the treatment depend.

The treatment frame specifies the basic parameters of the treatment,
including frequency and duration of sessions, duration of treatment,
scheduling and payment arrangements, issues of confidentiality, contact
between patient and therapist between sessions, contact with third parties, and the respective roles and responsibilities of therapist and patient
in the treatment, including the handling of emergencies and medication
management (Table 8–2).

In addition, the treatment frame will include parameters introduced on
an individualized basis to address specific behaviors likely to interfere with
the patient's or therapist's ability to effectively and productively conduct an
exploratory treatment; in the contracting phase, the therapist introduces
specific arrangements based on an understanding of the patient's psychopathology, personal history, life circumstances, and experience in prior
treatments. These may include, for example, parameters around such issues
as substance misuse or eating disorder symptoms, and self-destructive behaviors such as cutting, reckless driving, or unsafe sex (Table 8–3). The
need for behavioral control is introduced from the perspective of the need
to create and protect the necessary conditions for conducting an exploratory therapy.

The treatment frame is formally established and mutually agreed upon
by patient and therapist in the form of a treatment contract. This is not a

---

TABLE 8–1. Functions of the treatment frame and contract

Establish a mutual understanding of problem(s) to address in treatment.

Define the reality of the treatment relationship, organized in relation to the treatment goals and the respective responsibilities of patient and therapist.

Provide a consistent, "safe" place for the patient's dynamics to unfold.

Create a setting in which the patient's behavior in relation to the treatment can be explored in terms of enactment of conflictual object relations.

Help the patient contain and limit destructive and disruptive behavior.

Minimize secondary gains of illness.

Set the stage for exploring the meanings of deviations from the treatment frame and contract.

Create a framework for exploring the motivations for and meanings of destructive and disruptive behavior.

Support the therapist's ability to confront and limit destructive behavior while minimizing the patient's denial and externalization of conflict.

Help the therapist contain countertransference.

TABLE 8–2. Universal elements of the treatment frame and contract

---

Frequency and duration of sessions

Arrangements around scheduling and payment

Issues around confidentiality and contact with third parties

Intersession contact

Arrangements for handling of emergencies

Arrangements for medication management

Attention to the treatment goals

Patient involvement in structured activity (e.g., work, school, day hospital program, full-time childcare)

Roles of therapist and patient in treatment

---

written contract but rather a clearly and specifically described agreement between patient and therapist outlining the necessary conditions for treatment. The objective of the contracting phase is for patient and therapist to agree upon the *least* restrictive set of conditions needed to support a psychotherapeutic process.

In TFP-E, the treatment frame and contract serve multiple functions throughout the course of treatment. In the contracting phase, the treat-

---

TABLE 8–3. **Individualized elements that may be introduced into the treatment contract for transference-focused psychotherapy — extended**

Self-destructive behaviors, including minor self-harm

Behaviors destructive to others

Substance misuse

Eating disorder symptoms

Lying and other forms of deception

Lack of compliance with medication management of medical or psychiatric problems

Reckless behavior (e.g., dangerous sexual activity, driving while intoxicated)

Excessive phone calls, electronic communications, or other intrusions into the therapist's life

Destructive behavior in relation to therapist's practice (e.g., making excessive noise, defacing furniture, refusing to leave office when session is over, leaving trash in or taking periodicals from waiting area)

Boundary violations of the treatment relationship (e.g., stalking therapist or therapist's family members on social media, attempting to initiate social contact with members of the therapist's social or personal sphere)

Circumstances that interfere with patient's ability to continue in therapy, including inability to pay for treatment

Excessive secondary gain from illness that would interfere with patient's motivation to get well (e.g., arrangements about financial support from family members or social services)

---

ment goals, frame, and contract function to define and establish the reality of the treatment relationship, in which patient and therapist work together in a clearly defined fashion with the aim of helping the patient attain specific goals. This realistic relationship is the foundation of the developing therapeutic alliance and at the same time will invariably be distorted, to a greater or lesser degree, by the unfolding of the patient's conflictual object relations in the treatment. Establishing a mutually agreed-upon treatment frame in the form of a treatment contract lays the groundwork for the treatment that will follow, and establishing the contract is an important joint task for therapist and patient. Effective contract negotiation predicts a positive therapeutic alliance (Hilsenroth and Cromer 2007), a reduced rate of dropping out prematurely (Yeomans et al. 1994), and positive treatment outcome (Horvath et al. 2011). Although the contract may be modified at any point during treatment if needed, treatment does not formally begin until the treatment frame has been established and the patient and therapist have agreed upon a treatment contract.

The treatment contract is conceptualized in terms of universal elements that apply to all TFP-E treatments (described in Part 2) and individualized elements tailored to the clinical needs of the specific patient (described in Part 3).

Part 2

Universal Elements of the Treatment Contract

THE BASIC ELEMENTS OF THE TFP-E TREATment contract include universal and essential parameters that apply to the treatments of patients across the range of severity of personality pathology.

Logistics

The treatment frame defines the concrete arrangements of the treatment and the respective tasks of patient and therapist in their work together. In TFP-E, sessions ideally occur twice weekly (see the following subsection, "Frequency of Sessions"), and treatments typically last at least 1 year but rarely more than 4 years. Sessions are 45 or 50 minutes long, and patient and therapist sit across from one another, face to face, in comfortable chairs. It is often helpful to have regularly scheduled appointments that take place on the same day and time each week, but if this is not practical, a flexible schedule can work as well. What is important is that standard procedures for scheduling, rescheduling, and canceling appointments are explicitly established at the beginning of treatment, and that appointments are scheduled ahead of time and not on an as-needed basis, except in extraordinary circumstances. All therapy sessions are confidential, except when emergency situations occur or when the patient's or someone else's safety is at risk. Phone calls and other contacts between sessions are typically limited to those necessary for schedule changes and emergencies; patients are encouraged to discuss even pressing matters in session rather than calling or otherwise contacting the therapist between sessions.

All these parameters of treatment, along with the therapist's policies regarding payment of fees, insurance, and missed sessions, should be discussed explicitly with the patient before treatment starts. Discussion should also address what the patient can expect with regard to the therapist's standard procedures for returning phone calls or responding to electronic communications from patients.

From the perspective of the patient, clear and explicit discussion of the concrete, logistical aspects of the frame and introduction to the therapist's standard policies allow treatment to begin with the patient already fully informed about the agreement he is entering into; he can rely on the stability and predictability of the frame to provide a relatively safe setting within which to conduct the treatment. From the perspective of the therapist, a structured frame and standard procedures set the stage for approaching the patient's deviations from the frame as having underlying meanings and motivations, while providing the added benefit of calling the therapist's attention to any temptation to modify her usual approach, opening the door to the therapist's use of her countertransference as a source of information about what is occurring in the current clinical situation.

Frequency of Sessions: Twice Weekly Versus Weekly

TFP-E, like transference-focused psychotherapy (TFP; Yeomans et al. 2015), is a twice-weekly treatment. However, in some settings, it may be unrealistic or impractical to insist on twice-weekly sessions; indeed, in some health care systems, twice-weekly psychotherapy sessions are summarily disallowed. When this is the case, once-a-week TFP-E, though perhaps not ideal, may prove the best option for many patients with personality disorders.

Alternative options, notably dialectical behavior therapy (DBT) and mentalization-based therapy (MBT), should be carefully considered, however, especially for patients with more severe personality pathology. These treatments typically involve weekly individual sessions combined with weekly group meetings, and thereby provide more structure and contact with therapists than weekly individual sessions alone, and may be a good choice for many patients in systems that do not support twice-weekly individual psychotherapy. Once-weekly TFP-E, while clearly offering therapeutic potential, is qualitatively different from twice-weekly TFP-E, and tends to lead therapists to drift toward a more supportive stance and technical approach over time.

The positive impact of twice-weekly sessions in TFP-E goes beyond the increased dose per unit of time and additional support concretely provided by increased frequency of sessions, although the latter does have material impact on clinical process (Evans et al. 2017). In the treatment of patients with a borderline level of personality organization (BPO), a major tactical challenge is to contain the highly affectively charged, consciously experienced or enacted, conflictual object relations activated in the treatment, and the propensity toward action stimulated by this process. Twice-weekly sessions, in conjunction with a well-defined and mutually agreed-upon treatment frame and contract, provide the therapist and patient with a greater opportunity to bring these object relations into the treatment without overwhelming either patient or therapist. Twice-weekly sessions mean that the patient is not "left alone" for an entire week to manage (or fail to manage) his affective experience between sessions, and twice-weekly sessions provide the therapist with the time and breathing space, sometimes in short supply, needed to keep track of developments in the patient's life at the same time that she follows developments in the treatment.

In the treatment of patients with a neurotic level of personality organization (NPO), on the other hand, a central tactical challenge is to help the patient gain access to deeper affective experience. With these patients, greater frequency of sessions, in conjunction with analysis of defensive operations, allows for greater affective engagement on the part of the patient, because stably repressed, unconscious, conflictual object relations and associated affects can emerge in the treatment in a fashion difficult for most patients to attain in weekly sessions.

In sum, twice-weekly sessions 1) offer NPO patients increased opportunity to "open things up" and to be more immediately and affectively engaged in session, and 2) benefit BPO patients by increasing the opportunity for containment of affect and destructive behavior through additional contact with the therapist. Thus, twice-weekly sessions facilitate the therapist's ability to optimize the patient's level of affective involvement in his sessions so that experience is affectively charged, but not so overwhelmingly that it cannot be examined (see discussion of tactics in Chapter 11).

Introducing and Negotiating Universal Elements of the Treatment Contract

The process of establishing a treatment contract typically takes one or two sessions but may take longer in more complicated situations. In introducing the contract, it is recommended that the therapist avoid assuming the patient has accurate or realistic expectations of the treatment. The more specifically the therapist outlines the necessary conditions for treatment, the details of how patient and therapist will work together, and the rationale for both, the better positioned the therapist is to explore the meanings of any difficulty that the patient might later experience in participating in the treatment as agreed.

In the contracting phase, the therapist pays careful attention to the patient's participation in and reactions to what the therapist is proposing and to how she is explaining her rationale for setting the treatment up as she is. Is the patient seriously considering what is being proposed or is he providing superficial and meaningless agreement? It may be tempting to take a patient's ready agreement with the conditions of treatment at face value; for example, a patient may glibly assure the therapist that he will not have difficulty leaving work to come to midday sessions, or a young patient might assure the therapist that her father will happily support the treatment indefinitely. What is most helpful, however, is to shine a light on and explore in detail the issues involved and the patient's responses to the conversation. For example, the therapist might ask the following questions of the patient who will take time from work for his sessions: "Have you discussed this with your boss? What did you tell him and how did he respond?" "Is this common practice in your office or could it cause problems down the road?"

Assessing Motivation for Treatment

Thorough discussion of the treatment contract before beginning treatment enables the therapist to assess the patient's motivation for treatment and ability to work productively in the therapy, and also helps identify early difficulties that may emerge if treatment does begin. Some patients who seem potentially suitable in the assessment phase are unable or unwilling to agree to the necessary conditions for treatment outlined in the treatment contract. In this situation, the therapist will explore the patient's reluctance to agree to the conditions of treatment. If the patient is not able or willing to work within the constraints of the TFP-E treatment frame, he can be offered other forms of treatment, either with the current therapist or with another practitioner to whom the therapist refers him, perhaps in a different treatment setting.

It is necessary that the therapist resist pressures—which can come from the patient, from third parties, or from forces within the therapist—to initiate TFP-E without a proper contract in place following the guidelines outlined in this chapter. An analogy is the surgeon who does not operate without a sterile field and antibiotics, necessary conditions for a successful surgery. A TFP-E treatment initiated under conditions of "making an exception" is likely to fail.

Clinical Illustration 1: Contracting Around Limited Motivation for Treatment

Mr. F, a 35-year-old man functioning at a high BPO level with narcissistic and histrionic features, was "dying to get started and get to the bottom of my problems." However, when the therapist slowed things down and carefully went through the conditions of treatment with the patient, Mr. F explained that it all sounded "great" but he could not commit to consistently attending sessions—surely the therapist could appreciate that Mr. F needed to feel free to travel with his girlfriend when it suited him, and surely such a skilled therapist could handle the repeated absences and interruptions in the treatment that would result, and could work with the patient whenever he was in town. The therapist inferred an underlying wishful fantasy on the patient's part of being able to "have his cake and eat it too," a wish closely tied to his presenting complaints.

The therapist tactfully pointed this out to Mr. F and then explained that although he sympathized with the patient's wish, it was not realistic to begin treatment if Mr. F could not imagine attending consistently. After exploring with Mr. F whether he could consider being more flexible about curtailing his travel (he adamantly insisted he could not), the therapist restated that TFP-E is an ambitious treatment that requires consistent attendance over time. The choice was the patient's: either he could begin TFP-E at this time or he could continue to have the freedom to travel. The therapist went on to say that he would support either choice; if Mr. F was unable or unwilling to make the time commitment at this point, the therapist could offer the patient supportive therapy that would have a more flexible frame, as well as less ambitious treatment goals.

This vignette illustrates the therapist's assuming a neutral stance in relation to the patient's conflict about beginning treatment, even while taking an active stand with regard to the necessary and realistic preconditions for treatment.[1] The therapist—rather than allowing the patient to externalize his conflict about whether or not to begin in treatment by encouraging the patient to agree, for example, or enabling him to hold on to his unrealistic expectations by agreeing to begin without a clear understanding about attendance—implicitly encourages the patient to face his own internal dilemma and to make a decision grounded in reality.

When the therapist takes this neutral stance while carefully explaining the rationale behind the various elements in the treatment contract, it is rare for the patient to reject the therapist's proposal. The therapist does not take the patient's initial, superficial agreement with or rejection of the conditions for treatment at face value—for example, Mr. F's expressed wish to "get started"—but rather, ensures that the patient has carefully considered what his agreement entails. Because the patient's conflicts and feelings in relation to beginning treatment invariably touch on the core conflicts that interfere with functioning and bring the patient to treatment, the process of carefully establishing the contract sets the stage for exploring these conflicts once treatment begins.

Some patients with personality disorders view themselves as unable to take responsibility for their actions to the degree necessary to comply with the contract outlined by the therapist. Some feel they are too disorganized to maintain a schedule, too irresponsible or impulsive to live up to an agreement, or too depressed to consistently get out of bed to attend sessions or hold down a job ("If I could do that, I wouldn't need to be here!"). In our experience, many patients with personality disorders are capable of more than they or the people around them appreciate; the treatment contract encourages the patient to function at the peak of his potential.

However, if a patient with a personality disorder diagnosis is literally too disorganized to keep a schedule, too depressed with psychomotor retardation to get out of bed, or too impulsive to control his behavior in session, a complete psychiatric evaluation and medical management, perhaps in conjunction with cognitive-behavioral therapy (CBT), should be undertaken before reconsidering the patient's suitability for TFP-E.

The therapist's temptation to begin treating a patient in TFP-E without first having satisfactorily established the necessary conditions for treatment

---

[1]In this vignette, the therapist points out obvious realities and identifies logical conclusions for Mr. F. We emphasize that this stance is consistent with, rather than incompatible with, the therapist's maintaining a neutral stance. The therapist's interventions can be understood in terms of his confronting the patient's defensive denial of reality. In this example, the therapist remains neutral in that he does not encourage Mr. F to pursue treatment, and does not take the position that it would be a bad idea for Mr. F to do so. Instead, the therapist helps him realistically view his internal and external conflicts in relation to engaging in an intensive treatment.

is typically an early clue to countertransference difficulties and points to the likelihood of countertransference pressures becoming increasingly unmanageable over time. On the other hand, if the therapist is able in this setting to establish the necessary conditions of treatment by adhering to contract guidelines, this same patient may do well; many patients with personality disorders do poorly in unstructured treatments but are able to work productively with a contract in place (see also the section "Working With the Patient to Introduce a Framework for Anticipating and Managing Behaviors" later in this chapter). As illustrated in Chapter 9 ("Identifying a Focus for Intervention"), the latter constructive engagement occurs not simply because the contract limits behavior potentially disruptive to the treatment, but also because the contract provides a framework within which the therapist is able to productively explore these behaviors with the patient.

Once treatment begins, maintaining the treatment frame is an essential responsibility of both patient and therapist in TFP-E. When there is a disruption of the treatment frame or a deviation from the contract, reestablishing the frame and exploring the meaning of the disruption becomes a priority theme in the session.

Identifying Early Transference Developments

The treatment contract establishes the realistic relationship between patient and therapist. However, from their first moments of contact, this relationship will be distorted by activation of the patient's defenses and conflictual object relations. Because beginning treatment is stressful for most patients, and at the same time tends to stimulate conflicts around dependency, authority, and intimacy, the patient's character defenses and early transference predispositions are often immediately enacted in relation to the contracting process, influenced by the patient's personality style and core conflicts. For example, patients with more paranoid traits tend to feel controlled or to fear being exploited, patients with narcissistic traits expect special treatment and exceptions to the rules, and those with sadomasochistic traits can quickly become embroiled in subtle (or not so subtle) power struggles. More dependent BPO patients tend to quickly idealize the therapist, whereas more controlling patients may have difficulty flexibly negotiating the frame. Character defenses will be activated even in relatively well-adapted NPO patients during contracting. For example, a hysterical patient may be noticeably warm, flexible, and charming; a depressive one may be accommodating and ingratiating; and an obsessional patient may be efficient and businesslike.

In the contracting phase, the therapist makes note of transference developments and activation of core conflicts and defensive object relations in response to the therapist's explication of the preconditions for treatment, but abstains from making full interpretations until a contract has been agreed upon and treatment formally begins. Instead, the therapist might make a general statement about the patient's concerns, but then focuses on whether the patient can imagine working within the parameters of the treatment.

Clinical Illustration 2: Noting Early Transference Developments While Avoiding Interpretation

Mr. D, a high-BPO patient with paranoid traits who came to therapy at his wife's urging to address problems in his relationships with family members and coworkers, assumed that the therapist was recommending twice-weekly sessions because the therapist would benefit financially. The therapist responded by first acknowledging Mr. D's concerns: "I can see that you are suspicious of my motivations." She then went on to explain her clinical rationale for twice-weekly sessions: "I am making this recommendation because in my assessment, it is the most effective way to gain a deeper understanding of your difficulties and to attain your treatment goals. This would be much more difficult to do in weekly treatment."

When Mr. D remained silent, the therapist went on: "But I would add that I suspect this tendency of yours to be mistrustful plays a role in the difficulties that you describe in your relationships and that bring you to treatment. Your extreme caution when it comes to trusting others will no doubt be something we focus on in your therapy if we agree to work together. For now, though, I'm wondering if you feel able to agree to twice-weekly TFP-E treatment, or whether we would do better to consider other forms of treatment that are more adaptable to a once-weekly schedule."

At times, making exceptions to the rule of avoiding interpretations during the contracting phase is needed. In particular, when the patient's anxieties lead him to reject the contract out of hand and to change his mind about beginning treatment, exploring and interpreting the patient's anxieties may enable him to embark on treatment when he might not otherwise have done so. In this setting, the therapist may attempt to interpret the anxieties (typically linked to whatever transferences are being activated in the patient), with the expectation that this process may free up the patient to be more reflective.

Clinical Illustration 3: Incorporating Early Interpretation of Transference Anxieties in the Contracting Phase

Ms. E, a middle-aged woman who had two teenage daughters and was highly self-critical and functioning at an NPO level, presented with difficulty advancing at work in the setting of feeling conflicted about her professional ambitions. The patient immediately agreed to the frame as proposed by the therapist, without questions or requests for clarification, and the therapist in turn accepted her quick accommodation without questions or exploration. The next morning, the therapist discovered that he had received a voice mail from Ms. E, left late in the evening, canceling the next session because she didn't think the therapy was "going to work out." The therapist returned the patient's call and invited her to come in and discuss how best to proceed and how he could be of help. Ms. E agreed and came in to explain that when she heard the therapist outline the logistics of the treatment, it felt like "too much of a commitment." Until that point, she hadn't realized what she was "getting into."

When the therapist asked for clarification, what emerged was that the patient believed that committing to a regular twice-weekly schedule would make it impossible for her to be available to her daughters in the way that she felt she needed to be. Having grasped Ms. E's concern, the therapist pointed out the patient's latent belief that it was possible for her to meet her own needs only at the expense of her children, and that this was likely part of the picture in her difficulty to advance at work. Because Ms. E remained somewhat guarded, the therapist went on to suggest that it seemed she assumed he would be inflexible and had no interest in accommodating her schedule—as though he would accept a patient only if she were submissive and self-sacrificing.

At this point, Ms. E smiled, visibly relaxed, and asked if the therapist was able to schedule sessions in the evening when her husband was home. This was the beginning of a highly successful treatment, organized in relation to the patient's internal negotiations with a maternal representation that demanded total and singular devotion to her children.

Introducing the Treatment Frame

Introducing the treatment frame entails outlining for the patient the universal aspects of the treatment contract as they pertain, first to the patient's responsibilities, and then to those of the therapist (summarized in Table 8–4). Patient responsibilities include consistent attendance and adhering to the time frame of scheduled appointments, providing timely payment, and communicating freely and openly during therapy sessions.

TABLE 8–4. Patient's and therapist's responsibilities

Patient's responsibilities

  Consistent attendance

  Timely payment

  Making every effort to communicate openly and freely

Therapist's responsibilities

  Consistent attendance and attention to scheduling

  Listening attentively

  Making every effort to help the patient gain greater self-awareness and self-understanding

  Clarifying the limits of therapist's involvement, if necessary

---

Corresponding responsibilities on the part of the therapist are consistent attendance and attention to scheduling, listening attentively with the objective of helping the patient gain greater self-awareness and self-understanding, and clarifying the limits of her involvement.

Introducing the Patient's Responsibilities

Consistent Attendance. In introducing the patient's responsibilities in relation to attendance, the therapist communicates the importance and value of consistent attendance to the outcome of the treatment. In introducing the patient's responsibilities, the therapist might say something like this:

> It is your responsibility to consistently attend your sessions, and we will start and stop on time. If you have to cancel a session, please give me as much advance notice as possible. There may be times when you feel twice-weekly sessions are too much, or when you feel tempted to skip a session—perhaps because you're feeling bad or perhaps because you're feeling well. The temptation to skip a session or cut back is often a signal that something important is getting stirred up in the treatment that would benefit from exploration, so I encourage you to do all you can to come in even at times when you might prefer not to or when it seems inconvenient. What are your thoughts about this?

When a patient has difficulty agreeing to what the therapist is proposing in the contracting phase, rather than exploring the patient's objections and fears in depth as the therapist might once treatment has begun, the therapist makes a general statement about the patient's concerns but then again focuses on whether the patient can imagine working within the parameters of the treatment, such as follows:

> I can see that you are having difficulty with the idea of starting and ending our sessions according to a fixed allotment of time. I am aware that this is very much in contrast to how things worked with your previous therapist, who would extend sessions if you were late and routinely see you later in the day if something came up that made it inconvenient to come in at your scheduled hour. I understand that what I am proposing is more inconvenient, and I can imagine it might stir up a variety of uncomfortable feelings, some of which you may be aware of and some out of your awareness. These feelings will likely be important should we decide to work together, and in your therapy we will try to understand them more fully. However, we know that things fell apart in your last treatment, and your therapist told me that over time you rarely arrived on time, that you often missed sessions, and that she ended up feeling she couldn't handle the inconvenience you were introducing into her schedule. For these reasons, I encourage you to consider whether you feel able to work within the framework that I am proposing.

This kind of discussion not only increases the likelihood that the patient will attend consistently, but also sets the stage for an exploration of the meaning of the patient's behavior once treatment begins, should the patient have difficulty adhering to the terms of the contract.

Timely Payment of Fees.   Before beginning treatment, the patient must have a clear understanding of the therapist's fee, billing procedures, expectations for payment and for dealing with insurance, and charges for canceled or missed sessions. Every therapist should develop her own formal policies, which makes it less likely that the therapist will bend to early countertransference pressures and make exceptions. For example, the therapist might say the following:

> My fee is $150 per session. I will give you a bill on the first of each month or as soon as possible after the first, and I ask that I be paid by the middle of the month. I am reserving your two sessions for you each week. If you have to cancel a session, I ask that you give me at least 48 hours' notice.

The therapist should be sufficiently comfortable with her fees and procedures to communicate them clearly and unapologetically, implicitly conveying that her time, effort, and expertise are of value. This may be difficult for younger or inexperienced therapists who lack confidence about what they have to offer. With BPO patients, it can be especially important that the therapist remember that the patient is paying for the therapist's *time and effort,* and not for any particular outcome; the patient can neither reward nor punish the therapist monetarily on the basis of the gains made in treatment or the lack of them.

Once the frame and contract are in place and treatment formally begins, the patient's beliefs and attitudes toward the therapist's perceived investment in the treatment outcome and toward the therapist's requirement of payment for her services can then be explored for their transference implications.

Clinical Illustration 4: Difficulties That Emerge Without Following a Formal Fee Policy

Ms. G, a high-functioning narcissistic patient, who was in a variety of ways interesting to the therapist who saw her in consultation, explained that although money was "not an issue," she was having "short-term cash-flow difficulties." In response, feeling reluctant to put pressure on the patient, the therapist refrained from introducing his usual policy of asking for payment by the middle of each month.

In the ensuing months, Ms. G apologetically but repeatedly deferred paying her bill, assuring the therapist that the next month she would be able to pay. Initially, the therapist felt guilty about asking for payment; after all, the patient had anticipated a problem and he had not introduced a formal policy about the timing of payments. To introduce a policy now, several months into the treatment, felt uncomfortable. By the time Ms. G had failed to pay for 4 months of sessions and owed the therapist such a substantial sum that it was unclear if she would ever be able to pay, the therapist had begun to find himself distracted by his irritation with the patient around nonpayment. The therapist felt trapped in a situation destined to deteriorate—until Ms. G abruptly announced that she could not afford therapy, could not cover her debt to the therapist, and dropped out of treatment.

Had the therapist introduced his policy during the contracting phase, the scenario would have played out differently. The patient would have been forced to think more seriously about whether she could actually afford the treatment. If in fact she could not afford the therapist's fees, this would have been established and an alternative plan put in place; if she could afford the treatment, there would be opportunity for a discussion about how to accommodate the requirement to pay the therapist regularly given her cash-flow problems. Once they had come up with a plan, were she to be late in paying in any given month, the therapist could comfortably and neutrally refer to their initial discussion and her plan to ensure that she would pay as they had agreed.

Rather than getting into an uncomfortable discussion that could leave the therapist feeling he was trying to squeeze money out of the patient, or deviating from his neutral stance and encouraging her to find the funds to stay in treatment, or avoiding having that discussion by making ever-greater accommodations, the therapist could point to the patient's apparent change of heart and could explore the motivations involved in her deviation from their agreement. In essence, when he has contracted around payment before beginning treatment, the therapist is in a position to help the patient observe the internal conflict between the part of herself that wants to agree to pay regularly and be in treatment, and the part that is disrupting her opportunity to continue therapy rather than exploring the conflict between herself and the therapist. The issue is framed not in terms of payment per se, but rather as adherence to the treatment contract and as continuing versus interrupting the treatment. It is explored first in the light of what it means to the patient to pay or not to pay, and next in terms of the reality that as she clearly understood before they began, treatment cannot proceed without the patient making payment and agreeing to do so moving forward.

Clinical Illustration 4 *(continued)*: Recontracting Regarding Fees

Ms. G came back some months after her abrupt departure and agreed to recontract with the therapist around payment. When Ms. G made her first payment on time, the dynamics both enacted in and concealed by the earlier nonpayment emerged clearly in the patient's expressed expectation that an exception would be made for her, and in the difficulty that she had in tolerating the need to make a financial sacrifice to pay for her treatment. Underneath these revelations lay a hidden motivation to devalue and control the therapist. These became central dynamics and transferences that were successfully explored in depth in Ms. G's treatment, rather than simply enacted. The therapist's attention to contracting when Ms. G returned created a setting within which this could be accomplished.

Communicating Freely and Openly.   Once therapist and patient are able to reach agreement about the concrete logistics of treatment, the therapist encourages the patient to ask questions and also explains, if she has not already done so, the rationale for the treatment structure. This approach fosters a collaborative atmosphere and communicates that the therapist's approach is not arbitrary. Once the patient has agreed to the arrangements of treatment, the therapist goes on to explain how therapist and patient will work together in each session, as well as the specific tasks for which each of them will be responsible.

Patients with personality disorders enter therapy with all sorts of expectations about treatment, some based on previous personal experience, others based on the media or other external influences, and many of which are direct expressions of their defenses. For example, there may be a wish for magical caretaking or to be unconditionally loved and cherished; or a fear of being controlled, humiliated, or somehow exploited; or an expectation that a recovered memory or perfect insight will relieve all of the patient's difficulties.

Regardless of how "experienced" the patient, it is best to assume that he does not have a realistic understanding of what psychotherapy is. Furthermore, explaining to the patient how the treatment works, what his role is, and what role the therapist plays lays the groundwork for the developing treatment alliance, and also for the therapist's eventual exploration and interpretation of the meaning of the patient's difficulty in communicating openly and freely.

Each therapist should develop her own way of introducing the roles for patient and therapist in the treatment. As an example, the therapist might say something like the following:

> Your role in your therapy sessions is to speak as openly and freely as you can about whatever is on your mind, paying special attention to the difficulties that bring you to treatment. I am interested in anything you might be thinking, feeling, or doing while you are here. This can be a challenging task, to openly share your thoughts and feelings, and I will do what I can to help you. I am suggesting that we work in this way because it is the best way I know for us to learn about the thoughts, feelings, and behaviors underlying the difficulties that bring you here.
>
> At times, you may find that the thoughts you have in session seem unimportant or embarrassing, but I encourage you to share them even so. Similarly, if you have thoughts or questions about me, I encourage you to share them as well, even when they may not be the kind of thing someone would share in an ordinary social relationship. Things you find yourself thinking about as you are coming to or leaving your sessions may also be helpful to explore.[2] You will likely find at times that you are not comfortable being open, are tempted to withhold things, or do not know what to say. This is not unusual, but in fact, understanding whatever is interfering with your thinking and also communicating freely and openly when you are here are important parts of the therapy and help us better understand your difficulties.

---

[2]With NPO patients, there is potential value in their sharing of dreams and daydreams. Working with dreams in the treatment of BPO patients typically is not of particular value until the later phases of treatment. See Chapter 13 for further discussion.

With patients who have a history of impulsive or self-destructive behavior (see also later in this chapter the subsection "Working With the Patient to Introduce a Framework for Anticipating and Managing Behaviors" and the section "Contracting Around Specific Behaviors, Adjunctive Treatments, and Medication"), the therapist might add the following:

> Beyond the general rule of speaking freely in session, if something is happening in your life where you run the risk of harming yourself or others, or if something is happening that might affect the continuity of the treatment, then you should bring that up. For example, if you acted out sexually over the weekend, or if you were in trouble at work and risked losing your job, it would be important to raise that for discussion in the beginning of your next session.

Introducing the Therapist's Responsibilities

The therapist's central responsibility is to help the patient become more self-aware and to develop a more complete understanding of himself, his personality, and his difficulties, in order to help resolve his problems. The therapist's other responsibilities involve scheduling, limiting her involvement with the patient to the work of exploratory therapy, and maintaining confidentiality. Expressly articulating the therapist's responsibilities conveys the collaborative nature of the process and the reality that both therapist and patient are active participants in the therapy.

Consistent Attendance and Attention to Scheduling. The therapist discusses with the patient her procedures for scheduling and notifies the patient of both her scheduled times away and any unanticipated cancellations. The following is an example:

> I will meet with you twice a week on days and at times that we will figure out together. Each session will be 45 minutes long. I will tell you a month in advance when I am planning to be away from the office. I will always do my best to reschedule a session I have canceled if I am in the office other days that week. In the case of an emergency cancellation, I will call your cell number. I am committed to working with you on a regular, twice-a-week basis.

Listening Attentively and Helping the Patient Gain Greater Self-Awareness and Self-Understanding. The therapist's description of her role in the therapy is part of the process of helping the patient gain a general understanding of the nature of the therapy and of what goes on in each session. The therapist's description of her role will focus on her listening attentively and contributing to the patient's development of a

deeper level of self-understanding, with the overarching objective of helping the patient develop a greater awareness of the behaviors, motivations,
thoughts, and feelings that out of his awareness play a role in the difficulties that brought him to treatment. In addition, the therapist will provide
an explanation of how she decides when to speak, the nature of confidentiality, and the limits on the therapist's involvement.

For example, the therapist might say something like this:

> My responsibility is to listen attentively to what you are saying and to
> share my thoughts when I feel I have something to add that will help
> deepen our understanding of the patterns of thinking, feeling, and behav-
> ing that underlie your difficulties. There will be times when I talk a fair
> amount and other times when I will be relatively silent. You will also find
> that there will be times when I may not answer your questions. This is not
> to be rude or to discourage your curiosity, but rather to focus on what the
> thoughts and feelings behind your questions may be. Similarly, there may
> be times when you want my advice or guidance. This is only natural, but
> the form of therapy we are embarking on is meant to foster your own abil-
> ity to think about yourself and to make decisions for yourself. My role is
> to help you understand what it is that you want and what conflicts you
> have around what you want, rather than to tell you what to do. I want to
> stress that everything you tell me here is confidential; what we say here is
> a private matter between us. I will provide no information to third parties
> unless we first discuss it here and agree on it. In that case, I will ask you
> for a written authorization to release information. What questions do you
> have about what I have said?

With patients with a history of suicide attempts or other destructive
behaviors, the therapist would add this:

> The only exception to the confidentiality rule would be if you pose a threat
> to your life or someone else's, in which case I will be obliged to take what-
> ever steps are necessary to protect you or whomever else might be in-
> volved.

Clarifying the Limits of Therapist's Involvement.   Depending on the
patient's history and presentation, the therapist may want to more explicitly delineate the limits of her involvement with the patient—specifically,
that the therapy is restricted to verbal interaction in an office setting
during the established session times, except in the case of emergencies.
This explication is generally not necessary with NPO patients, who for the
most part take for granted these parameters of a professional relationship,
but it may be important with some BPO patients, particularly those who
have participated in prior treatments in which they relied on the therapist
for phone support or in which boundaries were not clear.

The therapist should explain the rationale for limiting phone calls. It is not merely that the therapist does not want to be bothered, but that the policy is intrinsic to how the therapy works. For example, a therapist might explain in this way:

> The work we do in this form of therapy takes place in our regularly scheduled therapy sessions and in the time frame that we have agreed upon. I know this is different from your last treatment, where you would routinely call your doctor when you felt distressed in the evenings and over the weekend. Although I understand that this was helpful for a time, I think you are here because you felt that your previous treatment could only take you so far. In general, the treatment I am suggesting does not always provide immediate relief in the form of my supporting you on the phone or even of my supporting you during your sessions. In fact, if I am put in the role of providing support or coaching, either on the phone or in person, it will interfere with my being able to best help you attain the long-term goals of this treatment: to help you think about and manage what is going on inside you, to help you function more independently and adaptively in the world, and to help you use your new knowledge to make good decisions for yourself. Having said this, I understand that there will likely be times when you want to contact me between sessions. Or there may be times when you leave a session feeling distressed. We should consider whether you feel you are motivated at this point for this kind of treatment. If you are, let's think about what you can do to help you best deal with your feelings at those moments when you are experiencing distress, and let's consider resources to which you may have access, both within yourself and in your outside life. For example, you might deal with the situation by using your DBT skills, calling a friend, going for a run, going to a meeting, or reading a book.

Part 3

Individualized Elements of the Treatment Contract

THE GOAL OF THE CONTRACTING PHASE IS to establish the least restrictive framework for the treatment. At a minimum, this phase entails establishing the treatment frame focusing on goals, logistics, and the roles of patient and therapist. For most NPO patients and many BPO patients, the universal parameters of treatment outlined in Part 2 of this chapter will be sufficient to create a safe framework within which the patient's conflictual object relations can unfold. For these patients, the contract will establish the treatment frame and organize the treatment, while helping patient and therapist explore the meaning of—and, if need be, set limits on—deviations from the agreed-upon treatment arrangements. Among these deviations are such behaviors as inconsistent attendance, inconsistent payment, chronic lateness, and failure to participate fully by communicating openly in session.

In contrast, when treating patients with more severe pathology, whose behavior may be overtly destructive or who derive significant secondary gain from their illness, as well as the sizable number of patients with personality disorders who present with a co-occurring diagnosis (e.g., substance misuse, eating disorder, or a chronic medical condition), the therapist may need to introduce additional arrangements in order to conduct the treatment and to enable the therapist to manage and explore destructive behaviors within the framework of TFP-E. In addition, if the TFP-E therapist is to be prescribing psychoactive medications, an agreement about how to handle medication management within the framework of TFP-E will be introduced as part of the treatment frame.

Common Behaviors That May Require Specific Parameters in the Treatment Contract

A variety of types of behavior may require the introduction of specific parameters into the treatment contract. Most obvious are self-destructive behaviors that are sufficiently dangerous to demand that the therapist intervene directly to attempt to control the patient's behavior, superseding and potentially making it impossible to do exploratory work. This group includes, for example, suicide attempts and gestures and cutting (all most commonly encountered in patients with borderline personality disorder), reckless driving or driving under the influence, unsafe sex, and unlawful activities. Also included are various forms of substance misuse and eating disorder symptoms.

For patients with potentially life-threatening medical or psychiatric chronic illnesses who have a history of noncompliance with their treatment, compliance with medical management may also be included in the contract as a precondition for TFP-E treatment. Less obvious but equally problematic are behaviors that are sufficiently gratifying to interfere with the patient's motivation to change—for example, leading a passive, parasitic lifestyle while extracting financial support from family or social services; or using the illness to control family, other social support, or the therapist. Finally, behaviors that have functioned as chronic and disruptive resistances in previous treatments will often require specific arrangements.

General Principles: Introducing Specific Parameters Into the Treatment Contract

During the contracting phase, the therapist takes the following steps in relation to specific behaviors that may require the introduction of individualized elements into the TFP-E contract:

1. Identify behaviors that require specific parameters through careful assessment and history taking (see the following subsection, "Identifying Behaviors That May Require Specific Parameters in the Treatment Contract").
2. Work with the patient to introduce a framework for anticipating and managing these behaviors—one that involves the patient's taking responsibility for the behavior, and removing the therapist from control of the patient's behavior (see the subsection, "Working With the Patient to Introduce a Framework for Anticipating and Managing Behaviors").
3. Work with the patient to eliminate life situations that provide excessive secondary gain, and ensure that the patient is employed or engaged in structured activity (see the subsection "Addressing Social Dependency, Secondary Gain, and the Importance of Structured Activity").
4. Consider holding a joint meeting with the patient and the patient's family or significant other during the contracting phase (see the subsection "Involving Third Parties").

Identifying Behaviors That May Require Specific Parameters in the Treatment Contract

A current or past history of self-destructive or dangerous behavior, substance misuse, eating disorder, or major medical or psychiatric illness—

any of which may require specific parameters—will have been identified and carefully assessed as part of the consultation. In negotiating the treatment contract, the therapist will discuss the management of these behaviors in the context of a potential treatment. The best indicators that specific behaviors are likely to emerge as a threat to or be unduly disruptive to treatment are the patient's behaviors in previous treatments and the patient's behavior with the current clinician during the assessment and contracting phase. Patients apt to engage in disruptive behaviors—such as chronic poor attendance, consistent lateness, harassing the therapist with phone calls, failure to pay the therapist in a reasonable fashion, or failure to leave sessions when time is up—often demonstrate these behaviors during the assessment and contracting phase. Similarly, behaviors that were disruptive in previous treatments are extremely likely to present in subsequent treatments.

Speaking With Previous Treaters

Before initiating the contracting phase with a patient who has a personality disorder, the therapist should have a clear view of previous treatments, including what the patient hoped to get out of the treatment and what he felt he was able to accomplish, how the patient viewed the therapist, how the treatment ended and whether the patient played an active role in it ending, what the major problems in the treatment were, and whether the patient believes he would do anything differently this time. It is important to obtain permission to speak with prior therapists, and to share any concerns raised in those conversations with the patient as part of the contracting process. If a patient refuses to provide permission for contact with a previous treater, it is best not to proceed until this issue can be resolved.

Working With the Patient to Introduce a Framework for Anticipating and Managing Behaviors

Contracting Around Treatment-Interfering Behaviors

In making the determination as to whether and how to contract around certain behaviors or sources of secondary gain, the therapist considers, on the one hand, the ideal of being as unrestrictive as possible and, on the other, whether each behavior under consideration is sufficiently severe or disruptive that proceeding with therapy is unreasonable without a specific plan or safeguards in place. This determination reflects the dangerousness of the behavior, the behavior's potential disruption to the treatment (including the degree to which it is likely to interfere with the therapist's ability to freely listen to the patient, to be emotionally available, and to maintain a neutral stance), and the extent to which the behavior could override whatever genuine motivation the patient may have to change.

If during the contracting phase the therapist identifies behavior that raises a potential threat to the treatment, the next order of business is to share this with the patient. As described in Clinical Illustrations 5–8, the therapist calls attention to the behavior in question, shares her concern that it poses a potential threat to treatment, and explains her rationale for why the behavior is not compatible with TFP-E. The objective is to appeal to the patient's sense of reason while at the same time demonstrating that the therapist is not being judgmental or arbitrary; **the therapist communicates that the issue is not the therapist's personal attitude toward the patient's behavior, but rather the therapist's assessment that the behavior poses a problem within the treatment frame of TFP-E.**

Having shared her concern and her rationale, the therapist listens to the patient's response. If the patient is receptive or curious, the therapist then invites the patient to suggest a concrete plan to limit disruptive behavior, or the therapist may take a more active role by suggesting a plan to the patient. In either case, therapist and patient discuss the specifics of arrangements for managing the identified behavior within the treatment until the two agree upon a clearly described plan that represents the minimal conditions for the treatment or they come to the determination that this is not possible.

Clinical Illustration 5: Identifying and Contracting Around Behavior Disruptive to the Treatment

Ms. K, a high-BPO patient, was seen in consultation several years after a lengthy previous treatment had ended. She was a 45-year-old homemaker diagnosed with narcissistic personality disorder with sadomasochistic features. She described having initially felt hopeful about that treatment, but ultimately she left it feeling disappointed; she remained plagued by the same interpersonal problems that had brought her to treatment almost a decade earlier.

Ms. K described her previous treatment and therapist, Dr. A, in bland, vague terms; she gave Dr. P, the therapist seeing her in consultation for

TFP-E treatment, permission to contact Dr. A. When he spoke to Dr. A, Dr. P learned that in all the years the patient had been in treatment with him, she had consistently been at least 5 minutes (and usually 10 minutes) late for her sessions, regardless of the time at which they were scheduled. Although Dr. A had raised this behavior as a problem, Ms. K persisted in arriving late. Dr. A explained to Dr. P that he had ultimately concluded that this was "the best the patient could do," and that his seeing her for a foreshortened session was better than not seeing her at all.

Ms. K arrived a few minutes late to her next meeting with Dr. P, and Dr. P raised the issue of the patient's consistent lateness in her previous treatment. The patient was dismissive, insisting that it wasn't a big deal and that often her sessions were "boring, and didn't help anyway."

Dr. P explained to Ms. K that although he understood that her lateness seemed unimportant to her, from his perspective, chronic lateness, even if only of a few minutes, was extremely important, and in his estimation had likely contributed to the disappointing outcome of her previous treatment. Dr. P went on to say that he suspected that by arriving late, she had kept important feelings out of the treatment; if she and Dr. P were to work together, figuring out how to bring those feelings into the new treatment would be an important objective.

Dr. P then shared his impression that if Ms. K was unable to modify her behavior and attend sessions on time, he anticipated another failed treatment, and he had reservations about beginning under these conditions. Dr. P suggested making consistent and timely arrival to sessions a condition of treatment. The patient agreed, and treatment began.

Ms. K again arrived a few minutes late to her next appointment. Dr. P identified the patient's late arrival as a priority theme, exploring how it had happened that she was late on the heels of their recent discussion. When the patient was dismissive, Dr. P reminded her of their discussion and of the agreement they had made, and commented that her behavior left him curious; he had made it quite clear that her continued lateness would interfere with the effectiveness of the treatment. In light of this clarification, how did she understand her lateness for this appointment? Ms. K demonstrated a visible flash of anger, which she denied and would not elaborate, saying simply that she would be on time in the future.

Ms. K arrived promptly to the next session. Her manner was initially subdued and then increasingly guarded; exploration of her attitude toward the therapist led to elaboration of her experience of Dr. P as controlling and untrustworthy, "playing" her while he harbored a hidden intent to frustrate or humiliate her. Identifying and exploring this affectively charged paranoid transference, which had been split off and enacted with the roles reversed in the previous treatment, was the beginning of finally understanding and ultimately resolving the patient's interpersonal problems.

This vignette illustrates the importance of controlling certain forms of acting out—not for the purpose of correcting the patient's behavior per se, but because such behavior functions as a fixed defense against the unfolding of conflictual object relations in the treatment.[3] In this example, the patient's behavior was neither dangerous nor overtly disruptive, but nevertheless threatened the successful outcome of the treatment by protecting Ms. K from experiencing pathogenic object relations in the treatment and in the transference; as long as she arrived late, she avoided feeling controlled and potentially frustrated and humiliated by the therapist. In this example, contracting around timely attendance marked the difference between a successful outcome and another treatment failure.

This example also illustrates the importance and value of developing a clear understanding of problems that have emerged in previous treatments, especially those that have disrupted treatment or led to a stalemate. It may be tempting to feel that past failures reflect the limitations of past treaters or treatment approaches, but more often than not, they also reflect the nature of the patient's personality pathology. It is advisable to structure the treatment contract with the expectation that the same behaviors will pose a risk to any new treatment that is initiated; unless the treatment contract accounts for past problems and structures the treatment to guard against them, it is likely that history will repeat itself.

Contracting Around Destructive Behavior

Some patients with personality disorders may rely on destructive behaviors to manage anxiety and depressive affect or to modulate mood states—for example, superficial cutting, periodic bingeing or purging, substance use, or anonymous sex. Some of these individuals may be motivated for treatment but find it difficult to agree to completely relinquish these behaviors at the outset. Although these behaviors may likely be disruptive to a TFP-E treatment if persistent over the long term, they may not be sufficiently dangerous or acutely worrisome to preclude beginning treatment. The therapist can share with the patient a concern about risks posed to the treatment by the behavior and ascertain whether the patient is motivated to establish the goal of relinquishing destructive behavior during the early phase of treatment.

In the contracting phase with patients in this group (or when recontracting with these individuals), it is essential to incorporate a plan for managing the behavior within the constraints of the treatment while the

---

[3]In psychodynamic lingo, this patient's lateness could be described in terms of *acting out as a form of transference resistance*—that is, the patient's behavior (acting out) defended against (resisted) emergence of the paranoid transference.

patient works with the TFP-E therapist to address underlying personality pathology and to identify the triggers and motivations for and meanings of the behaviors. If this approach is to work, any secondary gain that the patient may derive in relation to the therapist or the patient's family must be addressed—for example, by ensuring that destructive behavior does not lead to additional contact with the therapist or an opportunity to control the family.

Further, the patient must understand that the behavior in question, in the long term, is incompatible with TFP-E and ultimately guarantees a treatment failure; thus, the patient begins treatment with the agreement that TFP-E is being initiated on a trial basis, to see if the patient can make use of the treatment to control his behavior within an agreed-upon period of time. If during the early months of treatment, the patient fails to relinquish—or at least to significantly decrease—identified behaviors, discontinuing TFP-E and shifting to a behaviorally oriented approach is recommended.

Clinical Illustration 6: Contracting Around High-Risk Behavior

Dr. M, a specialist in the treatment of personality disorders, was contacted by Dr. A, who asked if he could transfer to Dr. M's care a patient he had been seeing in psychotherapy. Dr. O was a 38-year-old single male physician presenting with relationship problems. Dr. M had diagnosed the patient with histrionic personality disorder with sadomasochistic and narcissistic features organized at a middle to high borderline level.

Dr. A had been seeing Dr. O for the past 12 months in an unstructured, twice-weekly psychotherapy, using an "eclectic" approach. Initially, things had seemed to go well; the patient's depressive symptoms resolved and he "worked hard" in the therapy, in which he focused on his troubled childhood, while maintaining an idealizing transference. Several months into the treatment, Dr. O shared with Dr. A that when he felt anxious, he would go to bondage, discipline, and masochism (BDM) Web sites to find a woman to have sex with. Though he denied engaging in "dangerous" sex games, he shared with Dr. A that in recent months he had on several occasions engaged in unprotected intercourse during "adventures" of this type.

Over the ensuing months, Dr. A became aware of a pattern in which Dr. O would respond to an especially emotional therapy session by going home, finding a partner, and "hooking up." Dr. A felt uncomfortable with this turn of events; he tried interpreting the meanings of the patient's activities but found that his efforts had no impact on his patient's behavior. With time, Dr. A found himself avoiding affectively charged material in session for fear of precipitating what he described as "sexual acting out."

Dr. A acknowledged to Dr. M that he felt totally controlled by his countertransference at this point, which was expressed as worried preoccupation with Dr. O's behavior and, beneath his worry, profound feelings of guilt and shame; he viewed himself as participating in a treatment relationship that was potentially destructive to the patient but felt helpless to make it stop.

The patient, meanwhile, was becoming increasingly critical of Dr. A; he routinely complained that after a year of treatment, he was no better off than when he started, and began to request a new therapist. Dr. A shared with Dr. M that he felt "totally burned out" by this patient and his treatment and was happy to comply with this request. He hoped that Dr. M would agree to see Dr. O in consultation and consider treating him.

When Dr. M saw Dr. O in consultation, his assessment was that the patient had an overall favorable prognosis with TFP-E, but that the patient's propensity to manage his anxiety by periodically indulging in high-risk sexual behavior had disrupted his last treatment and no doubt had the potential to do so again. During the evaluation, Dr. M asked Dr. O about his sexual behavior; the patient spoke freely and also stated that it was his goal to get into a stable relationship within which he could safely enjoy BDM sexual activity.

Dr. M inquired about the previous treatment, and shared with Dr. O that Dr. A had been under the impression that the patient would respond to anxiety-provoking sessions by sexually "hooking up" and that at times he did not use condoms. Dr. O said that this was true, that he had been aware this was what he had been doing, and that he understood Dr. A was uncomfortable with BDM. Dr. M explained that from his perspective, the issue was not Dr. A's level of comfort with BDM, but rather the patient's high-risk behavior.

Dr. M went on to share his impression that Dr. O had a choice between two overall approaches to treatment. One was a behaviorally focused treatment focusing on anxiety management and behavioral control, with the goal of helping him both in managing his anxiety and in pursuing his sexual interests in a way that did not endanger his health or safety. Dr. M suggested that this approach would make sense if the patient felt it would be difficult for him to limit himself to relatively safe sexual encounters.

The other possible approach was TFP-E, which Dr. M said he considered to be the most likely to help Dr. O develop the kind of stable relationship he was seeking; this kind of treatment was twice-weekly and intensive, and could only take place if the patient could guarantee his own safety. The treatment would focus on the feelings and motivations behind Dr. O's interpersonal difficulties; in this form of treatment, Dr. M explained, the therapist helps the patient observe and reflect on the motivations behind his behavior, thoughts, and feelings, including pressure to engage in potentially dangerous sexual activity, and to explore his internal experience. However, the therapist's freedom to work in this way is predicated on the patient's being able to limit destructive behaviors.

Dr. O expressed interest both in working with Dr. M and in beginning TFP-E. He said that he sensed Dr. M knew what he was talking about, and he shared his anxiety that during the previous treatment, things had been "getting out of control." Dr. M explained to the patient: "TFP-E is at times anxiety provoking and can stir up strong feelings; it is an important part of the treatment to help you develop a greater capacity to manage and contain strong emotions. But this can only be done if you are able to control your behavior—to pay attention to and explore your impulses rather than act upon them."

Dr. M went on to suggest that they discuss a treatment contract, one that would protect Dr. O from putting himself at risk by helping him control his behavior and make good choices, and that at the same time would also protect the therapist's ability to calmly reflect on what was happening in the treatment and to help the patient explore his inner life. Dr. M said that from his perspective, this would mean their agreeing that as a condition for beginning and continuing the treatment, the patient would avoid unprotected sex, join a "safe" online BDM community to identify sexual partners, and meet regularly with his internist to be monitored for sexually transmitted diseases. He suggested that Dr. O spend time before their next meeting thinking first about whether he would be able to work within these parameters, and then about whether these were restrictions that he wanted to take on at this point.

The patient returned, agreed to the conditions outlined by Dr. M, and said that he wanted to begin treatment. Making use of Dr. A's earlier experience in treating the patient, and now beginning treatment with a suitable contract in place, Dr. M was able to help Dr. O explore the anxieties that he had been avoiding and enacting with his self-destructive sexual behavior—in particular, conflict over allowing himself to pursue his own needs and enjoy his autonomy and sexuality versus being forced to submit to another part of himself that wanted to keep him restrained, submissive, and self-destructive. This conflict manifested in the treatment through activation of the defensive object relation of a submissive, helpless self in relation to a dominating, controlling, and sadistic other. Although in his previous treatment with Dr. A, Dr. O had lived out this dyad in his sexual life and enacted it in the transference with the roles reversed (i.e., Dr. A ultimately felt controlled and helpless in relation to the patient), the new treatment contract enabled Dr. M to help Dr. O explore this object relation in the transference, focusing on the patient's wishes and his subtle efforts to either submit to or to control the therapist.

Focusing on Necessary Conditions for Treatment

When introducing limits on specific behaviors as part of the treatment contract, the therapist makes clear that the parameters she is proposing **do not represent a judgment about the patient's behavior but rather reflect an informed understanding of what is needed for a TFP-E treatment to be successful.** It is extremely helpful to patient and therapist alike to conceptualize this aspect of the treatment contract as creating and protecting the *necessary conditions for treatment.* In introducing the need to contract around behaviors in which the patient may be highly invested, insofar as they are "tried-and-true," often ego-syntonic mechanisms for managing distress, the therapist is respectful of the patient's autonomy, sharing the rationale for why such behavior is not compatible with TFP-E treatment and supporting the patient's freedom to make an informed choice. The therapist's approach is neutral and logical, based on what is needed to safeguard the treatment, and she does not otherwise take a position in relation to the patient's behavior. (For example, the therapist does not state that smoking marijuana daily is "bad for your health" but rather that it is not compatible with beginning a TFP-E treatment.)

In sum, effective negotiation of the treatment contract in relation to disruptive and destructive behaviors is predicated on the therapist's ability to maintain a neutral stance in relation to the patient's behavior and to avoid engaging in debate about the need for behavioral control, as well as on the patient's willingness to assume responsibility for managing his behavior.

Addressing Social Dependency, Secondary Gain, and the Importance of Structured Activity

It is common for patients with personality disorders to function below their abilities or level of education (Torgersen 2014), and for many, improved professional functioning will be a goal of treatment. However, some patients are neither employed nor attending school; they may be supported by stipends, investments, or assistance from family members. Others live on public assistance. The motivations driving such arrangements are heterogeneous, but patients with dependent, infantile, or passive traits, and those with narcissistic and antisocial traits, are especially predisposed to this kind of arrangement.

For example, Ms. V, a woman in her 30s who functioned at a high borderline level, had been unemployed since losing a job several years earlier and was supported by her affluent father. She explained that working was very "stressful" for her. Ms. V tended to feel easily overwhelmed, tearful, and unable to follow instructions or indeed to function at all, and much preferred to "spare myself another humiliation" by staying out of the workplace.

Another patient, who was organized at a low borderline level and had a narcissistic personality disorder with antisocial features, was collecting public assistance. Though she had done office work in the past, the patient explained that she didn't like "answering to anyone" and could collect almost as much from public assistance as she would be able to earn if she were to return to work.

Regardless of the motives driving a patient's dependent lifestyle, chronic dependence and unemployment pose a significant risk to treatment. This is both because secondary gains, be they emotional or financial, may override the patient's motivations to get well and because TFP-E focuses simultaneously on the patient's behavior in session and on his functioning in the world; therefore, a patient who is attending his therapy sessions but otherwise sitting at home avoiding rather than facing his anxieties and conflicts about functioning in the world will be able to avoid his conflicts in his treatment as well.

In our experience, with the exception of full-time students and those with full-time childcare responsibilities, patients with personality disorders will need to be engaged in structured activity if they are to benefit from TFP-E. Such activity can be tailored to the patient's current level of actual disability, with the expectation of increasing levels of responsibility over time. Some patients may only be able to participate in a day program, whereas others are fully capable of full-time work at a very high level. In between is a range of patients, from those who begin by participating in volunteer work to those who pursue job training, part-time work, or full-time work that may be below what they are ultimately capable of.

During the evaluation, the therapist takes a careful history of how the patient supports himself, how he manages his day-to-day functioning, and how he spends his time. For a socially dependent patient, the therapist does a thorough assessment of the patient's educational and work history, capabilities, understanding of what is holding him back from working, and motivation to work versus hanging on to a nonfunctioning lifestyle because of psychological and financial secondary gain. If the patient is not working, the therapist frames this as a threat to treatment during the contracting phase; and if patient and therapist confirm treatment is to begin, the contract includes parameters around structured activity and employment that are presented as a precondition of treatment.

Most patients agree to some sort of structured activity, at least within a circumscribed timeline. However, some patients, especially those who derive gratification from extracting money from family members, as well as those who are more antisocial, may ultimately be unwilling to contract around employment. In this case, the therapist should explain that engagement in structured activity and having financial independence as a goal are preconditions for the treatment, necessary if the patient is to benefit from treatment. Patients who adamantly refuse to participate in structured activity or to entertain the goal of relinquishing a dependent position are best told that TFP-E is not the proper treatment for them because one of its goals is autonomous functioning. Patients in this group can be referred for supportive treatment or general clinical management. If the patient otherwise has a good prognosis, the therapist can share her impression that the patient indeed might benefit from the treatment were he willing to pursue employment, and she can offer to see the patient in the future should he so choose.

In Video 3, "Contracting," Dr. Yeomans illustrates several aspects of the TFP-E contracting process with a patient with borderline personality disorder. Dr. Yeomans first addresses the patient's history of cutting and the TFP-E approach to this behavior. He then focuses on the need to engage in work or other structured activity in order to participate in the treatment. Dr. Yeomans does not accept the patient's initial rejection of his recommendations for structured activity, and instead tactfully explains to the patient his rationale for structuring the therapy as he is. Dr. Yeomans empathizes with the patient's sense that returning to work is beyond her abilities while simultaneously conveying his confidence that she is capable of living a productive life. In addition to illustrating contracting around self-harm and structured activity, this video highlights how the TFP-E therapist makes use of the shared diagnosis and psychoeducation during the contracting phase.

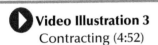 **Video Illustration 3**
Contracting (4:52)

Clinical Illustration 7: Contracting Around Secondary Gain

Ms. V (mentioned earlier in this subsection), single and in her 30s, had dependent personality disorder, had been unemployed for several years, and was supported by her affluent father. She expressed interest in beginning TFP-E. She presented with chronic depression, a long history of troubled relationships with men, and a wish to be married. She had failed several previous, rather lengthy treatments.

During the first contracting session, the therapist explained that if the treatment were to be effective, Ms. V would need to be engaged in some kind of structured activity. At the outset, it could be a part-time or even a volunteer position, but at least a half-time commitment was a precondition for treatment. The patient responded that working was very "stressful" for her in that she would feel easily overwhelmed, tearful, and unable to follow instructions or indeed to function at all, as indicated earlier. The therapist sympathized with her difficulty and stressed that this was something they would be working on together in the treatment.

Ms. V responded that she knew the therapist was right—she *should* be working—but that she didn't like deadlines or being told what to do. The therapist replied that this, too, was something important that they would work on in the treatment, but it was still the case that if she were not working, she would not benefit from the treatment. If Ms. V could not agree to find work within a few months' time, TFP-E was not the right treatment for her right now, and they could talk about other treatment options, such as supportive psychotherapy or CBT.

Involving Third Parties

It can often be helpful to involve the patient's family or significant other in the contracting phase, especially when a patient has more severe pathology. The meeting should take place with the patient present, and all parties should be made to understand that outside of emergencies, the content of the patient's communications with the therapist is to remain confidential. At the same time, the family is free to share with the therapist any information they feel is important.

A helpful rule of thumb is that if the family or a significant other is providing a primary source of support, be it financial or emotional, it is generally a good idea to have a meeting to include that person before the patient begins treatment. A family meeting is clearly indicated if a patient lives with or is financially supported by his parents, or if the patient's spouse or parents will be paying for the treatment. A family meeting is highly recommended when contracting with any patient who is at significant risk for destructive or self-destructive behavior; in our experience, it is extremely difficult for the TFP-E therapist to maintain a neutral stance with a destructive patient unless there is cooperation from the patient's support system.

A family meeting during the contracting phase can start off the therapy on solid footing and may serve to prevent potential problems down the road, including the patient's attempt to create a split between the therapist and the family, and the family's inadvertent support of the patient's efforts to circumvent aspects of the treatment contract. The goal of a family meeting during the contracting phase is to help the family understand what the treatment is about, what the treatment contract includes, what to expect, and how to handle the patient's behavior once treatment begins, as well as to discuss how payment will be handled. When the therapist is treating a patient at risk for destructive or self-destructive behavior, meeting with the family provides a needed opportunity to discuss how emergencies are handled within the frame of TFP-E, and to discuss the rationale behind limitations of the therapist's involvement. The therapist can also educate family and significant others about how they can best be of help to the patient in any emergency situation that should arise.

Contracting Around Specific Behaviors, Adjunctive Treatments, and Medication

Applying the general principles introduced above, we next present the TFP-E approach to contracting around specific behaviors: suicidality, co-occurring disorders (including substance use and eating disorders), and medication management (including noncompliance).

Suicidality and Parasuicidality

Patients with severe personality disorders may have a history of recurrent suicide attempts, gestures, or other forms of extreme, overtly dangerous, or even life-threatening forms of destructive behavior. This behavior manifests especially in those with borderline personality disorder, but also in some patients with narcissistic personality disorder or antisocial personality disorder, typically with a low or at times middle level of BPO.

DBT is a treatment specifically developed for treatment of parasuicidality, and patients for whom this is a primary complaint may do well with initial referral to DBT. However, many patients who present with chronic suicidality or self-destructive behavior have more ambitious goals than behavioral control; if the contract is tailored appropriately, some of these individuals can do well with TFP-E (Clarkin et al. 2007; Doering et al. 2010; see the section "Differential Therapeutics and Discussing Treatment Options" in Chapter 7). This approach is outlined in detail in the TFP manual (Yeomans et al. 2015), which describes a form of TFP-E developed specifically for treatment of borderline personality disorder.[4]

---

[4]For readers who work extensively with low-BPO patients, the cited TFP manual offers in-depth discussion of contracting and emergency management with severely disturbed populations.

The overall strategy for contracting around chronic and dangerous forms of destructive behavior is that the therapist and patient agree on a plan that enables the patient to manage self-destructive impulses without involving the therapist outside treatment hours. Rather, the patient manages his own behavior outside his sessions and then uses the sessions to explore the motivations driving his behavior and the object relations enacted in them, which often become tied to developments in the transference. The plan outlined in the initial contract involves the patient taking responsibility first for deciding whether he can control his impulses on his own (e.g., by using DBT skills or coping mechanisms, such as exercise or meditation, or by contacting social supports), and then, if he cannot, making a commitment to visit an emergency room or crisis team for evaluation of dangerousness. In the latter case, the TFP-E therapist consults with the emergency room physician, but the determination of dangerousness and the decision about disposition are made by the evaluating physician; such determinations are outside the therapist's control.

The therapist explains to the patient:

> The treatment I am recommending is predicated on your being able to control your own behavior, and on my helping you do that by exploring the feelings and conflicts that are motivating your behavior. For me to help you in this way, I cannot be involved in managing and controlling your behavior in the way that your previous therapists have done. My taking an active role to protect you from yourself will not help you learn how to be less self-destructive, and at the end of the day may even be counterproductive. So we have to decide together if this is the right approach for you.

This tactic is especially integral to the treatment of patients whose destructive behavior is supported by secondary gain derived from controlling or frightening the therapist; the TFP-E approach to contracting will reduce this motivation as a potential driver of destructive behavior. In this setting, once the contract is in place, it becomes the therapist's task to identify and explore with the patient the conflict between 1) the part of him that wants to make use of the treatment and establish a working relationship with the therapist, and 2) the part of him that wants to enjoy the sadistic pleasure of controlling and torturing the therapist at the expense of making productive use of the treatment.

Co-Occurring Disorders

In approaching the patient with personality pathology who also has a co-occurring psychiatric disorder, such as alcohol or drug abuse, eating disorder, affective illness, or anxiety disorder, it is essential to appreciate that TFP-E is not a treatment that specifically targets these disorders, which often co-occur with personality pathology. For the patient who presents for treatment of a personality disorder and also has co-occurring diagnoses, the strategy is to ensure that neither the co-occurring disorder nor its treatment precludes effective TFP-E treatment of personality pathology. This requires that in the consultative and contracting phase of TFP-E, co-occurring disorders are thoroughly evaluated and a strategy for treating co-occurring disorders is put in place before beginning TFP-E. In addition to medication management, evidence-based treatments for these disorders typically involve CBT or some form of supportive psychotherapy or peer counseling. The overall aim during the assessment and contracting phase with this group of patients is to determine the feasibility of putting together a treatment package that addresses both behavioral and structural pathology, while allowing the TFP-E therapist to preserve the stance and techniques that define TFP-E.

The specific strategy adopted in relation to co-occurring disorders will reflect the degree to which the co-occurring psychopathology is severe and refractory, as opposed to mild and responsive to treatment. Generally, thinking in terms of sequential treatment is best in more severe cases (e.g., substance dependence and eating disorders of moderate or greater severity; affective and anxiety disorders sufficiently severe as to significantly interfere with the patient's functioning and/or thinking). Specific treatment for the co-occurring disorder is initiated, and then the indications and the patient's motivations for TFP-E are reassessed. In milder cases, it is often feasible to treat personality and co-occurring disorders simultaneously, by integrating medication management into TFP-E and/or building a treatment package that addresses co-occurring disorders. Such a treatment package might incorporate a specific form of treatment delivered by a provider other than the TFP-E therapist—for example, a 12-step program or substance abuse counseling; treatment for eating disorders or nutritional counseling; psychopharmacological consultation or a short-term cognitive-behavioral intervention; or, for patients with sexual disorders or marital problems, couples or sex therapy. Integrating these modalities into the patient's care will become part of the overall frame of the TFP-E treatment.

In the mildest cases—for example, patients who engage in occasional binge drinking or weekend drug use—TFP-E contracting may control co-occurring problems sufficiently well so as to make it reasonable to begin TFP-E on a trial basis, with the understanding that identified behaviors pose a potential threat to the treatment and will be assessed in an ongoing fashion. If psychoactive medication is to be provided in the setting of TFP-E, procedures for integrating medication management into the treatment will be introduced as part of the treatment frame.

Substance Use

Many patients with personality disorders have a current or past history of substance abuse or dependency. Patients who are currently dependent on alcohol or other substances, or who are in the early phases of recovery, do poorly in TFP-E, and these patients should be referred to treatments that focus on detoxification, harm reduction, and/or sobriety and relapse prevention. In some cases, TFP-E can cause emotional stress and potentially increase the likelihood of relapse, especially for those in the early phases of recovery. For these reasons, TFP-E for patients with a history of substance dependence is recommended only when they are in stable remission. Depending on the patient's substance use history, the therapist should generally look for *at least* a 6-month period of abstinence and a structured recovery plan before considering beginning TFP-E. The therapist should include strict parameters that support relapse prevention, which most commonly involve the patient's consistent participation in a 12-step program or substance abuse treatment, possibly with adjunctive medication management, as part of the treatment contract. If a therapist has questions about the patient's reliability to cooperate with treatment, it can be helpful to involve a substance abuse specialist who can evaluate the patient before treatment begins and comment on the risk of relapse and, if treatment is initiated, perform random substance screening and work with the patient on relapse prevention.

More common than patients who present with actual substance dependence are those who abuse alcohol, cannabis, cocaine, prescription medications, opioids, or other illicit drugs. Contracting with these patients can be challenging, especially with patients whose social or professional circles openly sanction substance use. In our experience, individuals who routinely use substances to manage anxiety and distress are unlikely to do well in TFP-E unless they are genuinely motivated to curtail this usage. It is not imperative that patients in this group be completely abstinent before starting treatment (as illustrated in Clinical Illustration 8 later in this chapter), but they need to understand that 1) TFP-E is not a treatment for substance abuse, 2) significant substance abuse will preclude a positive outcome in TFP-E, and 3) TFP-E may in fact lead to exacerbation of substance-related problems.

If during the consultation or at any later point during treatment, substance abuse emerges as a central issue, it is often preferable to address this in a behaviorally oriented treatment before the patient begins or continues TFP-E. If the extent and clinical significance of substance abuse are at any point unclear, it can be helpful to meet with a family member or spouse to get a more complete history and share concerns, and to identify an outside party who is in a position to assess the patient's behavior and safety.

Eating Disorders

The TFP-E approach to eating disorders is essentially the same as with substance misuse. Patients with active and severe anorexia or bulimia are best treated with cognitive-behavioral treatment to stabilize symptoms before treatment of underlying personality pathology is considered. For those with milder symptoms and no history of significant medical complications, it may be possible to advantageously combine treatment of personality pathology in TFP-E with behaviorally oriented interventions for eating disorder symptoms. For example, it is reasonable to begin TFP-E while referring the patient to an eating disorders specialist or nutritionist who can monitor the patient's weight and work with the patient on abnormal eating behaviors.

Typically, the contract with the patient includes the condition that if her weight falls below a certain goal, if the frequency of purging surpasses a certain threshold, or if metabolic or dental complications develop, the therapist will interrupt the usual treatment to focus on eating disorder symptoms. Once these symptoms are stabilized, the therapist can then evaluate whether it makes sense to resume TFP-E. For patients with relatively mild symptoms—for example, occasional bingeing with or without purging, mild food restriction, or compulsive exercising—it may be sufficient to introduce the expectation that at the beginning of a session, the patient will raise the topic regarding any eating-disordered behavior as soon as it occurs; in addition, the patient should be expected to weigh herself at regular intervals or to have her internist do so, and to report weight measurements to the therapist.

Medication Management

Many patients with personality disorders come to TFP-E already taking medication; many of those who are not may benefit from medication trials for treatment of affective and anxiety disorders or for specific symptoms, such as paranoia, poor impulse control, or affect dysregulation. Still others may develop symptoms during the course of TFP-E that warrant psychopharmacological intervention. Many patients taking psychotropic medication will require adjustment of their regimens to optimize treatment response and minimize side effects, and even patients taking stable doses of medication require ongoing evaluation for long-term side effects and recurrence of symptoms.

Therefore, in the treatment of personality disorders, the therapist needs to identify and monitor the course of symptoms; and when patients are taking medication, the therapist needs to identify and monitor the response to it and any side effects that occur throughout the course of treatment. This applies regardless of whether the therapist is a physician, and whether the therapist or an outside consultant is prescribing and monitoring medication.

When discussing medication management with the patient, the therapist is more structured in her questioning and more directive in her interventions than is typical for the TFP-E therapist as a rule. When managing medication and tracking symptoms, the therapist will often set the agenda and systematically ask the patient to provide specific information, regardless of whether this is the affectively dominant issue. As a result, when a patient is taking psychoactive medication, it is necessary to have a framework within which to organize the integration of medication management into the therapy. This framework is introduced in the form of an agreement between therapist and patient about how discussion of medication management will be handled within the structure of the treatment. These arrangements, an integral part of the treatment frame, are part of the treatment contract and can be introduced in the context of the discussion of how therapist and patient will work together and the role of each in the treatment.

Although there are different ways to handle medication management within the structure of a TFP-E treatment, it is helpful to reserve the first few minutes of each session for discussion of medication-related matters. The therapist explains to the patient that he should use this time to bring up any issues or questions that he might have related to medication, including the status of his symptoms, side effects, and need for prescription renewals. The therapist also explains that she, too, will use the beginning of the session should she need to raise issues pertaining to medication.

This approach to medication management is analogous to the way that the therapist often discusses other specific behaviors included in individualized aspects of the treatment contract. For example, in Clinical Illustration 6, presented earlier in this chapter, Dr. M explained to his physician-patient Dr. O that should he deviate from their treatment contract and engage in unprotected sex, or if he felt pressure to do so, he should raise this as the first topic in his next therapy session, rather than following the usual procedure of sharing whatever was on his mind.

Noncompliance With Medication for Major Medical or Psychiatric Illness

For patients with a history of acting out in relation to medication prescribed for treatment of either chronic illnesses or a psychiatric disorder co-occurring with a personality disorder, it is sometimes advisable to contract around medication compliance, as in the following examples.

> A young woman with type 1 diabetes began TFP-E treatment with poorly regulated blood sugars and a history of potentially life-threatening hypoglycemic episodes, which she had used in the past to demand attention from both her family and her treatment team. Contracting for TFP-E included working closely with an endocrinologist and a diabetes nurse who would direct the patient's diabetes management; the therapist and patient also made an agreement that the patient would discuss with the therapist any occasions when she had purposefully or inadvertently mismanaged her insulin or had "lows," and that the TFP-E therapist, endocrinologist, and nurse would communicate freely about the patient's management.

> A middle-aged man with narcissistic personality disorder and a history of severe, protracted depressions with potentially lethal suicide attempts and poor compliance with antidepressant medication and mood stabilizers (which precipitated recurrence of suicidality), now affectively stable on maintenance medication, presented with interpersonal problems and requested TFP-E. In his previous therapy, this patient had devoted many hours to negotiating with the therapist about reducing or discontinuing his medication. The former therapist had felt compelled to repeatedly convince the patient of the necessity of taking his medication and to entreat him not to discontinue it, which he nevertheless did on a number of occasions, ending up in the hospital. The new therapist made it a condition of treatment that the patient meet regularly with a pharmacologist, follow the pharmacologist's recommendations, and cooperate with regular monitoring of antidepressant blood levels.

Recontracting After Treatment Begins

During the contracting phase, the therapist makes her best assessment, based on information available to her at the time, of the need to address in the contract any specific threats to treatment. However, it is not uncommon for maladaptive behaviors not previously present to manifest during the course of treatment, or for behaviors that were unrecognized or quiescent during contracting to reemerge and require limit setting and potential revision or elaboration of the treatment contract. The contract agreed upon by the patient and therapist before treatment begins is not a final agreement, written in stone; if need be, it can be modified or elaborated at any point during the treatment, using the same approach outlined for the initial contracting phase.

Clinical Illustration 8: Recontracting Around Alcohol Use

Ms. R, a 25-year-old graduate student functioning at a high borderline level, who presented with social anxiety in the setting of avoidant personality disorder with depressive and paranoid features, acknowledged "having a glass or two of wine" with her husband "to relax" in the evenings. The patient, who was quite guarded during the contracting phase, denied a history of alcohol-related blackouts or withdrawal and insisted that her drinking caused no impairment, or that it was or ever had been in any way a problem; in a quietly hostile fashion, she accused the therapist of a "conventional" attitude toward alcohol that was not shared by most persons in the patient's age group.

The therapist explained that he was not making a value judgment but rather that routine consumption of significant quantities of alcohol was incompatible with the treatment under consideration, which required a clear head and could at times stimulate anxiety and emotional distress. In fact, an objective of Ms. R's treatment would be to help her better tolerate and manage her emotions, and the use of alcohol to quell her anxiety could interfere with this process.

Ms. R assured the therapist that she rarely had more than a glass or two of wine at a time and abstained from drinking hard liquor. The therapist remained concerned but opted to proceed. He explained to the patient that he felt it made sense to initiate treatment under the circumstances, but with the caveat of concern about the potential for the patient's drinking to interfere with her capacity to make full use of the treatment; the therapist stated his concern about the risk of Ms. R's alcohol usage escalating during treatment if she were to use it to manage emotional distress. In light of this, the therapist requested that the patient apprise him of how much alcohol she was consuming and alert the therapist if she found herself drinking more. The patient consented, and the treatment began.

Several months into the treatment, Ms. R began arriving late to her 11:00 A.M. appointments. She acknowledged that she was having difficulty getting up in the mornings and that this was interfering with her completing her graduate course work. When the therapist inquired about her drinking, Ms. R acknowledged that it had escalated and that she and her husband were currently sharing several bottles of wine during the course of an evening. By this point, the patient no longer experienced the therapist as highly judgmental, as she had at the outset, and consequently was less guarded with him. When the therapist reminded Ms. R that they had agreed she would notify the therapist if she found herself drinking more, the patient responded that she hadn't said anything earlier because she had been afraid of the therapist's judgment and of the possibility of being "kicked out" of treatment.

For the first time, Ms. R then acknowledged that she herself felt concerned about her drinking; her wine intake was greater than it had ever been in the past, and she felt it was excessive, although she continued to insist that the therapist underestimated what was "normal." The therapist reminded the patient of their initial discussion about the incompatibility of alcohol abuse with the treatment, and asked the patient to consider the options about how they might best proceed. Ms. R rejected the therapist's suggestion that she attend Alcoholics Anonymous. Instead, she opted to begin by significantly curtailing her alcohol intake, with the understanding that if this failed, making the switch to sobriety would be the next step.

Ms. R spoke with her husband about cutting back on their drinking in general and about her decision to abstain from drinking on weeknights, asking him to support her in both decisions. She also began an internship that required an early start each day. In addition, for the first time, Ms. R agreed to try taking a selective serotonin reuptake inhibitor, which she found made it much easier for her to function socially during the day, and she began taking naltrexone, which helped her limit her drinking in the evenings.

This vignette highlights the need for therapists to actively question all patients in an ongoing fashion about substance use. The therapist took a flexible stance in relation to the patient's alcohol consumption, which escalated during the early months of treatment. Rather than taking a hard line early on, when the level of risk was not entirely clear, the therapist flagged alcohol as a potential problem and kept herself informed about the patient's usage. In this case, the patient's enlisting her husband's help in making a lifestyle change was sufficient to modify her alcohol consumption. Had the problem proved more refractory, the therapist was in a position to introduce more specific parameters around the patient's drinking, such as suggesting that the patient and her husband meet with the therapist together, or referring the patient to a substance abuse counselor or other form of treatment specifically targeting alcohol abuse. In more extreme cases—for example, if the patient were unable or unwilling to modify her behavior around alcohol—it could become necessary to interrupt treatment of personality pathology to focus on substance abuse treatment.

Key Clinical Concepts

- The treatment frame is an essential element in any form of psychotherapy, creating the setting within which the treatment is conducted.

- In TFP-E, the treatment frame is established in the form of a treatment contract.

- The treatment contract represents the necessary conditions for treatment.

- The treatment contract establishes the parameters of the treatment and the manner in which patient and therapist will work together.

- Contracting around specific behaviors and medication management enables the therapist to treat patients with complex comorbidities and to integrate other approaches into the overall framework of TFP-E.

- Treatment does not begin without a mutually agreed-upon treatment contract in place.

References

Clarkin JF, Levy KN, Lenzenweger MF, Kernberg OF: Evaluating three treatments for borderline personality disorder: a multiwave study. Am J Psychiatry 164(6):922–928, 2007 17541052

Doering S, Hörz S, Rentrop M, et al: Transference-focused psychotherapy v. treatment by community psychotherapists for borderline personality disorder: randomised controlled trial. Br J Psychiatry 196(5):389–395, 2010 20435966

Evans LJ, Beck A, Burdett M: The effect of length, duration, and intensity of psychological therapy on CORE global distress scores. Psychol Psychother 90(3):389–400, 2017 28261919

Hilsenroth MJ, Cromer TD: Clinician interventions related to alliance during the initial interview and psychological assessment. Psychotherapy (Chic) 44(2):205–218, 2007 22122211

Horvath AO, Del Re AC, Flückiger C, Symonds D: Alliance in individual psychotherapy. Psychotherapy (Chic) 48(1):9–16, 2011 21401269

Links P, Mercer D, Novick J: Establishing a treatment framework and therapeutic alliance, in Integrated Treatment for Personality Disorder: A Modular Approach. Edited by Livesley WJ, Dimaggio G, Clarkin JF. New York, Guilford, 2016, pp 101–119

Torgersen S: Prevalence, sociodemographics, and functional impairment, in The American Psychiatric Publishing Textbook of Personality Disorders, 2nd Edition. Edited by Oldham J, Skodol A, Bender D. Washington, DC, American Psychiatric Publishing, 2014, pp 109–129

Yeomans FE, Gutfreund J, Selzer MA, et al: Factors related to drop-outs by borderline patients: treatment contract and therapeutic alliance. J Psychother Pract Res 3(1):16–24, 1994 22700170

Yeomans F, Clarkin JF, Kernberg OF: Transference-Focused Psychotherapy for Borderline Personality Disorder: A Clinical Guide. Washington, DC, American Psychiatric Publishing, 2015

Section V

Techniques and Tactics of TFP-E

IN THE FOUR CHAPTERS IN THIS SECTION (Chapters 9–12), we describe 1) the *techniques* of transference-focused psychotherapy—extended (TFP-E)—that is, what the therapist does moment to moment in each therapy session; and 2) the *tactics* that the therapist uses to determine where, when, and how to intervene.

We begin with the tactics that guide the therapist as she identifies a focus for intervention, or priority theme, in each session. In TFP-E, the priority theme will typically reside in the *affectively dominant* object relations: those object relations organizing the patient's behavior, experience, and communications in session. However, when there are deviations from the treatment frame—when the patient is engaging in disruptive or destructive behavior or is failing to actively pursue the treatment goals—the therapist will identify these behaviors as the priority issue.

Once the therapist identifies a priority issue, this issue becomes the focus of intervention in the session. Then the therapist considers how to intervene in relation to the identified focus. In her interventions, the therapist will make use of the various techniques in the TFP-E toolbox, selecting and organizing her interventions systematically. The core techniques of TFP-E are exploratory interventions: clarification, confrontation, and interpretation, with special applications of these techniques to transference analysis. These interventions are made from a position of technical neutrality and are supported by analysis of countertransference. The tactics guiding exploratory interventions direct the therapist to begin with the patient's dominant experience in the moment, and then to open the patient's field

345

of view incrementally to include aspects of experience that are less accessible to consciousness, while supporting the patient's capacity for self-observation and reflection.

In addition to exploratory techniques, the TFP-E therapist makes use of supportive, or structuring, interventions to the degree that they are needed. The primary supportive techniques used in TFP-E are contracting and limit setting. Supportive interventions are employed to maintain the treatment frame and to contain destructive or disruptive behaviors, ensuring the necessary conditions for treatment.

The TFP-E therapist always addresses first any deviations from the frame, including destructive behavior or behavior disruptive to the treatment. If exploratory interventions fail to resolve the identified behaviors, then the therapist makes use of structuring techniques to set limits and to recontract if necessary. When the therapist makes use of limit setting or recontracting, she is choosing to deviate from technical neutrality.

In sum, the five basic *exploratory techniques* of TFP-E—what the therapist does moment to moment in each therapy session to promote the clinical process—are the following:

- Clarification
- Confrontation
- Interpretation
- Managing technical neutrality
- Countertransference utilization

In addition, these five basic techniques are the building blocks of higher-order exploratory interventions, notably:

- The interpretive process
- Transference analysis
- Working through

The five basic techniques are supplemented as needed to protect the clinical process by supportive interventions, most commonly these:

- Limit setting
- Recontracting

The *tactics* of treatment, guiding the therapist as to which material to address and how to organize her interventions, include the following:

- Contracting before beginning treatment
- Following a hierarchy of priorities to identity a priority theme, or dominant issue, in each session
- Using the tactics that guide the interpretive process and the process of working through to determine where, when, and how to intervene in relation to the dominant issue

We discuss principles for identifying a priority theme in Chapter 9. We cover clarification, confrontation, and interpretation in Chapter 10, and we discuss their application to the analysis of transference in Chapter 11. In the second half of Chapter 11, we discuss tactics guiding the use of exploratory techniques and help the therapist identify where, when, and how to initiate exploration. In Chapter 12, we discuss the use of supportive interventions and we complete the discussion of the interpretive process, focusing on managing technical neutrality, utilizing countertransference, and the process of working through.

Videos 4–7 are provided across Chapters 9, 10, and 12, with prompts for the reader to view in relation to pertinent text that discusses particular techniques and tactics in the videos. However, because the topics covered in Section V overlap by necessity to reflect the therapeutic process, these videos also demonstrate the integration of a variety of techniques to reflect a realistic clinical encounter; therefore, they can be viewed as a whole in conjunction with this entire section.

Identifying a Focus
for Intervention

ANY GIVEN THERAPY SESSION PRESENTS
the therapist with a wide array of possible issues to address. Some will be
embedded in what the patient is saying to the therapist; others in what the
patient is doing, or failing to do, in the treatment; and still others in the
atmosphere the patient is creating in session and the feelings she is stimulating in the therapist. Other important issues may be split off from the
patient's communications in session, reflecting the impact of dissociative
defenses on the patient's cognitive processes and communication. This
material may be expressed in the form of behaviors outside the sessions
that are potentially harmful to the patient, are disruptive to the treatment,
or potentially impede the patient's progress in the treatment.

Ultimately, the therapist must make an active choice regarding where
to focus clinical attention and therapeutic inquiry. This decision will have
great impact on how a session unfolds, and over time on the unfolding of
the entire treatment. We can think of this process in terms of identifying
a *priority theme*, or central issue, in the session (this concept of a priority
theme or central issue is similar to Bion's (1967) "selected fact").

Identifying a Priority Theme

In identifying a priority issue, the therapist using transference-focused
psychotherapy—extended (TFP-E) straddles two perspectives: one focus-

ing on the patient's internal experience in session, and the other on aspects of the patient's experience that may be split off from what she brings into the session but that are expressed in her behavior in relation to the treatment frame, treatment goals, and her general functioning outside sessions. To attend to the material the patient brings into the session, the therapist follows procedures for identifying the affectively dominant object relations, attending to the patient's verbal and nonverbal communications and the countertransference. To identify important aspects of the patient's functioning that may be split off from the material she brings into session, the therapist pays careful attention to the integrity of the treatment frame and contract and to what the patient does or does not bring into session with regard to her outside functioning, especially as it pertains to presenting complaints and treatment goals.

Hierarchy of Priorities Guiding Intervention

TFP-E is primarily an exploratory treatment. At the same time, we are mindful that in the treatment of personality pathology, the effectiveness of exploratory interventions is dependent on the integrity of the treatment frame and on the containment of dangerous or destructive behaviors in the patient's life (Yeomans et al. 2015). These requirements are reflected in the hierarchy of priorities for intervention.

Three Levels of Priority Themes

To identify a priority theme or central issue, the TFP-E therapist relies on a *hierarchy of priorities guiding intervention* (Table 9–1). We discuss each level of priority in further detail later in the chapter. Urgency of dangerous or disruptive behavior, psychodynamic factors central to treatment, and severity of personality pathology all influence the therapeutic focus on these priorities.

Priority Themes Across Degrees of Urgency

The hierarchy of priorities in relation to their relative urgency is as follows:

1. The therapist will always intervene first in relation to **emergency themes (Priority 1)**, if present. These include all behaviors that endan-

---

TABLE 9–1.　**Hierarchy of priorities guiding intervention**

Priority 1: Emergency themes, including dangerous behavior and threats to the continuity of the treatment

Priority 2: Integrity of the treatment frame, including attention to treatment goals

Priority 3: Affectively dominant object relations

---

ger the patient or others, or that threaten the continuity of the treatment, such as substance misuse, dangerous sexual practices, suicidal gestures, reckless driving, and cutting that is more than superficial.

2. Next, the therapist will attend to the **integrity of the treatment frame** (**Priority 2**). This includes adherence to the treatment contract negotiated before treatment commenced and attention to the mutually established **treatment goals**.

3. Finally, at those times when the frame is intact and there are no emergency themes, the therapist will focus directly on the **affectively dominant object relations** (**Priority 3**) that the patient brings into the session.

Priority Themes Central in Treatment

The hierarchy of priorities according to their relative centrality in the treatment is in reverse order to their relative urgency (discussed above).

Affectively Dominant Object Relations.　Priority 3, exploring the affectively dominant object relations, is the centerpiece of the treatment, the vehicle by which TFP-E promotes reflective and integrative processes within the patient. Identifying the dominant object relations is the first step in implementing the techniques that form the core of the treatment, and is also the ultimate outcome of pursuing Priorities 1 and 2. At the same time, although exploring the affectively dominant object relations is the central technical intervention of TFP-E, the effectiveness of these exploratory interventions is dependent on the integrity of the treatment frame and containment of destructive behavior on the part of the patient (see Chapter 12).

Integrity of the Treatment Frame.　In TFP-E, the treatment frame, negotiated in the treatment contract, represents the necessary conditions for treatment. Thus, if a patient is not adhering to the treatment frame, this becomes the priority theme in the session. Similarly, if a patient is consistently not taking obvious steps in her daily life to pursue the goals of treatment, this also becomes a priority. From this perspective, the therapist considers the treatment goals, once they have been mutually agreed upon in the contracting phase, as part of the frame of the treatment.

Dangerous Behavior and Threats to Continuity of Treatment.   Protecting the treatment from destructive behavior, if need be, is always the highest priority for intervention. If a patient is engaging in behavior that is overtly dangerous, prolonged efforts at exploration in the absence of behavioral cooperation are at best meaningless and at worst destructive. The gratification of engaging in destructive behavior while under the therapist's watch (best conceptualized as a form of *secondary gain*) can for some patients further fuel their destructiveness, even beyond the baseline that brought them to treatment in the first place.

Priority Themes and Clinical Process

The purpose of the treatment contract is to contain destructive behavior, support behavior change, and maintain the necessary conditions for treatment. Challenges to the treatment frame are ultimately understood in terms of enactment of and/or defenses against object relations activated in the treatment. For example, a patient with narcissistic personality disorder consistently cancels or skips sessions. This behavior can be understood as an effort to avoid the sense of humiliation associated in this patient's mind with having to accommodate to the therapist's schedule. Within the frame, deviation is the enactment of an object relation composed of a superior, devaluing patient in relation to a devalued, inadequate, and humiliated therapist, defending against its obverse: a superior, devaluing therapist and an inferior, humiliated patient. When the therapist addresses deviations from the frame, the objective is not to be rigid or to force the patient to comply, but rather to maintain the necessary conditions for exploration of the object relations associated with the deviation.

Once the contract has been established, the therapist frames any habitually destructive behavior in terms of deviations from the contract, invoking the patient's conflicts in relation to the treatment. For example, if a patient is cutting and this is a deviation from her treatment contract, the therapist focuses on what the patient is enacting in her behavior, often framed in terms of a conflict between a part of her that wants to be in treatment and receive help, and a part of her that wants to destroy that opportunity, and/or in terms of the object relation activated in the transference—for example, cutting as a refusal to submit to an arbitrary authority. In most cases, focusing on the contract will gradually lead to behavioral improvement (see Chapter 8). At times, the therapist may need to make use of limit setting in this process (see Chapter 12).

Priority Themes Across the Range of Severity

With neurotic personality organization (NPO) patients, the therapist is able to focus fairly consistently on identifying and exploring the affectively dominant object relations; issues of the frame—and even more so, emergencies—tend to take a back seat. In contrast, in the early phases of treatment with borderline personality organization (BPO) patients, deviations from the treatment contract are extremely common and often become the dominant vehicle for expression of the affectively dominant object relations in the session. As a rule, the more severe the patient's pathology, the more frequently intervention is directed toward maintaining the integrity of the treatment frame. As severity of pathology increases even further, emergency themes may become a priority, especially in the opening phase of the treatment.

Integration of Priorities in Treatment Focus

In sum, maintaining the integrity of the treatment frame and containing destructive behavior can be understood as playing a supportive and preparatory role in TFP-E, both by protecting the necessary conditions for treatment and by bringing conflictual object relations into the treatment, rather than allowing them to be split off and/or simply expressed in behavior. The objective in focusing on destructive behaviors and frame violations is not simply to extinguish them (although this is without question both important and necessary), but also to transform pathogenic, characterologically based behaviors into object relations enacted in the treatment and in the transference.

Priority 1: Attending to Emergency Priorities—Dangerous Behavior and Threats to the Continuity of Treatment

Whenever the therapist becomes aware that a patient is engaging in dangerous behavior or in behavior that immediately threatens the continuity of the treatment, attending to such developments automatically becomes the priority theme in the session (Table 9–2), superseding whatever else may be going on in the treatment or in the patient's life, as well as other potential deviations from the agreed-upon frame. Clinical developments in

---

TABLE 9–2.   Priority 1: Emergency themes — common presentations of dangerous behavior and threats to the continuity of the treatment

---

Threats to the patient's life: Potentially lethal suicide attempts, dangerous substance use

Threats to safety of others: Physically aggressive treatment of others, significant threats to harm others, stalking, neglect or abuse of children

Reckless behavior: Driving while intoxicated, engaging in potentially dangerous sexual encounters, engaging in physical fights

Potentially lethal suicide gestures: Overdosing, cutting of sufficient severity to require medical attention

Illegal activity: Shoplifting, blackmail, forgery

Threats to disrupt the treatment: Initiating plans to move to another city or part of the country; interviewing for a position that would make it impossible to attend therapy appointments; leaving current job, school, or structured activity without alternative plan

Threat of destroying financial viability of treatment: Losing job; threats to leave job; antagonizing family, spouse, or others supporting the treatment

---

which dangerous behavior becomes a priority theme are most common in the treatment of middle- and low-BPO patients, often representing the very problems that brought the patient to treatment. Some BPO patients with higher level pathology may also engage in destructive or self-destructive behavior that will become a priority theme. Occasionally, an NPO patient will engage in potentially dangerous behavior as well (e.g., a public figure who chooses to use illicit substances, or an academic who initiates an affair with a student), but these are relatively uncommon developments.

In many cases, dangerous behaviors that become an issue in treatment will have been included in the treatment contract, but it is also relatively common for new emergency priorities to present during the course of treatment. If new behavior that is not part of the treatment contract emerges in the course of treatment, the priority theme becomes evaluating this behavior and recontracting if warranted (see Chapter 8, "Recontracting After Treatment Begins"). Even when problematic behaviors have been addressed in the treatment contract, it is not realistic to expect that patients will be able or willing to immediately relinquish long-standing destructive patterns. Often destructive behaviors are a powerful source of gratification and/or secondary gain, and may also serve defensive functions (see Clinical Illustration 1 throughout this chapter).

Challenges to the treatment frame in the form of potentially danger-ous acting out, as well as the emergence of new destructive behaviors in the treatment, are relatively common, especially in the opening phase of work with low-BPO patients and, to a somewhat lesser extent, with mid-dle-BPO patients. In some patients, beginning treatment seems initially to accentuate dangerous behavior during the opening phase. Across the BPO spectrum, impulsive decisions that could abruptly disrupt the treatment are relatively commonly encountered—for example, the patient moves out of town so as to be unable to see the therapist or leaves a job so as to be unable to pay for treatment. When a patient announces such a "decision," this be-comes a priority theme. In these situations, in which the patient either en-gages in familiar destructive behaviors or pursues treatment-disruptive decisions, the therapist typically witnesses activation of a conflict between a constructive part of the patient that wants and seeks help and a destruc-tive part of the patient motivated to undermine the treatment.

Sometimes, patients openly report dangerous and disruptive behav-iors. At other times, dangerous behavior may be mentioned only in pass-ing or may have to be inferred by the therapist on the basis of what is omitted from the patient's discourse. As a result, the TFP-E therapist, es-pecially in the early phases of treatment with BPO patients, is mindful of needing to listen for indications that the patient is cooperating with the treatment contract and abstaining from dangerous or potentially treat-ment-disruptive behavior. If the therapist finds himself unclear about the patient's involvement in dangerous or disruptive activities, he should in-quire.

To the degree that a patient is able to achieve behavioral control and stay in treatment, the therapist will have an opportunity to explore the mo-tivations and meanings underlying destructive behavior, focusing on both their defensive and expressive functions. The overall tactical objective in TFP-E is to convert habitually destructive behavior into the conflictual in-ternal object relations organizing the behavior. However, in the setting of dangerous behavior, exploration is a viable and productive undertaking only to the degree that the patient is able to control the behavior; in our experience, it is rarely useful to speak about motivations and meanings as long as the patient continues to indulge in dangerous behavior.

For further discussion of the management of dangerous behavior in the treatment of patients with severe personality disorders, we refer the reader to Chapter 8 in this volume and to the transference-focused psychotherapy treatment manual (Yeomans et al. 2015).

Clinical Illustrations of Dangerous Behavior and Treatment-Disruptive Behaviors as Priority Issues

Clinical Illustration 1: Driving Under the Influence as a Priority Focus—Ms. P

Ms. P, a 23-year-old student functioning at a middle borderline level, with a diagnosis of borderline personality disorder with sadomasochistic traits and a history of superficial cutting, was in treatment with the goal of improving her affect regulation and stabilizing her relationships. In the middle of a session, Ms. P mentioned that she was "really tired"; she had been out "partying" the entire previous night. Ms. P had a history of driving under the influence (DUI), and her therapist, Dr. K, inquired whether she had been driving. Dismissively, Ms. P acknowledged that she had, but insisted, "I was totally in control; there were no problems, nothing happened. But don't worry, I won't do it again. So we really don't have to waste my therapy time today discussing it. I really want to talk about what my mom said to me about my dad."

Dr. K identified Ms. P's DUI, her dismissal of its significance, and her denial of the danger involved as the priority theme in the session: "You say it isn't worth discussing, but in fact there is nothing more important for us to discuss here today. Rather than a waste of our time, addressing your behavior—driving while intoxicated—and the danger it poses to you and to others, are the only things worth our speaking about."

Clinical Illustration 2: Quitting Work as a Priority Focus—Mr. G

Mr. G, a 35-year-old man with narcissistic personality disorder and functioning at a middle borderline level, presented with chronic difficulties with work and periodic anger outbursts, which had brought him to treatment at the insistence of his wife. Mr. G spoke about a number of issues during his session with Dr. Y, then casually announced that he planned to give notice at his job the following day. This was the first that Dr. Y had heard of Mr. G's plan; when she attempted to explore his decision, the patient glibly replied that the job was boring, he was tired of it, and he didn't like having to answer to a boss. His intention was to take an extended vacation to "refuel" before looking for another position.

It was clear to Dr. Y that Mr. G's plan to leave his job was the priority issue in the session insofar as it threatened continuation of the treatment. The therapist responded to Mr. G's "offhand" announcement by reminding him of their current arrangement for payment for the treatment:

"We've agreed that your wife will pay for half of your treatment costs and that you will pay for the other half out of your earnings. In light of this arrangement, it seems your current plan essentially means not only leaving your job but also ending the treatment. What are your thoughts about that?"

Priority 2: Maintaining Integrity of the Treatment Frame, Including Ongoing Pursuit of Treatment Goals

In TFP-E, the treatment contract establishes the necessary conditions for the treatment, and in the setting of more severe psychopathology, that contract helps the patient contain and limit destructive behaviors. Thus, if a patient is not adhering to the treatment frame, this typically becomes the priority theme in the session. Once the treatment goals have been mutually agreed upon in the contracting phase, they are considered part of the treatment frame; if a patient consistently fails to take obvious steps in his daily life to pursue the goals of treatment, this, too, becomes a priority theme.

We introduced the treatment frame, established in the treatment contract, and its functions in Chapter 8. The treatment frame can be seen as defining the reality of the relationship between patient and therapist, organized in relation to the responsibilities of each participant and the treatment goals. From the perspective of clinical process, the frame functions to create and protect a setting in which the patient's behavior, especially deviations from the frame and failure to pursue treatment goals, can be explored in terms of enactment of conflictual object relations. Thus, the frame serves the dual function of facilitating exploration of conflictual object relations embedded in the patient's behavior and, if need be, providing a structure within which the therapist can maintain the necessary conditions for treatment and help the patient limit destructive and disruptive behaviors.

Common Deviations From the Treatment Frame Across the Range of Severity

Deviations from the treatment frame come in many forms; some are relatively minor, common, and purely of symbolic meaning (Table 9–3),

TABLE 9–3. Priority 2: Integrity of the treatment frame—common presentations of deviations from the frame

The structure of the treatment: Irregularities with scheduling, attendance, payment

Active pursuit of treatment goals: Losing sight of treatment goals, or failures to take concrete steps toward attaining them

Structured activity: Inadequate efforts to establish and maintain structured activity

Free and open communication: Failure to discuss behavior outside the treatment; withholding, lying, or other forms of deception

Behavior in relation to the therapist's practice: Disruptive behaviors such as creating excessive noise in office or waiting area, refusing to leave the office when session is over, taking periodicals from waiting area, leaving trash or defacing office furnishings, harassing office staff

Respecting boundaries of the treatment relationship: Frequent phone calls requesting intersession contact, violation of agreements restricting electronic communication, attending sessions in intoxicated state, stalking therapist or family members on social media, efforts to initiate social or sexual contact with therapist, initiating social contact with members of therapist's social or professional circles

Special aspects of the contract: Various forms of high-risk self-destructive behavior, failure to adhere to agreements about management of substance misuse and eating disorder symptoms, noncompliance with medication for medical or psychiatric conditions, failure of patient or third parties (usually patient's family or spouse) to respect arrangements made to reduce secondary gain, violation of agreements on handling of emergencies

whereas others are extreme and potentially threatening to the safety of the patient or the continuity of the treatment. Frame deviations can be identified in the treatments of patients across the spectrum of severity of pathology, especially in the early phase of treatment. However, deviations become much more common, prominent, and central to clinical process as pathology becomes more severe.

In working with both BPO and NPO patients, therapists may encounter difficulties maintaining the structure of the treatment with regard to scheduling, attendance, or payment through such behavior as frequent cancellations, chronic lateness, frequent requests for schedule changes, frequent phone calls, or delays in payment. Generally limited to the treatment of patients along the BPO spectrum are deviations from special aspects of the treatment contract—for example, agreements about frequent phone calls or the handling of self-destructive behavior; across the range of severity, patients may have difficulty maintaining agreements pertaining to substance use or eating disorder behaviors. BPO patients in particular may, either purposefully or inadvertently, keep information about their day-to-day activities and functioning out of the treatment, violating the agreement of full and open communication.

Patients may also demonstrate *acting-out* behaviors in relation to the therapy or the therapist that become priority themes. These behaviors may include leaving trash in the therapist's waiting room, refusing to leave the office at the end of sessions, or initiating inappropriate or disruptive interactions with office staff. Outright lying (in contrast to omissions), attempting to initiate social contact or physical contact with the therapist, coming to sessions while high or drunk, and invading the therapist's privacy are examples of particularly destructive deviations from the treatment frame that are generally limited to patients in the mid- and low-borderline range. All these behaviors constitute frame violations; when present, they become a priority issue.

A commonly overlooked form of deviation from the treatment frame, encountered in patients across the spectrum of severity, is failure to actively pursue the treatment goals. The treatment goals are part of the treatment frame, and failure to keep them in mind will lend a superficial and meandering quality to the treatment over time; the treatment goals are the "North Star" of any TFP-E treatment. As a result, one of the therapist's tasks in identifying a priority theme is to maintain awareness of the treatment goals, even when the patient does not, and to attend to whether the patient is pursuing them in a reasonable fashion in her daily life.

Patients across the spectrum of severity may, at least for a time, neglect or lose sight of their treatment goals. However, NPO patients will, for the most part, naturally allow the therapist to appreciate how they are spending their time outside sessions, revealing whether they are actively pursuing their goals or failing to do so. In contrast, BPO patients often leave the therapist in the dark, with a shadowy or uneven understanding of their day-to-day functioning, which can cause the therapist as well as the patient to lose sight of the agreed-upon goals. A patient's failure to communicate in this setting may reflect purposeful omission. However, this failure can also reflect the impact of the patient's dissociative defenses on her communications to the therapist—it may simply not occur to the patient to raise certain issues or discuss certain events with the therapist.

Assessing the Integrity of the Frame When Considering Priority Themes

When considering a focus for intervention, at the same time that the therapist attends to the patient's internal experience, the therapist will also be careful to maintain an outward gaze, monitoring the status of the treatment frame and the patient's functioning. With this in mind, as the therapist sits with the patient, he will periodically ask himself questions: "Is the structure of the treatment intact?" "Is the patient adhering to the necessary conditions for treatment that we agreed upon?" "Is she abstaining from behaving in ways potentially disruptive to the treatment?" "Have I been hearing about her taking obvious steps to pursue her treatment goals?"

If the answer to any of these questions is no, this issue becomes the priority theme in the session. If the therapist is unclear about the answer to any of these questions—if he feels he lacks a clear sense of how the patient is functioning in domains related to the contract and treatment goals—he should inquire. For example, if the patient contracted around going to 12-step organization meetings, the therapist might say, "We contracted around your participating in daily meetings, but I haven't heard anything from you recently about this." Or if the patient has contracted about getting to work on time and the therapist is unclear how the patient is doing in this regard, the therapist might say, "We agreed that you would consistently arrive at your workplace on time, but I haven't heard anything from you for several weeks about how this is going."

Treatment Frame, Priority Themes, and Internal Object Relations Across the Range of Severity

Overt challenges to and tests of the frame are near-universal developments in the treatments of patients across the BPO spectrum, whereas NPO patients, for the most part, are able and willing to adhere to the treatment frame with minimal difficulty.

Borderline Level of Personality Organization

In the treatment of BPO patients, attending to the frame maintains the necessary conditions for treatment and keeps treatment grounded in the reality of the patient's daily functioning (as in the example above in which the therapist inquires about the patient's attendance at 12-step meetings), while bringing conflictual object relations into the treatment where they can be explored. When present, deviations from the frame that violate the contract or threaten to disrupt the treatment (and those that endanger the patient or others, as discussed earlier in the section "Priority 1: Attending to Emergency Priorities") become priority themes, regardless of what else the patient may bring into the session.

For example, while speaking about how upsetting it was to visit his mother, who had rapidly evolving dementia, a patient mentioned in passing that he had been so upset that he had gone out and "had a few too many." If the patient had a history of binge drinking and had contracted around limiting his drinking, his alcohol consumption would be the priority theme in session, regardless of how upset the patient might be about his mother. Problems in adhering to the structure of the treatment—for example, inconsistent attendance, arriving late, or delaying payment, as well as failure to attend to the treatment goals—are less urgent but also represent priority themes.

In the event that the therapist notes a deviation from the treatment frame, it is best for the therapist to respond without delay. Rather than "letting it go" and waiting for behaviors to become a pattern, it is preferable to mark such behaviors, even on their first occurrence. It is a common countertransference to be tempted to ignore or minimize the significance of deviations from the agreed-upon structure of the treatment, often until they become an overt problem. On the basis of our experience, it is far more advisable in work with BPO patients for the therapist to address deviations from the treatment frame early and consistently, because these behaviors typically represent the acting out of dominant object relations; to the extent that such behavior is not addressed, dominant object relations will be split off from the contents of the session.

The therapist can begin by simply calling attention to the patient's actions and pointing out that they represent a deviation from the agreed-upon structure of the treatment, while expressing curiosity. If the behavior recurs, the therapist should remind the patient of previous discussions and identify the deviation from the frame as a priority theme for exploration.

Typically, as the therapist focuses clinical attention on deviations from the frame or on the patient's failure to pursue treatment goals, the object relations embedded in or obscured by the patient's behavior (these behaviors are classically referred to as *resistances*) will emerge, most commonly in the transference. Thus, while attention to the frame helps control destructive behavior and ensures the necessary conditions for treatment of BPO patients, the overall tactical objective of attending to frame deviations is to convert pathogenic behaviors (often chronic expressions of personality pathology and related to patients' presenting difficulties) into object relations enacted in relation to the treatment (generally in the transference), where they can be explored.

For example, a patient may talk in his sessions about his problems with authority or his relationship with his wife while simultaneously failing to look for work as he agreed to do or while frequently missing sessions or leaving trash in the therapist's waiting room. In this situation, pursuing the seemingly relevant material that the patient is bringing into his sessions would likely be of little utility; as long as the frame violations persist, the patient's behavior is the priority theme and the affectively dominant issue. Often at these times, the experienced therapist will notice in the countertransference a sense of the patient's engaging in "empty talk," even if the content is manifestly meaningful. These moments are equivalent to what Bateman and Fonagy (2006) refer to as *pretend mode*.

Attention to the frame will immediately bring into the treatment the problematic and contradictory aspects of the patient's functioning (he says he wants to work but does not look for work; he says he wants to participate in the treatment but will do so only on his own terms), rather than allowing them to be split off from the content of his therapy sessions. Once these behaviors are brought into the treatment, discussions of problems with the boss or of marital difficulties become meaningful, because they are no longer abstractions but are concretely linked to the patient's behavior in the moment and in relation to the treatment and the transference.

Noting the patient's failure to look for work or to attend sessions regularly calls attention to the dissociation between the verbal content of his communications in session and his behavior outside (he is apparently indulging freely in the behavior he is talking about wanting to change). At the same time, focusing on split-off behaviors that represent a violation of the treatment contract will in most cases quickly call attention to how the central difficulties that brought the patient to treatment (in this case, an intolerance of being told what to do or of being held to an external schedule and "yessing" while ignoring those in positions of authority) are being activated in the therapy and in relation to the therapist. In our current example, the patient's failure to pursue work, or his failure to attend sessions regularly, would become a priority theme for intervention. Calling attention to the dissociative defenses organizing his attitude and behavior in relation to finding work, the therapist might say, "I've noticed you haven't said anything recently about pursuing work. We agreed on your finding employment as a condition of treatment, and you speak about being upset about not having a job, but I've heard nothing about any efforts on your part to secure work. What are your thoughts about this?"

In sum, in the treatment of BPO patients, attention to the integrity of the treatment frame and identifying deviations from the frame will direct the therapist toward a priority theme. BPO patients' reliance on action and dissociation means that they may not naturally bring problematic aspects of their functioning into the treatment, at least not purposefully. The therapist's monitoring of the treatment frame and goals, calling attention to deviations and holding the patient accountable, will enable the therapist to ground what goes on in sessions in the realities of 1) the necessary conditions for treatment and 2) the realities of the patient's daily functioning in relation to the treatment goals. At the same time, exploring deviations from the frame will function to transform chronic pathogenic behaviors (maladaptive personality traits) into object relations that can be explored in the treatment.

Neurotic Level of Personality Organization

The treatment frame is central in the treatment of NPO patients as well; however, its functions are more subtle, and deviations need not always be urgently addressed. In contrast to BPO patients, for whom nonadherence to the frame and to the agreed-upon contract is common and often extreme, patients with milder forms of personality pathology typically have far more subtle and symbolic struggles with the frame—most frequently, minor problems with scheduling, lateness, or payment. Also in contrast to BPO patients, NPO patients, for the most part, will naturally bring relevant aspects of their functioning into the treatment through their verbal communications and associations. As a result, behavior in relation to the frame plays a less central role in maintaining a close tie between aspects of an NPO patient's internal experience discussed in session and her day-to-day functioning and treatment goals.

For these reasons, the therapist may at times inquire about, but otherwise defer focusing on, deviations from the frame with the NPO patient, if the treatment is proceeding well and other issues are affectively dominant. On the other hand, if the therapist is having difficulty identifying dominant object relations or a priority theme in session, or if the treatment appears to be flattening out or stalling, the frame deviation is likely to become a priority theme.

Because deviations from the frame with NPO patients may be both objectively minor and ego-syntonic, it is especially important that during contracting, the therapist introduce the frame explicitly and in detail, so as to create a setting in which even subtle deviations from the frame can ultimately be viewed as having meaning. When there are deviations from the frame in the treatments of NPO patients, it is often the first sign of core conflicts being activated in the transference; focusing on these deviations will ultimately provide an opportunity to explore conflictual object relations as they are enacted in relation to the therapist.

The object relations linked to deviations from the frame in the treatment of NPO patients may be repressed. In this setting, the therapist can note the deviation but may have to defer exploration of the associated anxieties and defenses until they become more accessible to consciousness. For example, early in his treatment, an obsessional patient presenting with problems in his marriage missed several sessions per month. He would cancel at the last minute, feeling he needed to stay at his workplace to take care of matters that he viewed as time sensitive. When the therapist gently raised the possibility that perhaps the patient's behavior was meaningful or served a function for him, the patient maintained that his cancellations simply reflected the demands of his job. Meanwhile, the treatment appeared to be going well. Several months later, while between jobs, the patient felt pressured to consistently attend his sessions. At this point, he became acutely aware of fears of becoming "too dependent" on the therapist.

In this example, while not disruptive to the treatment, the frame deviation successfully protected the patient from awareness of central anxieties activated in the transference and linked to his presenting complaints. In work with NPO patients, therapists can think of a deviation of this kind as a latent priority theme, awaiting a time when it can be usefully explored.

Clinical Illustrations of the Integrity of the Treatment Frame as a Priority Issue

Clinical Illustration 1 (continued): Addressing High-Risk Behavior as a Deviation From the Treatment Frame — Ms. P

Ms. P, the student with borderline personality disorder introduced earlier in this chapter, had a history of responding to feelings of sadness or isolation by initiating sexual encounters with strangers whom she contacted via "hook-up" apps. Although sexual behavior of this kind was normative within her social group, it had on a number of occasions left her in potentially dangerous situations. During the contracting phase with Dr. K, with an eye toward optimizing both Ms. P's safety and Dr. K's ability to work comfortably with her, they had agreed that as a condition of treatment,

Ms. P would disconnect herself from hook-up apps and restrict her online sexual activity to men she met through legitimate dating Web sites.

Several months into her treatment, Ms. P came to a Tuesday session after a long weekend and started speaking about how miserable her weekend had been. She'd felt empty and sad; no one was around. She went on to say that she'd spent a lot of time in bed and on the Internet; she then smiled slyly at Dr. K as she told him that she'd been having fantasies about him—about meeting up with him, having an exciting night out together, and hooking up.

Mindful of the priorities of intervention, before pursuing Ms. P's thoughts about him, Dr. K opted to check in with her regarding the treatment contract. He told her that it sounded as though the weekend had been tough and had exposed her to painful feelings. He then commented that these were exactly the feelings that historically had prompted her to pursue potentially unsafe hook-ups. He inquired whether such behavior had been a temptation. Ms. P acknowledged that over the weekend she had indeed hooked up with a man whom she'd found through a questionable app; she had been reluctant to tell Dr. K because she knew it was a violation of her treatment contract.

Dr. K responded by reminding Ms. P that her abstinence in this regard was a precondition for treatment. TFP-E at times stirs up painful feelings; if she felt unable to manage those feelings safely, the two of them would have to reconsider whether this was the right treatment approach for her. Ms. P responded that she had been aware as the weekend began that she was failing to make plans (as she had taken to doing since starting the treatment) to help her manage her time when she was away from the structure of her class schedule. She knew that the contract had been helpful in restraining her sexual behavior, which she acknowledged could put her in danger. She had been thinking about Dr. K as she downloaded the app that she planned to use and was aware that this could be a problem in the treatment. After the hook-up on Sunday afternoon, she had called a girlfriend, who agreed to make herself available should Ms. P again find herself tempted to violate her arrangement with Dr. K.

Comments: In this example, Dr. K's attention to the treatment frame led him to inquire about Ms. P's behavior before pursuing her fantasies about him over the weekend. This choice entirely redirected the session. Dr. K's inquiry about the frame provided an opportunity to assess Ms. P's motivation to control her impulses, as well as her ability to do so, while revisiting the treatment contract, and also alerted Dr. K to the need to be attentive to these issues in upcoming sessions. If Dr. K had not followed the recommended hierarchy of interventions but had instead accepted Ms. P's invitation to explore her fantasies about him, this decision would have created a situation in which they talked about Ms. P's romantic and sexual fantasies about him, when in fact the dominant issue was her ongoing destructive behavior.

As Dr. K and Ms. P explored Ms. P's experience and behavior over the weekend, they were able to identify a conflict between a part of her that enjoyed feeling closer to Dr. K but found that threatening, and another part of her that wanted to undermine their relationship while maintaining that the only real interpersonal attachments are always destructive, dangerous, and hyperstimulating.

Clinical Illustration 2 *(continued)*: Addressing Deferred Payment as a Deviation From the Treatment Frame—Mr. G

Mr. G, the man introduced earlier with narcissistic personality disorder and who threatened to leave his job, requested to defer payment of Dr. Y's bill for a month while he got his feet on the ground in a new job. Dr. Y agreed, noting to herself that Mr. G was now working part-time and seemed, finally, to be settling down in the treatment.

Over the next few weeks, Mr. G continued to speak in an apparently meaningful way about himself and the difficulties in his marriage. Nevertheless, Dr. Y felt that the treatment had taken on a somewhat deadened quality, very different from the storminess of previous months. Mr. G's interactions with Dr. Y now seemed flat, leaving her feeling a bit detached and even bored in sessions. At the end of the month, Mr. G paid his earlier bill, but again maintained a 1-month balance, promising to settle up completely during the month but failing to do so. Dr. Y raised the issue, but Mr. G smoothly brushed her off while commenting on Dr. Y's being "so nice and so helpful."

Dr. Y inferred that nonpayment had become the dominant issue in the treatment. She chose to intervene by focusing on Mr. G's experience of the interaction between the two of them in relation to the deferred payment. In response to this inquiry, Mr. G was quite forthright in sharing his view of his therapist as weak and foolish, naive about the ways of the world, and vulnerable to exploitation. This led to an open, if somewhat intellectualized, discussion of Mr. G's "dog-eat-dog" view of human relations, marked by mutual exploitation and depreciation of the good.

However, in the following session, when Dr. Y finally set a limit, requiring Mr. G to pay his bill in full, the patient became acutely paranoid, experiencing her as victimizing, exploiting, and dominating him. This was the first step in a lengthy and successful exploration of his paranoid object relations, which lay at the heart of his difficulties in his marriage.

Comments: By withholding payment from Dr. Y, Mr. G was able to feel in control of his therapist, and as a result able for the most part to split off the paranoid object relations emerging in the transference. However, when Dr. Y ultimately set a limit on deferral of payment, these pathogenic object relations rapidly took center stage in the clinical process.

Protracted frame violations, like Mr. G's withholding of payment, can successfully keep out of the therapy the underlying conflictual object relations that are linked to presenting complaints and maladaptive personality functioning. The content of the sessions may then become a sterile landscape, dissociated from the patient's affective experience and life problems, while the affectively dominant object relations are acted out in relation to the frame but otherwise split off from the clinical material.

Clinical Illustration 3: Addressing Failure to Pursue Employment as a Deviation From the Treatment Frame—Ms. L

Ms. L, a 23-year-old unemployed woman, carried a diagnosis of avoidant personality disorder with depressive and borderline traits; structurally, she fell in the transitional area between NPO and high BPO. She had presented with chronic depression, self-criticism, self-deprecation, and a lack of assertiveness, with a pattern of often allowing others to take advantage of her.

Several weeks into her treatment with Dr. B, Ms. L came to a Monday session seeming anxious and initially saying nothing. When she did begin to speak, it was in a halting fashion, interspersed with silences in which she clearly felt uncomfortable. She described having felt "awkward" with her boyfriend over the weekend; usually, she felt no inhibitions with him, but on Sunday, had felt herself to be "acting weird" and "sounding stupid." She sheepishly acknowledged that when they spoke on the phone on Sunday night, she purposefully disconnected the call and then pretended it was an accident; there had been some silences between them, and she was fearful that in the silence she would say something "weird" or meaningless.

Ms. L went on to say that she had recently found herself feeling awkward talking to others, which she thought was because she was spending so much time alone. Her family had gone out of town 5 days earlier, and since then she had essentially stayed home, speaking to no one. The more time she spent alone, the more "weird" and "awkward" she felt. She went on to say that she was supposed to go out to dinner with her boyfriend and his father but she wanted to cancel; she was sure the father would find her disappointing, not smart enough, and not living up to his expectations, even though he had been very taken with her in the past.

Listening to Ms. L, Dr. B identified two salient issues. First, Dr. B heard Ms. L describing an object relation of a self that is weird or stupid, unwanted, and not living up to the expectations of an object that is powerful, desirable, critical, and potentially rejecting, associated with feelings of shame and inferiority. This object relation, which often colored Ms. L's general experience of herself in relation to others, was closely linked to her central difficulties and treatment goals, and seemed to be specifically activated now in relation to the boyfriend, his father, and Dr. B.

Second, Dr. B heard something else embedded in the material: Ms. L was not engaged in structured activity and was spending too much time alone. This had been a significant problem in the past, and as part of the initial treatment contract, they had agreed that she would find part-time work, something she had been dragging her heels on for unclear reasons, while she applied to graduate school. Ms. L's description of her behavior over the past 5 days made clear that she was not adhering to the agreed-upon treatment frame, at a cost to herself.

In choosing between focusing on the dominant object relations in the material and deviating from the treatment frame, Dr. B noted that the treatment contract was a higher-priority issue; even though it was tempting to take up the opportunity to explore Ms. L's dynamics, currently enacted in the transference and with her boyfriend, Dr. B opted to intervene first in relation to the frame. Dr. B began by pointing out that Ms. L seemed to be having difficulty with so much unstructured time alone, yet they had agreed that by now she would have found work or at least be actively looking for a job. Pursuing this theme, Dr. B inquired about Ms. L's efforts to find work and her attitude toward doing so. Ms. L responded that she had gone so far as to update her résumé, print it out, and post it online; however, she felt paralyzed about taking the next step of walking into businesses, such as retail stores, to inquire whether they needed help. When she anticipated doing so, she became confused and panicky, getting stuck on details such as whether she should have her résumé in hand or put it into an envelope. She anticipated that she would seem stupid, awkward, or weird, and no one would want to hire her.

Comments: In this example, Dr. B chose to intervene first at the level of the treatment frame. What emerged was that the same object relations present in the session were also active in relation to the patient's difficulty pursuing employment. This enabled Dr. B to link Ms. L's problems pursuing work to her discomfort with her boyfriend, and also to her experience in relation to Dr. B in the session. Had Dr. B focused immediately on Ms. L's experience of herself in relation to her boyfriend and therapist, the patient's failure to pursue employment would likely have been further delayed and could potentially have slipped into the background, with the risk that the content of sessions would become dissociated from her day-to-day life and functioning and from the treatment goals.

Clinical Illustration 4: Timing in Addressing Lateness as a Deviation From the Treatment Frame—Ms. S

We return now to Ms. S, the 50-year-old married volunteer research assistant introduced in Chapter 6 in relation to strategies of treatment. Diagnosed with depressive personality with dependent features and functioning at a neurotic level, Ms. S presented with problems with self-esteem and social isolation.

Six months into the treatment, Ms. S began consistently arriving 3 minutes late to her sessions, each time making a brief apology. At first, Dr. C was struck by Ms. S's perceived need to apologize for such minor lateness. Over time, Dr. C reasoned that the late start, though likely meaningful, was in no way interfering with the treatment; there were currently more active priorities, and the treatment was going well. Ultimately, Dr. C stopped paying attention altogether to both the lateness and the habitual apology.

Meanwhile, for many months, sessions had been focusing on Ms. S's view of herself as excessively aggressive, intrusive, and greedy. Somewhere along the line, Dr. C became aware of a vague feeling of stagnation in the therapy. Simultaneously, Dr. C noticed that Ms. S had taken to slouching as she entered and exited the office, as if to make herself smaller. When Dr. C called attention to this behavior, what emerged was that the slouching reduced Ms. S's anxiety in regard to an object relation activated in the transference, that of a powerful, aggressive, and intrusive maternal self in relation to a vulnerable, innocent, childlike therapist.

It occurred to Dr. C that Ms. S's lateness, similar to the slouching, functioned to reassure Ms. S and to defend against fears of being aggressive and intrusive with Dr. C. When Dr. C suggested this to Ms. S, the patient acknowledged that this suggestion made sense, though she had not thought about it. As she then began to arrive early to her sessions, Ms. S disclosed feeling increasingly anxious, worrying that she was somehow excessively aggressive and intrusive, even perverse, in her interest in Dr. C.

Comments: This example illustrates that with NPO patients, even minor or subtle deviations from the frame are often of psychological significance and may be the first sign of developments in the transference. At the same time, if things are going well in the treatment, the therapist may take more time to address minor deviations from the frame than would be typical in the treatment of BPO patients. In the treatments of NPO patients, often the object relations embedded in and defended against by chronic behavior in relation to the treatment frame can be explored initially outside the transference; Dr. C delayed pursuing Ms. S's lateness until the transference assumed affective dominance, as heralded by the patient's change in posture, and perhaps in addition by something not fully articulated in Dr. C's countertransference.[1] In this case, Dr. C's decision to bring in the lateness facilitated the emergence of Ms. S's deeper

---

[1]The therapist's sense of things stagnating in the treatment often serves as a prompt to initiate exploration of relatively minor but chronic deviations from the frame in the treatment of the NPO patient.

anxieties—of herself as perversely intrusive—as a focus of exploration in the treatment.

Priority 3: Intervening at the Level of Affectively Dominant Object Relations

Definition of Affectively Dominant Object Relations

As discussed in Chapter 5, the overarching strategy of TFP-E is to explore the object relations organizing the patient's experience and behavior in each session; we refer to these object relations as the *affectively dominant object relations*. As the patient interacts with the therapist, speaking openly and freely in her therapy session or failing to do so, one or two relationship patterns will typically emerge in the clinical material as salient, and these affectively dominant object relations are by definition linked to the central conflict that is active in the session and organizing the clinical material; affect activation is a signal of conflict. Thus, focusing on the affectively dominant object relations directs clinical attention to an area of conflict and serves as an entry point into conflictual aspects of the patient's internal world that are linked to presenting symptoms, subjective difficulties, and maladaptive behaviors.

Once identified, the affectively dominant object relations emerge in the mind of the therapist as a unifying theme for the session, a nidus at the center of the complex web formed by the patient's communications, experience, and behavior. The clinical material then seems to fall into place, and the session, even if manifestly disjointed or chaotic, will take on a degree of coherence in the mind of the therapist. In the treatment of BPO patients, the affectively dominant object relations are often enacted in the transference. In the treatment of NPO patients, the affectively dominant object relations are frequently enacted outside the transference.

Focusing on affect is a central tenet of psychodynamic treatments in general (Diener et al. 2007). Affects are tied to people's most powerful motivations: wishes, needs, and fears; and most forms of dynamic therapy direct the therapist to "follow the affect"—that is, to intervene in relation to material with which the patient is emotionally engaged. What is specific to TFP-E is that when the therapist thinks of focusing on affects, he is interested not only in encouraging the patient to be aware of and more fully experience her emotional experience, but also in facilitating exploration of the object relations that in the TFP-E model are by definition linked to these affect states. With this in mind, in each TFP-E session, the therapist works to identify the object relations that represent the most emotionally salient material in the session.

In TFP-E, emotional salience and affective dominance are often flagged by the expression of affect; however, this is not always the case. *Affective dominance* does not invariably mean "a lot of affect," but rather affective investment or *emotional salience*. Sometimes affective dominance is marked by the *absence* of expected affective expression or by *contradictions* between content and affect, both signaling the activation of defenses such as suppression, repression, denial, or dissociation. Alternatively, affective dominance may be expressed predominantly through *action*, entirely dissociated from affective experience. For example, a patient may report having been put on probation at work while appearing indifferent or perhaps even smiling; another may speak about feeling enraged with his wife in a flat, emotionless tone; and still another may report having achieved a long-sought-after success without any display of affect whatsoever.

Attending to the Three Channels of Communication

To identify the affectively dominant object relations, the TFP-E therapist attends to the *three channels of communication*: the patient's verbal communication, the patient's nonverbal communication, and the therapist's countertransference (Table 9–4). Verbal channels tend to be most informative in the setting of repression-based defenses, whereas when splitting-based defenses predominate, the patient's nonverbal communication and the countertransference tend to be the dominant channels for communicating the affectively dominant object relations. Table 9–5 shows manifestations of affectively dominant object relations across the range of personality pathology, as discussed further in the text. As described in Chapter 6, in the treatment of BPO patients, the affectively dominant object relations are typically enacted in the transference, whereas in the treatment of NPO patients, they may be less evident in the transference and instead communicated in descriptions of interpersonal interactions and self states.

In Video 4, "Identifying the Dominant Object Relations," Dr. Yeomans attends to the three channels of communication to identify the dominant object relations in a female patient with histrionic personality disorder. In this video, Dr. Yeomans also demonstrates the exploratory interventions and interpretive processes of TFP-E described further in Chapters 10–12. At the beginning of the video, the patient demands that Dr. Yeomans advise her as to whether or not to accept a proposal of marriage from her boyfriend.

Rather than providing advice, Dr. Yeomans maintains a neutral stance and uses the opportunity to elaborate the object relations organizing the patient's experience of herself and Dr. Yeomans in the transference. Dr. Yeomans begins by highlighting the patient's dominant self-experience, one in which she views herself as weak and victimized. He then calls her attention to a contradictory aspect of her self, expressed in her behavior but split off from her dominant self experience, in which she is far more powerful than she acknowledges. This video illustrates the process of naming the dominant object relations activated in the transference (the first step in transference analysis), and how the TFP-E therapist works with role reversals, putting words to the patient's dominant self experience before addressing ("confronting") object relations that are enacted and denied. In addition to illustrating the process of identifying and naming the dominant object relations, Dr. Yeomans is able, in an empathic, noncritical fashion, to confront more aggressive aspects of the patient's behavior. This video also highlights how the TFP-E therapist maintains a neutral, containing, and exploratory stance in relation to the patient's demands and elevated affect.

 Video Illustration 4
Identifying the Dominant Object Relations (4:35)

Verbal Content

The content of the patient's verbal communications often is the most direct and accessible way in which conflictual object relations emerge in a therapy session, especially in the setting of repression-based defenses. In listening to the content of the patient's communications, the TFP-E therapist will be especially attuned to relationship patterns embedded in the patient's descriptions of interpersonal interactions, including comments that the patient may make about interactions with, or experiences of, the therapist.

When a patient comments directly on her experience of the therapist (e.g., sharing impressions of how the therapist is treating her or may feel about her), the object relations–enacted relationship patterns activated in the transference typically have affective dominance in the session. In the absence of direct communication about the relationship with the therapist, the dominant object relations can emerge in verbal content through descriptions of interpersonal interactions and relational patterns outside the transference. Most typically, the same relationship patterns will be repeated in the patient's verbal communications, in different contexts and

TABLE 9–4. Priority 3: Affectively dominant object relations— three channels of communication

Patient's verbal communication: Descriptions of interpersonal interactions and self states, references to relationship with therapist, evidence of omissions, dissociation between or associations among different elements in discourse

Patient's nonverbal communication: Tone of verbal communication, body language and facial expressions, attitude toward material, overall atmosphere in the session

Countertransference: Therapist's private emotional responses and associations to patient's verbal and nonverbal communications and life situation

TABLE 9–5. Identifying affectively dominant object relations (ADORs) across the range of personality pathology

Splitting-based defenses	Repression-based defenses
ADORs are typically enacted in transference.	ADORs may not be evident in transference.
Nonverbal communications and countertransference are often dominant conveyors of ADORs.	Verbal communications are typically dominant conveyors of ADORs; these include descriptions of interpersonal interactions and free associations, daydreams, fantasies, and descriptions of self states.
A single salient ADOR organizes and dominates clinical material.	ADORs may be identified in a complex interplay of defensive and impulsive object relations around a particular conflict.
Frequent role reversals occur in ADORs.	Patient stably identifies with one side of ADOR, often childlike self in relation to parental object.

perhaps in different configurations, throughout the course of the session, pointing to affective dominance. Often these will be descriptions of interactions in which the patient took part, but sometimes the dominant relationship pattern described will not involve the patient directly. In either case, the therapist will assume that the patient is at some level identified with one or both positions in the object relation.

In work with NPO patients and in the setting of repression-based defenses, the patients' verbal communications are typically the central conveyor of their affectively dominant object relations. In such a case, in addition to attending to descriptions of interpersonal interactions in order to identify the dominant object relations, the therapist will need to pay careful attention to the patient's free associations and descriptions of self states; any description of self will be tied to an affective experience and either explicitly or implicitly tied to the representation of an object.

As the therapist listens to the patient's verbal communications, he will ask himself, "What are the different relationship patterns that the patient is describing in this session? How do they fit together? Which side of a given object relation is the patient most consciously identified with?"

As the dominant object relations begin to come into focus, the therapist will ask the patient, "How were you experiencing him [the other person] in that interaction? What is your image of yourself in relation to him? What were you feeling?"

Nonverbal Communication

Sometimes dominant object relations will be communicated most clearly through the patient's nonverbal communications. This is especially true in the setting of splitting-based defenses, which often lead the patient to communicate in action those aspects of her experience that she does not communicate in words. In such a case, the therapist attends to what the patient *does* in session, including how she says what she says, as well as to the general atmosphere in the room. The therapist will note in particular the patient's body language, facial expression, and eye contact, as well as the quality of her speech. The therapist will ask himself, "Is she speaking especially quietly or loudly, quickly or slowly, and is her tone flat or expressive?" The therapist will also note the patient's attitude: "Is she communicating openly and freely, or is she hesitant, silent, or guarded?"

Finally, the therapist considers whether the patient's nonverbal communications are congruent or discrepant with the content of her verbal communication. Discrepancies between nonverbal and verbal communications reflect the impact of the patient's defensive operations on her communications, and when these discrepancies occur, the therapist's attention will be directed toward the affectively dominant object relations. Nonverbal communications often reflect the object relations currently active and enacted in the transference; however, the patient may not be fully aware of her behavior and/or associated thoughts and feelings about the therapist until the therapist calls attention to them.

To transform the patient's nonverbal communication into an image of the object relations activated in the session, the therapist can ask himself,

"If I were observing this session on videotape, how would I describe the patient's overall way of being in the session and of relating to and interacting with me? Does she seem relaxed, does she speak freely or seem tentative or fearful, is she conveying warmth, or does she appear angry or frustrated? Is she attentive and engaged or is she dismissive? Is she controlling or eager to please?" The therapist can also consider these questions: "How is the patient treating me?" "How is she responding to or making use of my interventions, or is she ignoring them?"

Countertransference

In the same way that the therapist attends to the patient's nonverbal and verbal communications, taking them in and then reflecting on what they communicate about the patient's internal situation, the therapist also attends to his own countertransference (see Chapters 5 and 12 for additional discussion of countertransference). As described in Chapter 5, in TFP-E, we define *countertransference* as the therapist's total emotional reaction to the patient—the entirety of the feelings, thoughts, and object relations activated in the therapist as a result of interacting with the patient. In the setting of splitting-based defenses, the countertransference is often the first clue to the object relations organizing the transference, directing the therapist to the affectively dominant object relations.

As the TFP-E therapist listens to and interacts with the patient, the therapist will have a steady flow of reactions to the patient. Some reactions will be very powerful and prominent, and some so subtle that they are barely noticeable or may even be overlooked until discussed with a third party. Regardless of the content and quality of the countertransference, the therapist will make an effort to attend to and make note of his internal reactions to the patient while *containing* them. When we speak of containing countertransference, we refer to a process wherein the therapist refrains from reflexively acting on whatever is stirred up in him by the patient, instead reflecting on his internal experience vis-à-vis the patient.

The objective of the therapist, in making use of countertransference as a channel of communication, is neither to ignore (deny, repress, reject) nor to act on his reactions to the patient, but rather to consciously register those reactions and think about their implications. *Containment* implies the capacity to fully experience an emotion without being controlled by it or having to immediately turn to action to discharge the feeling. The therapist's task is to allow himself to respond freely *internally* to the patient, and then to move into the position of an observer in relation to his own reaction; the therapist will "listen to" and reflect on his countertransference and then make use of it to inform his understanding of what is going on within the patient and in the clinical process—that is, he uses his countertransference to further his understanding of the object relations currently active in the treatment.

Attention to the countertransference will inform the therapist's understanding of what may be going on inside the patient and in the transference, either within the patient's awareness or outside it. Countertransference tends to play an especially central role in conveying the affectively dominant object relations in the setting of splitting-based defenses. A patient's use of projective identification and omnipotent control, in particular, tends to activate complementary countertransferences in the therapist (i.e., the object relation is enacted in the mind of the therapist, with the therapist identified with the patient's objects).

To make use of the countertransference, the therapist can ask himself these questions: "What are the feelings stirred up in me by the patient and the clinical situation?" "What are the object relations embedded in my emotional experience?" This kind of introspection and reflection on the therapist's part enables him to empathize both with the patient's dominant experience and with more conflictual aspects of experience that the patient is defending against by way of projective mechanisms. That is, patients will often project conflictual aspects of their internal world into the therapist, opening up the possibility of the therapist's use of his experience of and reflections on what the patient has been projecting in order to make inferences about the patient's internal situation in the moment and the affectively dominant object relations. For example, a therapist who finds himself chronically concerned about being criticized by a particular patient and somehow feeling guilty that he is at fault can use that countertransference to make inferences about the patient's internal situation and chronic unhappiness.

Clinical Illustrations Identifying Affectively Dominant Object Relations Using the Three Channels of Communication

Clinical Illustration 1 (continued): Affectively Dominant Object Relations in the Transference With Role Reversal—Ms. P

Ms. P—the 23-year-old student organized at a middle borderline level, with a diagnosis of borderline personality disorder with sadomasochistic traits and a history of DUI—had settled into her treatment with Dr. K. In a Friday afternoon session, she was crying as she discussed a recent breakup, describing her anguish in agonizing detail. She told Dr. K that she was "desperate" and implored him to agree to speak with her over the weekend, "to provide support" as her former therapist had done. She went on to say that she knew this was a violation of their agreement about intersession contact, but she was at the end of her capacity to endure—she was heartbroken, and she needed him.

When Dr. K did not respond immediately to Ms. P's request, she started to whimper; it was all over, she declared—no one cared for her, Dr. K was heartless and uncaring, and she would be all alone this weekend, helpless. At this point, she paused, looked up at Dr. K, and then announced that given the circumstances, she might as well take her own life. Her tone was calm and threatening. When Dr. K tried to further evaluate Ms. P's state of mind to determine whether she needed to go to an emergency room, she became cagey; her responses were vague and noncommittal, seemingly purposefully frustrating Dr. K's efforts, but Dr. K detected a subtle look of pleasure in her eyes. In the countertransference, Dr. K made note of feeling controlled, frustrated, angry, and helpless.

Dr. K identified the affectively dominant object relation as composed of someone powerful, callous, and withholding who derived a sadistic pleasure from controlling and inducing suffering in a needy person who was anxious and powerless. This object relation initially emerged with Ms. P in the victim role and with Dr. K viewed as sadistically withholding when he did not immediately respond to her request that they speak over the weekend. The roles quickly flipped with Ms. P's threat, leaving her to derive sadistic pleasure from controlling and frustrating Dr. K.

Comments: This vignette illustrates the role of action (or *acting out*) on the part of the patient (the suicidal threat) in enacting the affectively dominant object relations. As can be anticipated in the treatment of patients with severe personality disorders, the affectively dominant object relations are enacted in the transference, with role reversals. Dr. K's attention to the countertransference (he felt controlled and frustrated) and Ms. P's nonverbal communication (her attitude as he tried to evaluate her was one of obvious pleasure) enabled him to identify the sadistic and controlling part of Ms. P, initially projected into Dr. K, that had a pattern of destroying all her intimate relationships.

Clinical Illustration 2 *(continued)*: Affectively Dominant Object Relations in the Countertransference—Mr. G

Mr. G, the 35-year-old man with narcissistic personality disorder who was functioning at a middle borderline level, was currently working part-time. His income was supplemented by funds provided by his wife and parents.

Mr. G began a session by complaining, "I can't get a break! All my wife does is criticize me and complain.... I asked her to help with the payment on my car; it's overdue. She *refused*—told me to pick up a shift at Starbucks! Can you believe it? It's not my fault I can't find a decent job!"

This and related complaints about his wife were repeated in Mr. G's verbal communications throughout the first half of the session, along with expressions of frustration, self-pity, and hostile derision of his wife. In the nonverbal channel, Mr. G's tone was hostile and derisive, and his facial expression communicated disgust.

In the countertransference, Dr. Y noted a marked absence of sympathetic feeling toward Mr. G in the moment; she found it difficult to empathize with his frustration or with his underlying sense of humiliation. In fact, as she listened to Mr. G's complaints, Dr. Y was struck by the coldness and contempt she experienced toward Mr. G in her countertransference, an attitude that she did not often experience toward her patients. Reflecting on this, she noted that the hostility and lack of empathy that characterized her attitude toward Mr. G in the session seemed to correspond exactly with Mr. G's description of his wife's attitude toward his distress.[2]

Dr. Y identified as the affectively dominant object relation a hostile and contemptuous figure in relation to a frustrated, diminished, and enraged other, with the entire relationship colored by feelings of mutual hostility and derision. Dr. Y noted Mr. G's identification with both sides of that object relation—that is, not only with the diminished, enraged figure, but also with the more dominant, contemptuous figure, expressed in his hostile verbal derision and lack of empathy in relation to his wife. These internal object relations shrouded the session in a general level of confusion and an atmosphere of hostility. Further, although the current focus was on Mr. G's hostile and mutually derisive relation with his wife, it was quite evident from the overall tone of the session—imbued by Mr. G's attitude toward Dr. Y, as well as the countertransference—that the same object relation was active in the transference as well. Dr. Y suspected that the situation in the session might be related to her having mentioned in their previous session that Mr. G was late with his payment.

Comments: This vignette illustrates the central role often played by the therapist's countertransference in identifying the affectively dominant object relations in the treatment of patients with severe personality disorders. The example also clearly illustrates the powerful impact of a single object relation, seemingly organizing every aspect of the patient's experience and behavior in the session—in the transference, the countertransference, and in Mr. G's account of his relation with his wife—with multiple role rever-

---

[2]This is an example of a complementary identification in the countertransference, often reflecting the patient's use of projective identification, in which the therapist is identified with the patient's internal and external objects (see Chapter 5).

sals. This caricature-like and extreme object relation emerges clearly from the clinical material as the affectively dominant one in the session.

This vignette also makes apparent Dr. Y's internal processing—listening to the patient's complaints about his wife, noting his derisive and hostile attitude and body language, and in particular maintaining awareness of the unfamiliar level of hostility and contempt she felt in the countertransference. Dr. Y put together communications from each of these three channels to identify the affectively dominant object relations in her mind.

Clinical Illustration 3 (continued): Affectively Dominant Object Relations in the Complex Interplay of a Conflict—Ms. L

Ms. L, the 23-year-old woman with avoidant personality disorder who was looking for work before starting graduate school (introduced earlier), was now working part-time in retail. She had presented with chronic depression, self-criticism, and a lack of assertiveness, and often allowed others to take advantage of her. She had recently been speaking in her sessions about an ongoing problem at her job; she had been hired to work 20–25 hours per week on a regular schedule but had been repeatedly called in at the last minute to cover open hours, and often ended up working 40 or more hours weekly. She was clear in her own mind that this was not what she wanted, and she had been able to acknowledge, with some help from Dr. B, that her boss was being inconsiderate and exploitative. At the same time, Ms. L had felt compelled to do as her boss asked, even canceling her own plans at the last minute to go into work, and had been reluctant to complain. She worked the longer hours even though the job was relatively uninteresting to Ms. L and unrelated to her chosen profession; she could easily have found another position or lived off her savings before beginning her graduate program a few months later.

Dr. B commented on Ms. L's apparent need to accommodate her boss's requests. Exploration of her conscious motivations for her behavior resulted in discussion for the first time of Ms. L's general sense, in virtually all relationships, that her status was conditional; she accommodated others because she believed herself to be in constant risk of being cast out. She went on to explain that even in her family, she felt this way, much as she knew she was loved. She linked this chronic self state to her early years, when she was separated from her parents and lived with her grandparents. Ms. L's manner and attitude toward Dr. B in describing this material was childlike, earnest, eager to please, and somewhat timid. In the countertransference, Dr. B felt protective of Ms. L.

Ms. L's verbal descriptions of her exchanges with her boss and of her chronic self state of being only conditionally accepted, as well as the timidity she exhibited in the session, enabled Dr. B to identify the affectively dominant object relation: an unworthy, unwanted, submissive child self attempting to maintain a connection with a disinterested and potentially rejecting parental object, associated with anxiety and painful feelings of being unloved. As well, Dr. B identified a different object relation enacted in the transference: a wished-for relationship between a dependent, trusting child self and an attentive and protective caregiver, which was communicated through nonverbal channels and the countertransference.

Comments: This vignette demonstrates a relatively complex cluster of object relations composed of 1) a defensive, somewhat idealized object relation (a dependent self and an ideal caregiver) enacted in the transference; and 2) a dissociated, more conflictual object relation (a disinterested caregiver and a cast-out, unwanted, inadequate self) enacted with the patient's boss, as well as implicitly expressed in the transference via the patient's timidity in session. The verbal channel of communication played a central role relative to the patient's nonverbal communication and the therapist's countertransference in conveying the affectively dominant object relations, and the affects and representations that characterized the two dyad components were relatively complex and well integrated in comparison to those of the previous two case illustrations, involving patients with more severe personality pathology.

Also reflective of a higher level of personality organization is the partial layering of Ms. L's experience in the transference. Rather than the simple dissociation seen in typical BPO structures, in this example, one object relation is clearly defensive, supporting repression of another object relation that is more threatening—with both object relations derived from a central conflict in relation to dependency.[3]

Clinical Illustration 4 *(continued)*: Affectively Dominant Object Relations in Verbal Communication—Ms. S

Ms. S, the 50-year-old married volunteer research assistant who had been diagnosed with depressive personality with dependent features and was functioning at a neurotic level, was introduced earlier as having presented with problems with self-esteem and social isolation. She had now been in treatment for several years and had begun presenting original scholarly work at local conferences. In session, she described her familiar anxiety before giving a talk, anticipating that she would sound ridiculous and make a fool of herself. She added that her anxiety had recently begun to relate to her appearance as well.

---

[3] The combination of repression and dissociation illustrated here is characteristic of patients falling on the border between high BPO and NPO.

After a pause, Ms. S commented that she had bought some expensive clothes for herself. She had done it on an impulse; never previously had she done anything like this. In the store, she thought the clothes looked great, but when she put them on at home and looked in the mirror, she felt she looked ridiculous; such beautiful garments should be worn by a more attractive, younger woman, not a frumpy old lady like her.

She then noted that she hadn't had a chance to tell Dr. C about her recent talk in another city. She'd been nervous, but it seemed to go well. Ms. S then added in an understated way that after the presentation, a leading scholar had asked her to lunch. He was a powerful man, she said, and also physically attractive, in his 40s. She couldn't believe that he wanted to spend time with her. At lunch, she was "totally bowled over" when he raised the possibility of an academic collaboration. That reminded her of something: for the first time, her husband had asked to look at her most recent manuscript. He had seemed genuinely interested in her ideas and proud of her. But she could never be sure with him; perhaps he was secretly making fun of her.

As Ms. S spoke, she became increasingly animated, ultimately flushing as she described her luncheon with the younger academic, quite a departure from her familiar subdued presentation. In the countertransference, Dr. C felt happy for the patient and proud, with a sense that Ms. S was coming into her own.

In reflecting on the clinical material, Dr. C noted to herself that Ms. S was describing two separate object relations. The first was organized around an ego-syntonic view, familiar to Ms. S and at this point clearly defensive, of herself as inadequate, inferior, unworthy of positive attention, and cut off from those who were more desirable and powerful. This object relation was associated with feelings of smallness and potential humiliation. The second object relation was organized in relation to a less familiar experience of herself and was associated with a fair amount of anxiety. In this object relation, Ms. S enjoyed being in the limelight; she experienced herself as able to take pleasure in attention and admiration from others who were powerful and desirable. This object relation was highly affectively charged, associated with feelings of power, intense pleasure, and excitement.

Dr. C identified this latter object relation as affectively dominant in the session. At this moment, Dr. C was less clear about what was dominant in the transference. Ms. S's attitude toward Dr. C seemed on the surface to be one of shyness combined with happiness at sharing a good feeling, as she might have toward a friend and confidant, or perhaps toward a desirable man. Dr. C wondered if Ms. S's excitement in session might in part be linked to repressed, conflictual wishes to be admired by Dr. C.

Comments: This vignette illustrates the role of verbal communication, and in particular of free association, in conveying affectively dominant object relations in the setting of repression-based defenses and a neurotic structure. Expressed in Ms. S's narrative and associations is a central conflict, associated with a series of defenses, anxieties, and conflictual wishes slowly emerging in the clinical material. Dr. C also hears a clear and stable layering of the relevant object relations, pointing both to the familiar, defensive object relation, and to the patient's newer, higher conflictual sense of herself emerging in the treatment and linked to anxiety. This complex structure is markedly different from the earlier Clinical Illustrations 1 and 2, involving the identification of dominant object relations in the setting of more severe personality pathology.

When the Therapist Cannot Identify Dominant Object Relations

We have illustrated that when determining a focus for intervention, the therapist will first work to identify the affectively dominant object relations in the session by attending to the three channels of communication: the patient's verbal communication, the patient's nonverbal communication, and the countertransference. If the therapist finds that he is unable to identify dominant object relations, it can be helpful for him to step back and consider, "What is going on in the transference? How is the patient behaving in session, and what is the general atmosphere in the room?"

If this approach does not bear fruit, a helpful second step is for the therapist to focus on the patient's participation in the treatment. In considering what might be missing to account for the absence of an apparent organizing theme in the patient's communications or whether there is a seemingly unfocused quality to the session, the therapist can consider these questions: "Is the patient adhering to the treatment frame?" "Is she meeting whatever special conditions were introduced as part of the treatment contract?" "Is she taking action in her life to pursue the treatment goals?" "What are the object relations enacted in or warded off by her behavior?"

Key Clinical Concepts

- The TFP-E therapist straddles two perspectives: one focusing on the patient's internal experience in session and the dominant object relations, and the other on the patient's functioning outside the sessions.

- The hierarchy of priority themes directs the therapist to identify emergency priorities, evaluate the integrity of the treatment frame, and identify the dominant object relations.

- Attention to the hierarchy of priority themes ensures that the exploratory process remains tied to external reality and to the patient's functioning in the world.
- Attention to the treatment frame and treatment goals anchors the treatment in the realities of the patient's life.
- The affectively dominant object relations serve as an entry point into exploration of the patient's internal world.
- To identify the dominant object relations, the therapist attends to the patient's verbal communication, nonverbal communication, and the countertransference.

References

Bateman A, Fonagy P: Mentalization-Based Treatment for Borderline Personality Disorder. New York, Oxford University Press, 2006

Bion WR: A theory of thinking (1962), in Second Thoughts. London, Heinemann, 1967, pp 110–119

Diener MJ, Hilsenroth MJ, Weinberger J: Therapist affect focus and patient outcomes in psychodynamic psychotherapy: a meta-analysis. Am J Psychiatry 164(6):936–941, 2007 17541054

Yeomans F, Clarkin JF, Kernberg OF: Transference-Focused Psychotherapy for Borderline Personality Disorder: A Clinical Guide. Washington, DC, American Psychiatric Publishing, 2015

10

Intervening I

Exploratory Interventions and the Interpretive Process

WE ORGANIZE OUR APPROACH TO THE
therapist's exploratory interventions under the heading of the *interpretive process* (Levy and Inderbitzin 1992; Sandler et al. 1992). The interpretive process can be conceptualized as a series of interventions, each building on the next, used by the therapist as she works with the patient to explore the patient's subjectivity. Our discussion of the interpretive process spans three chapters. Here, we focus on the exploratory interventions of clarification, confrontation, and interpretation proper; in Chapter 11, we focus on the transference analysis and other tactics guiding the interpretive process. In Chapter 12 we complete our coverage of exploratory interventions with discussion of countertransference utilization, managing technical neutrality and the process of working through.

To make a distinction, the classical approach to interpretation also focuses on the sequential steps of *clarification*, *confrontation*, and *interpretation*, with the overall objective of promoting insight and self-understanding (Auchincloss and Samberg 2012). For purposes of continuity we have retained these terms but introduce modifications, both in our technical approach to interpretation and in our understanding of its objectives. Regardless of the patient's dominant defensive style or the nature of the conflicts being explored, the objectives of the interpretive process are to help the patient identify, contain, reflect on, and contextualize conflictual aspects of experience while deepening his capacity for self-awareness, self-understanding, and self-acceptance (Caligor et al. 2009).

The Interpretive Process

We divide our discussion of the interpretive process into component parts: clarification, confrontation, and interpretation proper. Each component stands on its own as a type of exploratory intervention that serves specific functions in the treatment of personality disorders. Whereas clarification and confrontation focus on the *what* of the patient's experience, interpretation focuses on the *why*. Table 10–1 lists the exploratory interventions of the interpretive process, along with their purpose and the therapist's tasks.

Focusing on Experience in the Here and Now: Defining the Interpretive Process

In the clinical setting, the flow of exploratory interventions and their impact on clinical process will differ to some degree, depending on whether the current conflict and associated object relations are organized in relation to splitting-based or repression-based defenses. As a rule, as pathology becomes more severe, the focus of attention and intervention shifts toward the earlier phases of the interpretive process, in which clarification of the patient's dominant experience and confrontation of the impact of role reversals and splitting on his subjectivity serve important functions when it comes to helping patients cognitively contain, reflect on, and contextualize conflictual object relations. In contrast, when repression-based defenses predominate, greater emphasis is placed on the role of exploration and interpretation proper; in these situations, clarification and confrontation are more typically viewed through the lens of setting the stage for interpretation and the working through of unconscious conflict (for further discussion of working through, see Chapters 12 and 13).

As discussed throughout this book, in transference-focused psychotherapy—extended (TFP-E) we direct our interventions primarily toward the patient's moment-to-moment experience in each session and his cur-

---

TABLE 10–1. Exploratory interventions: purpose and tasks

The impact of the interpretive process on self experience is progressive and cumulative, building on the following interventions:

Intervention and purpose	Therapist's tasks
Clarification initiates a process of the patient's self-observation.	Asking for explanation of consciously experienced and described material that is vague or unclear.
Confrontation leads to the patient's increasing self-awareness.	Calling attention to contradictions or omissions, often preconscious, denied, or rationalized, in material that has been clarified.
Interpretation proper functions to deepen the patient's self-understanding.	Offering a hypothesis about why the patient may be experiencing or doing things as he is; making sense of manifestly irrational elements in confronted material by invoking unconscious motivations, anxieties, and personal meanings in the here and now driving defensive operations.
Working through promotes integrative processes and results in the patient's progressive levels of self-acceptance.	Repeatedly interpreting an identified conflict, in different contexts and over time (see Chapters 12 and 13 for further discussion).

---

rent functioning in his daily life. The focus of the interpretive process in TFP-E is on the patient's experience in the here and now; although the patient's past history is always an important piece of the puzzle, working in the here and now is the primary driver of personality change in TFP-E, supporting the structural and dynamic shifts that lead to personality integration.

Thus, although we may freely characterize the patient's experience in terms of objects from early life—for example, "It seems you are experiencing me as a rejecting mother"—we view this as a *descriptive* rather than an *explanatory* statement, very different from "You are experiencing me as rejecting you because your mother rejected you" or even "…because you felt rejected by your mother." This latter kind of intervention, essentially a reconstruction, generally does not function to deepen the clinical process in TFP-E and can detract from exploration of the patient's current conflict.

In contrast, once a conflict has been elaborated and the patient is beginning to tolerate awareness of conflictual aspects of his internal experience, it often becomes helpful to think about how all this may have come to be, and to link core conflicts to the patient's early history. As a result, it is well within the middle and into the advanced phases of treatment and in the process of working through that we most typically and usefully bring the patient's early life into the interpretive process. In this setting, forging ties between past self and present self helps to promote and solidify change.

Clarification

Clarification is the most basic and frequently employed exploratory intervention in TFP-E and is the first step in the process of interpretation. Clarification entails the therapist's seeking clarification of the patient's subjective experience. Areas of vagueness are addressed until both patient and therapist have a clear understanding of what has been said, or until the patient feels puzzled by an underlying contradiction in his thinking that has been brought to light. The material to be clarified may be an aspect of external reality, of the patient's history, or of his internal experience that he brings into the session.

Clarification serves the dual function of eliciting and elucidating information while helping the patient bring out new elements in his communication that may have been obscure, with the objective of obtaining the fullest possible appreciation of the patient's experience and behavior. Clarification is an intervention shared by many different forms of psychotherapy insofar as it helps therapist and patient attend to the details of the patient's conscious experience. In TFP-E, clarification initiates the process of self-observation and introspection that is the vehicle of the entire interpretive process.

Clarification can be a single intervention but is more often a back-and-forth process between therapist and patient that involves systematic inquiry, until both patient and therapist have a clear understanding of what has been said or is being enacted, or until the patient feels puzzled by an underlying contradiction in his presentation. The process of clarification typically involves the therapist's requests for specifics and details, and perhaps the therapist's sharing of her own difficulty in fully following what the patient is saying or in understanding what he is doing. Clarification may also involve asking for examples to illustrate what the patient is describing, or restating what the patient seems to be describing and asking for feedback as to the accuracy of the therapist's understanding.

The therapist will ask for clarification in relation to material that is unclear, vague, or somehow incomplete, qualities that often signal the impact of defensive operations on the patient's communications and on the clinical process. As a result, *clarification tends to direct clinical attention toward an area of defense and conflict, while staying at the level of the patient's dominant conscious experience*; clarification is purely elucidative, fleshing out the patient's experience as clearly and specifically as possible. Clarification does not involve addressing psychological material not currently within the patient's awareness. In TFP-E, clarification is always the first step in identifying and defining the affectively dominant object relations.

The following are examples of clarification:

Therapist: You told me you and John had an argument yesterday. Can you take me through what exactly happened between the two of you?

Therapist: You said you had a great weekend. Can you tell me more?
Patient: I just had a lot of fun.
Therapist: Can you give me an example of what you did that was so much fun?

Therapist: You said you were lonely. Can you tell me more about what "lonely" feels like?

Therapist: You said you've not been feeling very well. Can you tell me more about how you've been feeling?
Patient: I've been feeling really down on myself.
Therapist: In what way?
Patient: Well, I am really unhappy with my appearance, and now I'm going into the weekend feeling like my boyfriend doesn't really care whether I'm there or not. He could easily replace me with someone else.
Therapist: So it sounds like you're feeling unattractive and not like someone your boyfriend would really care about or find special? Is that an accurate description of how you're feeling?

Clarification and Severity of Pathology

In the treatment of patients functioning at a neurotic level of personality organization (NPO), the therapist will in general find the patient's communications relatively easy to follow and sufficiently specific, for the most part. However, repression-based defenses will introduce subtle omissions and areas of vagueness, or they may lead to inconsistencies in the patient's verbal communications that call for clarification (Caligor et al. 2007). Thus, as part of the interpretive process, clarification initiates a process of exploration in NPO patients by drawing attention to an area of defense and conflict and asking the patient to examine his experience more completely and specifically.

Clarification plays a more central and complex role when splitting-based defenses are organizing the clinical material. In the setting of splitting-based defenses, it is common for a patient's communications to be vague, superficial, incomplete, and difficult to follow; it is also common for the TFP-E therapist to feel confused as to what a patient functioning at a borderline level of personality organization (BPO) is trying to say or what he is describing, and often the patient will find himself confused as well. Facts and events may be incompletely or vaguely described, representations may be shadowy or poorly differentiated, and affects may be superficial and poorly integrated. In this setting, the process of clarification entails helping the patient more clearly and specifically attend to and articulate his external and internal experience; ultimately, this process will help the patient think more specifically about—and use less denial in relation to—his external reality and behavior, and help him observe and put words to his internal experience.

Clinical Illustration 1: Clarification With an NPO Patient

> Mr. Y: My divorce is finally going through. Julia has pushed me hard to get it finalized. I guess I was dragging my heels…not that I meant to, but I couldn't get going—it just didn't happen.
>
> Dr. B: I'm not sure I understand. What didn't happen or what couldn't you get going?
>
> Mr. Y: I had to meet with the lawyers, face the issue of custody for Nina, our youngest. I didn't want to think about it, didn't want to make it real.
>
> Dr. B: What is it that you don't want to make real?
>
> Mr. Y: That phase of my life is over…. Now I'm only "partial custodian" for Nina. Meanwhile, she lives with Julia and I'm the outsider…. It feels like there's this wonderful family I used to be part of and now I'm outside it. [*The patient becomes tearful.*] I know so much of it is my fault—I could have been so much better. I really can't blame Julia.

Comments: In this brief vignette, the therapist on two occasions asks for clarification, helping Mr. Y move from his general statement about dragging his heels to a specific description of his pain at losing his family, which he links to an internal experience of feeling excluded from a loving relationship because of his own deficiencies. In this situation, the therapist might decide to continue with the process of clarification—for example, asking to hear more about how the patient blames himself. This process might lead the therapist to suggest to the patient a description of the affectively dominant object relations—ideally, in words that the patient has himself introduced. For example, the therapist might say: "It sounds like you feel sad, almost like a child who has been cast out of his family because he didn't try hard enough, wasn't good enough, while it seems as if in your eyes, at this moment, Julia is merely doing what she has to do. Does this sound accurate?"

Clinical Illustration 2: Clarification With a High-BPO Patient

> Ms. J: I've been getting into work late. In the mornings, I'm paralyzed.
>
> Dr. C: I'm not sure I understand what you mean.
>
> Ms. J: I'm paralyzed—can't get out of bed, my body doesn't move.
>
> Dr. C: Can you tell me more?
>
> Ms. J: Well, I make coffee, read the paper...like I'm in slow motion. And I feel very depressed.
>
> Dr. C: I'm confused. What did you mean when you said you were late because you were paralyzed and couldn't get out of bed?
>
> Ms. J: Well, what I mean is, I *feel* paralyzed. I do get out of bed. But I move very slowly through my routine. I have no control over it. I'm aware that this will make me late, but it's like I can't move any faster. I guess I should get there on time.
>
> Dr. C: What is the arrangement with your boss about when you should get to work?
>
> Ms. J: Oh, Hal wants me there early. But I guess I don't feel like I care.
>
> Dr. C: So it sounds like Hal is telling you he wants you to be there on time, but that's not something you really care to do?
>
> Ms. J: Yes, I really don't care if I'm late, especially if I'm tired, but he makes such a big deal of getting in early. I can't tell if he's mad.
>
> Dr. C: So it sounds like, from your perspective, he's telling you what to do, maybe even bossing you around?
>
> Ms. J: Yes, and I don't like it.

Comments: In this vignette, the patient is notably vague and difficult to follow, and Dr. C must be quite active to clarify what exactly the patient is trying to say. In the countertransference, Dr. C is aware of her own irritation, with both the patient's communication style and her tardiness at work, imagining Ms. J's boss as likely irritated with her as well. Dr. C's interventions clarify the events that Ms. J is describing, as well as her boss's stated expectations, which the patient does not initially make clear.

At the end of this process, Dr. C is in a position to propose a way to think about the object relation organizing Ms. J's experience regarding her "paralysis." In this example, Dr. C went on to say, "What strikes me is that Hal's telling you what to do seems to leave you feeling paralyzed or in slow motion, as if something is forcing you to get to work late and make him mad. Is that how it feels on the inside?" Ms. J responded, "Yes, exactly. I know it sounds kind of crazy.... I don't like being told what to do."

Many BPO patients may assume that it is not necessary to provide a clear explanation of their experience; some patients take for granted that the therapist will automatically and magically understand, whereas others may obfuscate because they are fearful of truly being "known" or understood. Still others may be vague because it allows them to avoid thinking about aspects of their behavior or experience that are conflictual and that would be painful or upsetting to examine. For any of these reasons, some BPO patients may become angry or annoyed when the therapist asks for clarification, or if the therapist indicates anything but total, immediate, and automatic understanding, regardless of how vague the patient's communications may be.

When BPO patients are vague and unclear, a therapist may end up feeling that she should have followed what the patient said more closely, and that her failure to do so represents a failing on her part rather than an aspect of the patient's communication and defensive style calling for exploration. The risk is that the therapist will feel inhibited in relation to asking for clarification—a countertransference pressure that the therapist should resist, because it is important that the TFP-E therapist feel free to ask for clarification whenever she is unclear about the patient's communications. In the event that the patient responds negatively to requests for clarification, the clinical focus shifts to the patient's experience of the therapist in the moment—that is, to clarification and exploration of the object relations currently activated in the transference.

Clinical Illustration 3: A High-BPO Patient Responds to Requests for Clarification

A high-BPO patient with narcissistic personality disorder responded with irritation to his therapist's repeated request for clarification in relation to his vague and somewhat evasive description of his extramarital escapades. The patient responded with a hostile outburst: "We just went over this! Why do you keep asking me to explain what I'm saying? Aren't you listening to a word I say? Or is it that you don't trust that I'm being straight with you?"

The therapist responded by pursuing clarification of the object relation organizing the current interaction: "Can you tell me more about those feelings—either that I am disinterested, not fully attending to our conversation, or that I am suspicious of you, not fully trusting you to tell me the truth?" This line of inquiry uncovered the dominant issue in the session, which, as it turned out, was not the patient's extramarital affair, but rather an object relation activated in the transference characterized by one person disinterested and dismissive, the other suspicious and deceptive, with the relationship as a whole colored by mutual mistrust and devaluation.

Comments: In this vignette, the patient's vague and evasive style leads the therapist to ask for clarification. In response to the therapist's ongoing efforts to clarify the patient's communications, the patient becomes irate. Here, the process of clarification has led to crystallization of the affectively dominant object relations in the transference; as a result of the therapist's ongoing efforts to clarify what the patient is saying, it becomes clear that the most immediate communication of the affectively dominant object relations is in what the patient is doing rather than what he is saying (i.e., in what he is enacting with the therapist rather than in his descriptions of his sexual life). By attending to the patient's outburst, the therapist is able to identify and articulate the hostile object relation organizing the patient's evasive behavior with the therapist (and no doubt enacted in his intimate relations as well), a relationship in which one person is disinterested and dismissive and the other is suspicious and deceptive. This object relation is organizing the patient's experience of himself and the therapist in interaction, with the patient at some level identified with both sides of this object relation characterized by mistrust and hostility.

Summary

Clarification entails focusing on an area of vagueness or confusion and asking for further detail until both patient and therapist have a clear understanding of what the patient has been describing. Clarification is the most basic and commonly employed intervention used by TFP-E therapists in working with patients across the spectrum of severity. It is a process that elaborates the patient's dominant conscious experience, creating a psychological space in which the patient can observe and think about what he is doing and experiencing, while feeling that the therapist is interested in the details of, and ultimately "gets" or understands, his experience (Britton 1998; Steiner 1993). Clarification initiates a process of self-observation and introspection that characterizes the entire interpretive process.

Because splitting-based defenses by definition introduce significant vagueness, superficiality, and discontinuities into the patient's discourse, clarification tends to play a more central role in the treatment of BPO patients than it does in the treatment of NPO patients.[1] Across the spectrum of severity, clarification functions as the first step in the interpretive process, providing a clear and specific understanding of the patient's experience that is shared by therapist and patient, and often drawing clinical attention to an area of conflict. Clarification makes it possible to elaborate and describe the self and object representations organizing the patient's conscious experience.

To review, the therapist uses clarification to achieve the following:

- Approach material through the patient's subjective experience.
- Elaborate the patient's dominant experience.
- Initiate a process of self-observation and introspection.

The process of clarification often brings to light inconsistencies, omissions, or areas of confusion in the patient's narrative and subjective experience to which he did not previously attend. In this way, clarification leads quite naturally to the next phase of interpretive intervention: *confrontation*, discussed below.

Confrontation

Confrontation involves the therapist's calling attention to aspects of the patient's internal experience and verbal and nonverbal communications that are discrepant. In confrontation, the therapist invites the patient to step back and observe, and then to pull together and reflect on, aspects of his experience, communications, and behavior that do not fit together.

---

[1]Because vagueness serves defensive functions in the setting of splitting-based defenses, the process of clarification with BPO patients often functions as a form of confrontation (discussed in the next section of this chapter). This accounts in part for the negative reactions that may be elicited in some BPO patients in response to clarification (e.g., the patient with narcissistic personality disorder described earlier in Clinical Illustration 3).

The objective of confrontation is to encourage the patient to reflect on internal inconsistencies that he would naturally overlook.

Despite the unfortunate aggressive connotations of the word, we have chosen to retain the term *confrontation* for purposes of historical continuity. In TFP-E, confrontation is always done thoughtfully, with tact and from a perspective of neutral inquiry; it is helpful to think of confrontation not as a form of aggression, but rather as an invitation to reflect. (However, note that confrontation is apt to "go against the grain," increasing the patient's awareness of internal inconsistencies in his verbal and nonverbal communications that have been ego-syntonic.)

Confrontation may involve addressing contradictions or discrepancies within the patient's verbal communications in session or between the patient's verbal communications in session and in previous sessions. Confrontations often focus on nonverbal communications that the patient is denying. For example, the therapist may call attention to discrepancies between the patient's verbal and nonverbal communication when the patient smiles as he discusses painful material, or between the patient's dominant experience and his nonverbal communication when he accuses the therapist of being critical while the patient himself is behaving critically toward his therapist.

In contrast to clarification, which focuses on the patient's dominant conscious experience and asks for elaboration of how the patient sees it, confrontation involves expanding the patient's awareness by introducing a new perspective, one outside the perspective habitually assumed by the patient. As a result, confrontation is a more advanced intervention than clarification, in that it requires more of the patient in terms of the cognitive flexibility necessary to take himself outside his dominant experience in the moment to consider alternative perspectives. Confrontation calls attention to aspects of the patient's experience and verbal and nonverbal communications that he is denying, or to contradictions among them. In essence, *confrontation brings to the patient's awareness the subtle or not-so-subtle inconsistencies, contradictions, and omissions, introduced by his defenses, that he is denying* (Etchegoyen 1991); when the therapist makes a confrontation, she is initiating a process of exploring defense and conflict.

In contrast to interpretation (discussed later in this chapter in the section "Interpretation Proper"), confrontation entails sticking closely to the patient's conscious and preconscious experience and observable behavior; the objective of confrontation is self-awareness, in contrast to self-understanding, which is an objective of interpretation. The confronting therapist is not introducing new material. Rather, she is introducing a new perspective on material that has already been elaborated through a process of clarification. Confrontations draw the patient's attention to attitudes, ideas, and behaviors that are fully conscious (or in the case of behavior, fully observable), assumed by the patient to be perfectly natural in and of themselves (i.e., they are ego-syntonic, rationalized, or denied), but that are discrepant with other attitudes, ideas, or behaviors of the patient. In confrontation, the therapist calls the patient's attention to something that is evident but that defensively the patient is not attending to or is denying the significance of. As we illustrate in the vignettes that follow, confrontation promotes self-awareness by focusing on habitual, defensive ways of thinking, feeling, and behaving that are ego-syntonic and making them ego-dystonic—observable, and in some sense remarkable, to the patient—calling for further understanding.

The following are examples of confrontation:

Therapist: You've told me many times that you wish you were able to get more attention from men. So I'm a bit surprised to hear that when the guy you were interested in texted you last night, you didn't respond. What are your thoughts?

Therapist: I am struck by your description of feeling childlike in your interactions with your peers at work; when you describe the details [clarification] of what happened in the meeting, it sounds like everyone agreed you handled things in a masterful and assertive fashion.

Therapist: You describe yourself as afraid of confrontations, yet in your review, your boss commented on your need to go easier on the junior partners. How do you put that together?

Therapist: You said you had a tough weekend, but you were smiling as you told me this. What are your thoughts about that?

Therapist: You are describing yourself as a great student, but in our initial meetings you told me that you have been on academic probation. Can you help me understand?

Therapist: I understand that you feel I am critical of you; at the same time, you have spent most of this session criticizing me and the way I have handled your treatment. It's as if at the same time that you are viewing me as critical of you, you are—out of your awareness—behaving critically toward me.

Therapist: Are you aware that whenever I have started to speak today, you have interrupted me?

Therapist: You seem very comfortable here today and optimistic about our work together. Yet I wonder if you can recall how you felt last time you were here: hopeless and despairing, that this is the wrong treatment approach for you, and that things will never improve in your life.

Confrontation and Neutrality

The effectiveness of confrontation, and of the interpretive process in general, rests on the therapist's maintaining a neutral stance and containing (in contrast to acting on) her countertransference (Levy and Inderbitzin 1992). The desired outcome of confrontation is that the patient will struggle within himself with the discrepancy between two contradictory views, both of which he understands to be his own. An effective process of confrontation will help the patient step out of his dominant experience in the moment to hold two contradictory perspectives in mind.

If the therapist is not neutral, there is a risk that confrontation will degenerate such that the patient sees it one way, and the therapist sees it differently or is telling the patient he should see it differently. In this situation, the patient holds fast to one perspective while projecting the other onto the therapist. This development can be counterproductive, functioning to further rigidify the patient's dominant view rather than to create the internal dissonance and perspective-taking on the part of the patient that is the objective of confrontation.

It is the therapist's perspective, emerging from her stepping back from the immediate therapeutic field to view the total situation and observe both sides of the patient's conflict, that defines her neutral stance and that enables her confrontations to promote reflective processes in the patient. In essence, the therapist wants to help the patient develop the capacity, in areas of conflict, to step out of his dominant, ego-syntonic experience to entertain other perspectives that are dissociated, denied, or simply ignored. In the same way that the neutral therapist observes the different sides of the patient from the position of a neutral third party, the therapist wants to help the patient develop his own capacity to step back and observe the different sides of himself.

Clinical Illustration 4: Confrontation and Neutrality

A patient described her latest fight with her boyfriend. She complained that he had been selfish and withholding. From her perspective, all she needed was a hug. As soon as he hugged her, she knew she would be able to listen to him. But without that expression of physical affection, she felt unable to hear his side of things. From her perspective, what she asked for "was so simple," and yet he "stubbornly" refused to comply. Why, she wondered, did he have to be so selfish and controlling?

From a position of neutrality, the therapist offered a confrontation, inviting the patient to broaden her perspective by calling attention to the implications of aspects of her behavior that she was denying. The therapist said, "I hear that you felt John's behavior was selfish and withholding, and that you felt controlled by him. At the same time, I'm trying to imagine how he felt when you told him you couldn't listen to him unless he gave you a hug, even though he might not have felt like hugging you."

The patient responded, "So you're telling me it's my fault?" The therapist responded, maintaining a neutral stance and standing outside the situation, hoping to promote the patient's capacity to observe herself and reflect: "I'm not thinking about fault or blame here. Rather, I'm wondering if when this happens, you and John aren't kind of in the same boat. Could it be that at the same time that you experience him as withholding and controlling, he experiences you in the same way, when you refuse to discuss things with him until he hugs you?"

Comments: In this vignette, the patient is initially locked into her own view of the exchange with John. From her perspective, it is he who is selfish and withholding, he who doesn't listen. In the moment, the patient demonstrates no empathy for John's experience of their interaction, and she is seemingly unaware of the ways in which she is enacting the very behavior and attitudes that she criticizes in him. From a position of neutrality the therapist avoids taking sides ("Who is at fault?") and instead steps outside the dyad of the patient and her boyfriend to see them as a system in which the two mirror each other's behavior and attitudes. The therapist's objective in offering a confrontation is to help the patient step out of her own experience to observe herself, to consider John's perspective, and ultimately to step back and view the entire system, as the therapist has done.

The therapist begins by articulating the patient's experience of John as selfish, withholding, and controlling, communicating empathy for the patient's situation. The therapist then attempts, gently, to open up the patient's perspective to help her empathize with John. The patient's initial reaction is to feel attacked and criticized, and to reject the therapist's comments. In response, the therapist maintains her neutral stance, holding her ground while trying to contain the patient's affect. The therapist further encourages the patient to broaden her perspective to consider how John might be experiencing things, and to be more reflective in relation to her own behavior.

In Video 5, "Interpretive Process: Borderline Level of Personality Organization," this vignette is presented along with the therapist's additional work with the patient. While maintaining an empathic perspective, Dr. Caligor first uses clarification to articulate the object relation organizing the patient's current experience with her boyfriend. Later, Dr. Caligor offers a trial confrontation, calling the patient's attention to aspects of her own behavior, dissociated from her dominant experience, that seem to mirror her boyfriend's frustrating behavior. After Dr. Caligor explores with the patient the polarized views she holds of her significant others, who are seen either as idealized caretakers or painful and frustrating disappointments, Dr. Caligor calls the patient's attention to her idealization of Dr. Caligor herself. At this point, Dr. Caligor offers a transference interpretation, suggesting that perhaps the patient needs to rigidly idealize the therapist in order to avoid experiencing the same frustration and disappointment that the patient feels in her other relationships. This video illustrates the interpretive process with a BPO patient, the neutral observing stance of the TFP-E therapist, and how the therapist works to gradually help the patient first, to open her perspective and ultimately, to empathize with her boyfriend. This clip also illustrates activation of dominant object relations in both the patient's interpersonal life and in the transference, and how the TFP-E therapist is able to shift fluidly between the two.

 Video Illustration 5
Interpretive Process: Borderline Level of
Personality Organization (8:56)

Confrontation and Severity of Pathology

Confrontation is a central intervention in the treatment of personality pathology across the range of severity. Because confrontation calls attention to the impact of defense on the patient's experience, the nature of confrontations will to some extent be different in the setting of splitting-based versus repression-based defenses. In addition, differences between the psychological capacities of NPO and BPO patients lead to a more complex role for confrontation in the treatment of BPO patients.

In TFP-E, confrontation focuses attention on the impact of defenses on the patient's subjective experience, and in the process, it supports the patient's capacity to entertain alternative perspectives in the setting of psychological conflict. This capacity is to some degree compromised in all patients with personality disorders (such is the nature of "defensiveness") but is compromised to a much greater degree in BPO patients, especially as pathology becomes more severe along the BPO spectrum.

In terms of clinical process, we think of confrontation as creating ego-dystonicity in relation to habitual defensive operations—a necessary condition for later stages in the interpretive process involving exploring and reflecting on the personal meanings motivating defenses. Across the spectrum of severity, denial and rationalization support other defenses by helping the patient overlook or rationalize the subtle or not-so-subtle omissions and inconsistencies in his experience and behavior that have been introduced by habitual defensive operations. It is only after this denial has been diminished—that is, after defenses have become to some degree ego-dystonic as a result of repeated confrontation—that the patient becomes truly curious about the internal processes responsible for these inconsistencies and is able to work in a meaningful way with the anxieties motivating defense. At this point, or at these moments, the patient becomes able to make use of interpretation proper, which involves exploration of internal motives and meanings.

The Role of Confrontation With NPO Patients

NPO patients are generally capable of introspection at baseline. Reality testing is stable, and even though their experience can become more concrete in the setting of conflict and defense, NPO patients generally retain the capacity to entertain alternative perspectives and to appreciate the constructed nature of psychological experience, even in the setting of conflict. As a result, in the treatment of NPO patients, repeated confrontation often leads relatively quickly and smoothly to defenses becoming ego-dystonic, clearing the way for interpretation proper.

For example, in Video 6, "Interpretive Process: Neurotic Level of Personality Organization," Dr. Caligor treats a 40-year-old man with obsessive-compulsive and dependent features who presented with marital problems. Dr. Caligor explores a recent interaction between the patient and his wife that left the patient feeling painfully rejected. Dr. Caligor clarifies the patient's experience of that interaction, articulating the object relation organizing the patient's experience and highlighting what is for the patient a painful, repetitive interpersonal pattern. After exploring this pattern with the patient, Dr. Caligor tactfully calls the patient's attention to aspects of the exchange with his wife that he is not attending to, pointing to behaviors that perpetuate relational problems. After the patient reflects on his withdrawal and passivity, associating to a longstanding fear of his own aggression, Dr. Caligor offers an interpretation. She suggests to the patient that perhaps his passivity and withdrawal are defensive, enabling him to avoid being confronted with angry feelings, which he fears will drive others away. In addition to illustrating the interpretive process with an NPO patient, this clip highlights how dominant object relations in NPO patients often manifest in the form of a repetitive relationship theme. During the process of confrontation, the therapist tactfully confronts ego-syntonic aspects of the patient's behavior that perpetuate this relationship pattern. This clip also illustrates the potential value of the NPO patient's associations in elaborating underlying anxieties and conflicts, and the capacity for self analysis often demonstrated by NPO patients.

 Video Illustration 6
Interpretive Process: Neurotic Level of
Personality Organization (6:30)

Clinical Illustration 1 *(continued)*: Confrontation With an NPO Patient

We return now to Mr. Y, the patient undergoing a divorce and consequently mourning the loss of his family. He had been describing his state of mind: "It feels like there's this wonderful family I used to be part of and now I'm outside it. [*The patient becomes tearful.*] I know so much of it is my fault—I could have been so much better. I really can't blame Julia."

At this juncture, the therapist might begin with further clarification, helping the patient more fully elaborate his current attitude toward the ending of the marriage, one colored by self-blame and a protective attitude toward his wife. While Mr. Y was in the moment swept up in sadness and self-recrimination, Dr. B was aware that Mr. Y was enacting a view of himself in relation to his wife (with Mr. Y as a childlike figure cast out by a fair-minded mother figure because of his deficiencies)—and that this view, although painful, was only a part of the picture. Dr. B maintained awareness that this view was entirely discrepant with other things that Mr. Y had reported in the past about his wife's behavior in the marriage, including a history of infidelity that the patient was in the moment apparently denying, minimizing, or ignoring.

Dr. B opted to confront the patient's current view, calling attention to views he had shared in the past. "You are saying that you don't blame Julia for the dissolution of the marriage, because in many ways you could have been a better husband and father. I have no reason to doubt that you could have behaved better, but at the same time I'm struck by your attitude."

Dr. B paused and waited for Mr. Y's reaction: "What do you mean?"

Then Dr. B continued: "Well, it's almost as if you choose, or in some way need, to hold yourself entirely responsible for the dissolution of the marriage and to spare her any responsibility. After all, you've told me in the past that the marriage started to fall apart because she had an affair. But it's as if that reality is entirely off your radar as you speak with me today. Instead, it is as though your deficiencies are entirely to blame. What are your thoughts about that?"

In response to Dr. B's intervention, Mr. Y was reflective, able to make use of the confrontation to feel perplexed by his current, somewhat one-sided view, and curious about why he would organize his experience in this way. Dr. B noted that as they continued to explore Mr. Y's thoughts and feelings in the session, Mr. Y became anxious. He began to talk about his worries about being alone and lonely; in his associations, Mr. Y found himself wondering about the strength of his long-term friendships and questioning whether others would stand by him. In the countertransference, Dr. B felt vaguely guilty and worried that he had perhaps pushed Mr. Y too soon.

Comments: In this vignette, the therapist, after clarifying Mr. Y's current experience of himself in relation to the marriage, contrasts that view with a very different view of the marriage that Mr. Y presented at another time. Neither view is new and neither one is more "real" than the other—the point is that each has felt true, and yet they are frankly discrepant. In calling the patient's attention to the discrepancy, Dr. B is both introducing an alternative perspective to Mr. Y's current one and inviting him to feel curious about and reflect on his internal experience (e.g., why Mr. Y would experience things in this way at this moment; why he would deny the obvious reality that regardless of his failings, his wife Julia also played a role in the demise of the marriage).

As discussed later in the section "Interpretation Proper" in this chapter, the patient's current view of himself as culpable and rightly cast out by a fair-minded maternal figure is a defensive object relation protecting him from awareness of underlying object relations that are conflictual. In a neurotic structure, confrontation calls attention to defensive object relations so that over time they become less convincing to the patient and less effective at defending against underlying object relations and associated anxieties, which become more accessible to conscious awareness.

The Centrality of Confrontation With BPO Patients

Confrontation serves a variety of more specialized functions in the treatment of BPO patients, supporting and helping to consolidate capacities that may be fragile in the BPO patient in the setting of interpersonal closeness and in areas of conflict. The therapist may be called on to help stabilize the patient's reality testing, to support his capacities of self-observation and introspection, to introduce the consideration of alternative perspectives, and to support the capacity to reflect on internal states. In addition, confrontation of splitting proper helps the patient better contextualize dissociated aspects of his experience.

With BPO patients, interpretation proper is often deferred, especially in the earlier phases of treatment, until clarification and confrontation have stabilized these capacities, developments that both improve the patient's functioning and enable him to make use of more advanced phases of the interpretive process. The eventual focus on interpretation proper will involve an exploration of personal meanings and unconscious motives.

Clinical Illustration 2 *(continued)*: Confrontation With a High-BPO Patient

We return to Ms. J, the patient who had been describing her current difficulty getting to work in the setting of struggles with her boss. As a result of a process of ongoing clarification, what had emerged was that the patient was feeling "paralyzed" by her resentment in relation to her supervisor, Hal, whom she viewed as bossing her around and treating her dismissively. Ms. J was having difficulty both making it into work and functioning once she got there. She felt unable to follow instructions, became easily overwhelmed and confused, and was often tearful.

It was clear to Dr. C that Ms. J was immersed in a polarized, highly negative view of herself in relation to Hal, which had generalized to her experience of the job in general. Ms. J described herself as "in a negative spiral." She said, "Everything is falling apart" and she might "have to quit." Dr. C, meanwhile, was well aware that Ms. J's current attitude, although one she had held toward many other bosses and positions in the past, was entirely discrepant with how she had been feeling in her current position until recently.

Dr. C decided to confront the patient's dissociation of her current view from how she had felt until recently: "I understand that there are problems with Hal—that he doesn't seem to value you and leaves you feeling bossed around—and that you are having great difficulty getting to work and doing your job once you get there. You describe very familiar experiences, both of being paralyzed in the mornings, and—if you are able to drag yourself in to work—of feeling overwhelmed and inept, unable to think straight or follow instructions. [These were experiences that Ms. J had repeatedly had at previous jobs and that had been explored at length in earlier sessions through the process of clarification, with Dr. C helping Ms. J to elaborate the specifics of her experience while in these states.] At the same time, there is something that really gets my attention; I'm wondering if you would be interested in hearing my thoughts." Ms. J indicated that she would.

Dr. C continued: "It seems to me that your experience with Hal and at the job, though certainly not unfamiliar, is entirely discrepant with how you were feeling in this job for some time, up until last week. It's like black and white, night and day. Up until last week, you were feeling really good; you believed that Hal valued you highly. You were motivated—jumping out of bed, always the first one into the office, and happy to work on your days off and in the evenings. It's not that either experience is necessarily good or bad, right or wrong, but rather that the two are so entirely discrepant, and that you went from one to the other overnight. What are your thoughts about this?"

Comments: In this vignette, the therapist begins by restating the patient's current experience as it has been clarified. At this point, she contrasts Ms. J's current experience of herself in the workplace with an entirely discrepant view that until recently organized her experience of the exact same setting. As in the case with Mr. Y, and as is even more apparent because of the highly split nature of Ms. J's experience, both views are polarized, with neither view more accurate than the other. The point is that both, though mutually contradictory, have felt true at different times. The therapist is calling Ms. J's attention to the contradictory nature of her experience and inviting her to reflect on it, to develop greater perspective on how unstable it is and how distorted it must be.

Confrontations of this kind in the setting of a borderline structure can fulfill a variety of functions. Introducing an alternative view helps the patient take herself out of a monolithic, lost-in-the-moment, and concrete view of her current experience, one that involves both distortion and rigidity; this shift will improve her reality testing in relation to her currently highly split experience of herself in the workplace by helping her cognitively bridge the split between more idealized and paranoid perspectives. In addition, to the degree that the therapist's confrontation highlights that the patient has held totally contradictory views of the same set of circumstances, and that she has had similar experiences in the past, the therapist is tacitly highlighting the internal, constructed quality (as opposed to the concreteness that comes with splitting) of psychological experience, an awareness that opens up the possibility of greater flexibility and integration.

Supporting reality testing and supporting an appreciation of the internal and subjective nature of psychological experience are functions played by confrontation in the treatments of BPO patients that are less relevant in the treatment of patients with higher level personality pathology, in whom these capacities are more fully developed and more stable. In the treatments of both NPO and BPO patients, confrontations function to introduce alternative perspectives and greater flexibility into patients' thinking in an area of conflict.

The vignette of Ms. J illustrates confrontation of splitting (or idealization/devaluation) in the treatment of a high-BPO patient. We would be remiss, however, if we were to address confrontation in the treatment of BPO patients without specifically commenting on confronting projective identification (often described in TFP-E in terms of calling attention to *role reversals*). Confrontation of projective identification is one of the more central and powerful exploratory interventions made by the TFP-E therapist in the treatment of BPO patients: the therapist calls attention to the profound contradiction between the patient's dominant self experience and her observable behavior, something that would be evident to any third party but remains dissociated from the dominant conscious experience of the patient and is denied. The use of projective identification tends to be highly disruptive in the interpersonal lives of BPO patients, as well as in their transferences; to the extent that the patient can begin to make use of the therapist's confrontations to broaden her perspective to include observation of her own behavior, her reality testing in interpersonal settings will begin to improve (remaining split but less chaotic and confusing). Often this will be reflected quite quickly and directly in the patient's interpersonal relationships, which may become less stormy. A similar shift may be seen in the patient's treatment as things settle down in the transference.

For example, at some point when Ms. J was complaining about her boss, she shared an anecdote in which he asked her to complete a task; in response, she "had a panic attack, told him I couldn't do it, and went home for the day." Later in the session, Ms. J described her boss as controlling, demanding, and dismissive of her. Dr. C took that opportunity to wonder out loud: "I hear that Hal can be controlling and disrespectful of you. I also understand that when you're overwhelmed and anxious, you become unable to function and have to leave the office. When he asks you to do something and your response is to say that you can't do it and then to go home for the day, I wonder whether it seems to him that you are treating him much as you feel he treats you—in a rather disrespectful and controlling way. What are your thoughts about what I am suggesting?"

Summary

Confrontation entails calling attention to contradictions or discrepancies in the clinical material that reflect the impact of the patient's defenses on his communications in session; in making a confrontation, the therapist is in essence confronting denial and rationalization of subtle (neurotic defenses) or not-so-subtle (splitting-based defenses) distortions in the patient's subjectivity that have been introduced by his defenses. From the perspective of the interpretive process overall, confrontation makes the patient aware of things he is doing, thinking, and feeling that have largely been out of his awareness (or that he has been aware of but that seemed unremarkable to him), and causes him to consider that there is something curious (i.e., potentially ego-dystonic) about them; as a result of confrontation, the impact of defense on the patient's experience becomes increasingly ego-dystonic over time, a shift that is noticeable to the patient. At the same time, the effectiveness of defenses is diminished, allowing underlying anxieties to become more accessible. These shifts are necessary preconditions for exploring the anxieties and wishes motivating defensive operations—the final stages in the interpretive process.

To review, the therapist uses confrontation to achieve the following:

- Invite the patient to step back and observe aspects of his communications and experience that are discrepant.
- Call attention to defensive distortion or denial of external and internal reality.
- Invite reflection on contradictions typically overlooked, rationalized, or denied.
- Expand awareness by introducing a new perspective on the familiar.
- Create ego-dystonicity in relation to habitual defensive operations.

Interpretation Proper

Interpretation proper builds on clarification and confrontation and is the final phase of the interpretive process. Whereas clarification and confrontation focus on the *what* of the patient's experience, interpretation focuses on the *why*. Interpretation involves making a link between the patient's conscious or observed behavior, thoughts, and feelings, elaborated through clarification and confrontation, and the unconscious factors that may be underlying them. When the therapist offers an interpretation, she is presenting the patient with a *hypothesis* about unconscious psychological motives and meanings that may help make sense of aspects of the patient's words, behavior, and experience that on the surface appear illogical or maladaptive. Interpretations are *explanatory*, addressing the observations highlighted in the process of clarification and confrontation and suggesting why the patient may experience things as he does or may behave in a certain way (Sandler et al. 1992). Interpretations imbue with meaning the therapist's observations of behavior or statements that may seem illogical or random.

However, even while they are explanatory, interpretations are very much *not* statements of fact, but rather are hypotheses—conjectures offered by the therapist, or at times by the patient himself, as part of a process of ongoing inquiry. When a therapist makes an interpretation, she does so tentatively, in the spirit of open inquiry and of sharing one possible way that someone might put things together, while maintaining awareness that there are always alternative ways to understand the clinical data. An interpretation can be viewed as a symbolic narrative that pulls together data within an organized frame of reference; an effective interpretation promotes flexible management of conflict within a framework of personal meaning and self-understanding.

Whereas clarification and confrontation focus on conscious and preconscious material, interpretation involves bringing to the patient's awareness aspects of his inner life that are *unconscious*, actively defended against and inaccessible to consciousness because they are in some way anxiety provoking or unacceptable to the patient (Auchincloss and Samberg 2012). Because interpretation explores the personal *meanings* motivating the patient's behavior and organizing his internal experience, the patient's capacity to make use of this final level of intervention in the interpretive process is predicated on his capacity to observe and reflect on his internal experience, and to be curious about the nature of that experience (LaFarge 2000). An interpretation helps the patient make sense of his experience and behavior, deepening his understanding of his inner life, with the longer-term objective of helping him to gain greater perspective on, and to more effectively contain and contextualize, conflictual aspects of experience. (See Chapters 12 and 13 on working through.)

The following are examples of confrontation:

> Therapist: You've told me many times that you wish you were able to get more attention from men and that you think of yourself as undesirable [*a defensive self representation*]. Yet when John, a man you have just met and found attractive, texted you this morning, rather than being pleased and inferring that he might want to ask you out, you assumed he couldn't possibly be interested in you and instead merely wanted your girlfriend's number [*confrontation*]. Now I'm not saying you are necessarily right or wrong; that's not my point. What I am struck by is your assumption. It is as if you find it difficult to even imagine that a man you are attracted to might be interested in you, as if entertaining such a possibility would make you anxious. It's as if, deep down, a part of you believes that you don't deserve to be the one getting his attention, especially when you imagine that your girlfriend would also like to hear from him—as if you believe that to pursue his interest, and in the process to compete with your girlfriend, would make you selfish or somehow not a good person [*interpretation*].

Therapist: I understand that you feel I am critical of you; at the same time, you have spent most of this session criticizing me and the way I've handled your treatment. It's curious that at the same time you view me as critical of you, I think someone watching our interaction might in fact feel that you are behaving critically toward me [*confrontation*].

Patient: Well, that's how it might look, but I'm only criticizing you because you deserve it and because you are always so critical of me.

Therapist: I understand that this is how it seems to you. It's as if we are locked into a relationship of someone powerful and angry who is criticizing someone else who is forced to absorb the other's critique. It's as if at some level, to avoid the inevitable criticism you anticipate, you turn the tables; without even being fully aware of it, you become the critical one yourself [*interpretation*]. Does what I am saying ring at all true?

Therapist: You seem very comfortable here today and optimistic about our work together. Yet I wonder if you can recall how you felt last time you were here: hopeless and despairing, that this is the wrong treatment approach for you, and that things will never improve in your life. In fact, at one point you said things felt so bad that you were considering suicide.

Patient: I hadn't been thinking about it, but yes, I was quite down. But I'm feeling much better now. It isn't really important how I felt last time. It's over—no need to dwell on it now.

Therapist: I'm struck by how discontinuous these two experiences of yourself and of your treatment are. It's as if you feel, as you did last time, that all is lost and I [the therapist] have nothing to offer—or as you do today, you feel hopeful and that all is well, that I will be able to lead you to safe harbor. When you're in the negative, hopeless state, that's all there is and you can think of nothing else, and on the other, positive and hopeful side, the negativity is lost to you [*confrontation*].

Patient: That's true; it's how it feels. Choppy. But when I'm feeling good, I really don't want to think about the bad times.

Therapist: Yes, I can see how powerful those wishes are. I wonder if it's because you worry that if you were to remember the negative feelings—for example, your doubts about me and my ability to help you—your optimism would crumble; you would once again be swamped with negativity. It's as if the only way to protect the positive feelings is to totally sequester them from any hint of negative feelings or doubt [*interpretation*]. What are your thoughts about what I am saying?

Interpretation and Severity of Pathology

Across the spectrum of severity, interpretation focuses on the anxieties or "dangers," the wishes and the fears, that motivate defensive operations (see Chapter 3). In the treatment of BPO patients, interpretation typically entails exploring the anxieties that drive splitting, addressing the question "What is the patient protecting himself from or avoiding when he relies on splitting-based defenses?"

In the treatment of NPO patients, the process of interpreting entails exploring the anxieties that drive repression (i.e., those associated with expression of unconscious, conflictual motivations; see also Chapter 3) and addressing the question "What does the patient fear will happen if he were to experience things more fully and openly?" Interpretation plays a central role in the treatment of patients with higher level personality pathology, whereas clarification and confrontation play more central roles in the treatment of BPO patients, especially in the early phase of treatment.

Clinical Illustration 1 *(continued)*: Interpretation With an NPO Patient

As introduced earlier in this chapter, Mr. Y was mourning the loss of his family as a result of his divorce from Julia. Dr. B had confronted Mr. Y's defensive view of himself in relation to his wife: he as deficient and responsible for ending the marriage and she as blameless; he as childlike and she in a maternal role. Dr. B had suggested that it seemed Mr. Y was more comfortable in the moment holding himself entirely responsible for the dissolution of the marriage than he was to have Julia share responsibility, even though there was clear indication that it had been a complicated situation.

As therapist and patient continued to explore Mr. Y's thoughts and feelings in the session, Mr. Y became increasingly anxious, and he began to worry about being lonely. In his associations, Mr. Y found himself wondering about the strength of his longtime friendships and questioning whether people would stand by him. In the countertransference, Dr. B felt vaguely guilty, worrying that he had perhaps pushed Mr. Y too hard too soon, and he found himself empathizing with Mr. Y's view of himself as a lonely child. Meanwhile, Mr. Y continued to focus on his own deficiencies while keeping Julia in a maternal, relatively powerful, and benign (i.e., defensively idealized) position in his mind.

Taking into account Mr. Y's anxiety and associations in response to his interventions, Dr. B inferred that Mr. Y's views of himself as childlike and deficient and of his wife as powerful and blameless were serving defensive functions, protecting Mr. Y from profound feelings of loss and isolation. Using his previous knowledge of Mr. Y and his history, Dr. B hypothesized that Mr. Y's idealizing Julia and blaming his own deficiencies for the dissolution of his marriage seemed to protect Mr. Y from fully experiencing the loss of Julia, allowing him to deny its irrevocability and to hold on to her in some way in his mind. Underneath that conflict, at a deeper level even further from Mr. Y's awareness, the defensive object relation seemed to protect Mr. Y from feeling angry at Julia; if it was all about *his* deficiencies, then he had no cause for anger except toward himself.

On the other hand, the possibility that he had cause to be angry seemed to tap into long-standing, unconscious fears deep inside Mr. Y about the power of his aggression toward women. Mr. Y and Dr. B would come to understand that expression of Mr. Y's aggression was associated with the deep anxiety that his hostility was so overwhelmingly powerful that it would drive everyone away, leaving him entirely alone.

Dr. B decided to begin with an interpretation of the dynamics that were more accessible and closely allied with Mr. Y's current concerns. He commented, "It seems that our discussion of how you protect Julia has left you feeling more alone. It's as if when you begin in your mind to allow her to share responsibility for the marriage falling apart, it makes things worse for you, somehow more painful and isolating."

Mr. Y responded thoughtfully to Dr. B's intervention, confirming Dr. B's observation, and he asked Dr. B how he understood it. Dr. B went on to offer a suggestion, in the form of a more complete interpretation, that might explain Mr. Y's experience: "Well, it makes me wonder if perhaps one of the reasons you might see things as you do, blaming yourself and protecting Julia, is to hold on to a secret hope that the two of you might someday reunite. That is, if it's your fault, maybe you can fix it, and someday there might be a chance of reuniting. On the other hand, if you allow yourself to come to a more realistic appraisal of the two of you as a couple, it's as if, in your mind, things end more completely."

Mr. Y responded by saying that this was not something he had ever thought about before, but in listening to Dr. B, he thought what he was saying made sense; he did feel that he had been "holding on" at some level.

In the sessions that followed, Mr. Y continued to work through the ending of the marriage and the breakup of his family. His persistent tendency to focus on his own deficiencies and to place Julia in a maternal, relatively powerful position was an ongoing focus of attention.

After several weeks, Mr. Y came into a session to describe his frustration with himself. He was now observing himself more carefully and reflectively than he had in the past. He had noted that whenever there was a point of contention between Julia and himself, he would concede. As Dr. B and Mr. Y worked together to clarify Mr. Y's experience at these times, what emerged was that Mr. Y would often start to see Julia as treating him unfairly, and he would feel that he had a right to be angry. In that frame of mind, he would attempt to set limits on her demands, but as soon as he opened his mouth, he would quickly become anxious and back down; it was as if he felt compelled to give in, even though this was not what he wanted to do. "It's like I can't help myself," he said. As soon as Mr. Y started to push back, he found himself slipping once again into feeling like a deficient child in relation to a powerful woman who was morally unassailable; he felt paralyzed and isolated.

Dr. B suggested to Mr. Y a way of understanding his experience: "I'm struck by the way that as soon as you feel at all angry—or even that you have a right to be angry or that you want to assert yourself with Julia—you become anxious and you back down. As we've discussed, at those moments, your view of yourself shifts; you suddenly become little, childlike, and deficient, overwhelmed by the feeling that everything is your fault." This restatement of material that had been clarified served to highlight and confront the defensive object relation.

Mr. Y responded by sharing his frustration: "Yes, it's weird, I know, and also frustrating. It makes it difficult to act like an adult. I just get panicked about ending up alone, kind of desperate. It makes no sense."

Dr. B noted that Mr. Y's defensive view of himself was becoming ego-dystonic ("weird"), and at the same time, the anxieties warded off by the defensive object relation (fears of isolation) were emerging into consciousness. In light of these developments, Dr. B thought that Mr. Y might be in a frame of mind to make use of exploration of the unconscious motives and conflicts underlying the familiar defensive object relation. Dr. B proceeded to offer a suggestion that might explain this pattern of Mr. Y's, making an interpretation that linked Mr. Y's observed behavior and his conscious experience (he can't assert himself; he feels isolated and alone) to unconscious forces outside his awareness.

Dr. B observed, "I'm struck by how in the setting of conflict with Julia, your mind goes directly to the fear of ending up alone [the anxiety motivating the defense—an object relation of a small child and an absent parent, associated with feelings of painful isolation], and the result is that you feel like a small, frightened child." Dr. B paused, and Mr. Y looked at him expectantly. Dr. B decided to go on: "It's as if you can't bear to see yourself as having any power—or for that matter, even to see yourself as an adult—in the setting of conflict with Julia. I know it sounds paradoxical, but it makes me wonder if you need to make yourself small because at bottom, you are afraid of being *too* powerful. It's as if you worry that if you are powerful, you might do something destructive, or something ugly might come out of you that could drive Julia and everyone else away and leave you isolated. As if in your mind, your only choices are to be a child and maintain connections with others, or to be an adult and entirely alone."

Comments: In this vignette, Dr. B builds on clarification and confrontation to offer interpretations that might explain Mr. Y's tendency to feel like a deficient child in relation to his wife, a blameless maternal figure. As a result of the earlier interventions, which entailed ongoing exploration of the defensive object relation (a deficient child and a blameless maternal figure; self-criticism and regret), the underlying anxieties motivating defense began to emerge. These anxieties, having to do with fears of loneliness, isolation, and loss of attachments, were expressed in Mr. Y's associations and affective experience in session. As mentioned in the final paragraph of the vignette, Mr. Y's anxiety can be conceptualized in terms of an object relation of a small child and an absent parent, associated with feelings of painful isolation. Dr. B's interventions were timed to follow Mr. Y's lead; only as the anxieties beneath the defensive object relations—fears of loss, isolation, and aggression—started to emerge did he begin to offer interpretations.

It can be tempting but is rarely therapeutic to offer very early interpretations with the NPO patient. For example, in the initial session described in this final vignette, Dr. B might have immediately linked Mr. Y's idealization of his wife to fears of his own aggression. This intervention would have been accurate but unhelpful, directing the clinical focus toward material both far removed from Mr. Y's dominant concerns at the moment (i.e., to aggression rather than loss) and deeply repressed. Premature interpretations often lead to empty intellectual speculation, in contrast to a better-timed interpretation that leads to an authentic affective experience and deepening of the clinical material.

Alternatively, premature interpretations may be met with outright rejection from the patient. In the case of Mr. Y, it was his recognition of and frustration with his difficulty in being assertive that signaled to Dr. B that Mr. Y's conflicts in relation to aggression were at that moment more accessible than they may have been in the past, presumably as a result of repeated cycles of clarification and confrontation completed in the preceding sessions.

In his interpretations, Dr. B elaborated two different ways of thinking about how being childlike and idealizing Julia might protect Mr. Y from underlying feelings of loss. The first of these was in relation to dissociation and denial of Julia's behavior, and the second in relation to repressive defenses around unconscious aggression. Both interpretations functioned to help Mr. Y become aware of aspects of his internal experience that were unconscious.

The ultimate objective of Dr. B's interpretations, however, was not to uncover unconscious anxieties and motivations, but rather to help Mr. Y better contain and contextualize them. To elaborate further, the goal of an interpretation—for example, the one Dr. B made in relation to unconscious aggression—is not per se to make Mr. Y aware that he is angry, but rather to help him develop a broader perspective that will enable him to contextualize and contain the angry parts of himself within his overall conscious sense of self, so that they become part of a whole rather than taking over in the moment.[2] Thus, the goal of Dr. B's interpretations is to enable Mr. Y to tolerate angry feelings, with the understanding that experiencing hostility does not mean that he is *only* angry, and does not need to imply an inevitable, permanent, and excruciating loss, even if he may feel that these things are true in the moment.[3] These changes will enable Mr. Y to be more comfortable with himself as a powerful adult and will lead to his capacity to deepen his relationships with women, who can now be experienced in a more complete and complex fashion that includes their flaws.

Similarly, the objective of earlier interpretations—focusing on Mr. Y's denial of loss—would be for him to become able to tolerate feelings of loss without at the same time feeling condemned to be entirely alone forever as an unbearable punishment for his deficiencies or aggression.

Dr. B and Mr. Y spent several months working through Mr. Y's conflicts in relation to loss, isolation, and aggression; these conflicts re-emerged periodically throughout the rest of the treatment as part of an ongoing process of working through. They were quite clearly linked to Mr. Y's early history—both his experience with a depressed, withdrawn, and unavailable mother and his identification with a hostile, rather sadistic father. In his approach, Dr. B deferred focusing on these relatively clear and accessible developmental links until after the core conflicts had been elaborated in the here and now; at that juncture, making links to the past helped Mr. Y make sense of and symbolically manage these conflictual aspects of his experience and, in the process, better contain and contextualize them, while building a better-integrated narrative of himself through time. Possible developmentally based narratives entertained by Mr. Y and Dr. B to more fully understand Mr. Y's conflicts in relation to aggression and loss included the fear that it was his rage at his mother that had driven her away, and perhaps accounted for her depression as well, in addition to the fear that the angry parts of himself made him one with his sadistic father, whom he hated.

Clinical Illustration 2 *(continued)*: Interpretation With a BPO Patient

We return to Ms. J, who had entered a downward spiral at work, feeling paralyzed by her resentment of her boss. Dr. C confronted her radically contradictory, dissociated views in relation to her workplace—namely, the fact that her current images of her boss, herself as a worker, and her work-

---

[2]This final outcome of the interpretive process results from repeated cycles of clarification, confrontation, and interpretation, or the process of working through (see Chapters 12 and 13), which leads to progressively greater flexibility of defenses, increased levels of emotional insight, and, ultimately, the capacity to contain and contextualize conflictual aspects of experience within an overall sense of self.

[3]See Caligor et al. (2007) for further discussion of the impact of interpretation and mechanisms of change in the treatments of NPO patients.

place in general were all negative, whereas until recently, all had been exceptionally and entirely positive. Dr. C asked Ms. J for her thoughts about this.

Ms. J's initial response was to be rejecting of Dr. C's comments; she responded that there was "nothing to think about" and attributed the shift in her perspective entirely to Hal's (her boss's) bad behavior. Ms. J was upset with Hal for having "messed everything up"; she'd been so happy, had felt for once that she was valued and special, and now it was all spoiled (i.e., she located the problem in Hal and did not identify a problem within herself).[4]

However, as Ms. J and Dr. C continued to explore the specifics of Ms. J's experience, Dr. C persisted in drawing Ms. J's attention to her observation that it wasn't just Hal or Ms. J's experience of Hal that had shifted, but in fact Ms. J's entire view of herself as a worker, along with her actual ability to function in the work setting, had also abruptly changed.[5] Furthermore, Dr. C reminded Ms. J that she had had similar experiences in the past in other work settings.

All these interventions [*confrontations*] were directed toward helping Ms. J step out of her immediate experience in the moment to look at it from a broader perspective (i.e., to help her shift from a concrete to a more reflective state of mind). As they continued to explore Ms. J's experience at work, she began to acknowledge an awareness of the extreme, "all-or-nothing" quality of her experience. She wondered out loud, "Is it that way for everyone?"

Dr. C responded that in fact it was not that way for everyone, but certainly Ms. J was not alone, and that the somewhat unstable, black-and-white kinds of experiences that they had been looking at reflected instability in her view of herself and her view of others. Dr. C went on to say, "It's as if you have two ways of experiencing things with Hal, all good or all bad. When it's all good, you're valued, you feel competent, and you're able to function, while Hal, even if he's difficult, seems supportive and appreciative, and as though he sees you as special. Conversely, when it's all bad, he takes you for granted or, even worse, he sees you as useless; you feel overwhelmed and unable to follow even simple instructions, and then you feel like an absolutely hopeless mess. One side is associated with all very positive emotions, the other all negative." Ms. J acknowledged that she knew this was true; she felt Dr. C's description was extremely accurate, although she hadn't thought of things in those terms before. She wondered why this always happened to her.

Based on her knowledge of Ms. J and her history, Dr. C inferred that Ms. J's splitting seemed to be motivated by both paranoid and depressive anxieties related to the fear of losing an idealized relationship—paranoid

---

[4]This is an example of defensive *externalization*.

[5]This pairing of the shift of Ms. J's view of Hal with the shift in her view of herself emphasizes that within our model, any object representation implies a corresponding self representation.

fears, on the one hand, that aggressive attacks or excessive frustration coming from somewhere outside herself could too easily destroy the possibility of such an ideal relationship, and depressive anxieties (see Chapter 3), on the other hand, that her own aggression could be responsible for damaging such a relationship. However, these constructs were at this point merely general hypotheses that Dr. C was entertaining within herself; Dr. C did not feel that Ms. J was in a sufficiently reflective frame of mind to make use of this kind of conjecture—and sharing these thoughts carried the risk of intellectualization and distancing Ms. J from her more immediate affective experience. As a result, Dr. C decided to continue to focus on confrontation of the split and unstable nature of Ms. J's experience, with the aim of promoting greater reflectiveness and helping her gain greater perspective, as well as a deeper appreciation of the extent to which the origins of her difficulties resided within herself.

In the next few sessions, Ms. J began to comment on the abrupt shifts she was noticing in her relationship with Brian, a man whom she had just begun to date. Ms. J agreed with Dr. C, who pointed out the similarity to the experience Ms. J described with Hal. As Ms. J described her experience with Brian in detail [*clarification*], she seemed increasingly able to think about the shifts she experienced as not simply about Brian's behavior or her own, but also as impacted by her ability to read his behavior and her difficulty in knowing "what was really going on." She was often able to reflect on her experience at this point, without needing the prompting of a confrontation from Dr. C; thus, Ms. J was becoming increasingly self-observant and reflective, capable of stepping back a bit from her immediate experience with Brian and noting the extreme quality of her emotions—either she was "feeling fine," or she found herself in bed "weeping hysterically." She began to wonder, seemingly in earnest, "Why do I do this? What is wrong with me? Why can't I have the two pieces meet in the middle?"

Dr. C noted Ms. J's increased reflectiveness and her effort to cognitively bridge the split between her idealized and persecutory views of her relationship with Hal. She seemed able, in the moment, to hold on to an understanding that the problem on the table had to do with her internal states and experience, not simply the material exchange with Hal or with Brian. Accordingly, Dr. C thought it worth venturing a trial interpretation to see if Ms. J was in a frame of mind to make constructive use of a more abstract intervention. Dr. C commented, "Well, you're asking good questions. I think we're talking about what goes on inside you, how you experience things—not just what happens *to* you or what happens between you and Hal. Do you follow?" Ms. J nodded, and Dr. C continued, "I think the question you're raising is, why would a person divide her experience into something either all positive or something all negative? What would motivate a person to do that?"

At this point, Ms. J piped up: "Do you know?" This ready, somewhat passive and childlike response from Ms. J—seemingly inviting Dr. C to take her hand and feed her an answer, rather than having to grapple with the question herself—made Dr. C somewhat uneasy. Nevertheless, Dr. C decided to offer the interpretation first and then link the same dynamics to the transference that Ms. J seemed to be enacting in the moment.

Following the directive to address paranoid anxieties (fear of destruction of self or the good object by forces outside the patient) before depressive anxieties (fear of loss of the good object or self as a result of one's own destructiveness; see Chapter 13), Dr. C went on to offer an interpretation: "Well, I don't know for sure, but I do have a thought that might be helpful, if you're interested." Again, Ms. J indicated that she was. "Well, you've made clear that when things fall apart, it feels really, really bad, so you would think you'd give this whole thing up and find a middle ground where you wouldn't have to go so low. But you haven't, so there must be something that leads you to perpetuate this pattern. One thought I've had is that it may be about trying to hold on to that very special feeling that comes with a positive relationship—for example, how you felt in the beginning with Hal or with Brian, when everything seemed so wonderful and you were perfectly happy in yourself. Maybe the hope of being able to have and sustain that feeling keeps it all going. If you were to accept a more middle-of-the-road view, you'd be less vulnerable to those really negative experiences, but you'd have to give up the hope of that wonderful thing on the other side, and that may be really hard to do. It's like hoping to be a child forever, with an adoring parent who takes perfect care of you and treats you as special; even though you know that's no longer possible, that you're all grown up—it's hard to give that up."

Comments: In this rather lengthy vignette, we attempt to illustrate the process of repeated clarification and confrontation that typically precedes interpretation of unconscious motivations in the treatment of BPO patients. In the setting of borderline pathology, the interpretation of unconscious motivations and meanings is the final intervention in a protracted series of interventions, a series that gradually becomes shorter and more efficient as treatment proceeds and the patient becomes more reflective. Early in treatment, interventions that promote self-observation and reflectiveness are the highest priority, while exploration of unconscious meanings is often deferred. Thus, Dr. C did not move quickly from confrontation to interpretation. Rather, she continued to work with Ms. J at the level of ongoing clarification and confrontation, waiting until she sensed that Ms. J was thinking about internal states and was genuinely perplexed by and curious about them, before offering an interpretation of paranoid anxieties that motivated her wish to preserve the ideal relationship through splitting. The therapist can think of this process in terms of the centrality of focusing on the *what*, in contrast to the *why*, in the treatment of personality disorders.

In the treatment of middle- and low-BPO patients—those with more severe pathology than Ms. J—the period of treatment focusing on clarification and confrontation tends to be even more essential, central, and protracted. With these patients, clarification takes on a key function in its role of helping to contain intense affects stirred up in the treatment, and particularly in the transference (see Chapter 11 for a thorough discussion of transference interpretation). In addition, the process of clarification introduces a perspective of observation into the treatment, helping the patient begin to look at and subtly distance himself from his immediate experience in the moment.

With ongoing confrontation of her use of splitting-based defenses, focusing on idealization–devaluation and exploration of the paranoid anxieties motivating her defenses, Ms. J began to split less consistently and less broadly. There were moments of better integration, which now began to expose her to depressive conflicts. At that point, when Ms. J moved away from a more integrated experience of herself and her world and toward a split view, Dr. C interpreted the shift as an effort to get away from the pain of seeing herself as acting aggressively toward better-integrated, essentially positive images of others. Splitting at this juncture was understood as an effort to circumvent the pain and guilt of taking responsibility for her provocative and often hostile treatment of Hal and Brian, both of whom Ms. J now experienced in a way that was overall more complex and realistic.

Summary

Interpretation proper is the final phase of the interpretive process, following after clarification and confrontation. Clarification and confrontation focus on what the patient says, does, and experiences in an area of conflict, while inviting the patient to reflect. Interpretation builds on these earlier interventions, inviting the reflective patient to explore motives and personal meanings that may underlie and drive the repetitive behaviors, thoughts, and feelings that have been clarified and confronted. Whereas clarification and confrontation address aspects of experience and behavior that are accessible to consciousness, interpretation also considers unconscious mental processes, focusing on understanding the drivers of the patient's experience and behavior in an area of conflict.

Although interpretations are explanatory hypotheses, they are very much *not* statements of fact. Thus, when a therapist makes an interpretation, she does so tentatively, in the spirit of open inquiry and of sharing one possible way that someone might put things together. An interpretation helps the patient make sense of his experience and behavior, deepening his understanding of his inner life, with the longer-term objective of helping him to gain greater perspective on, and to more effectively contain and contextualize, conflictual aspects of experience.

To review, the therapist uses interpretation to achieve the following:

- Link observed behavior, conscious thoughts, and feelings with unconscious factors that may be underlying them.
- Posit hypotheses about unconscious psychological motives and meanings.
- Suggest *why* the patient does things as he does or experiences things in a certain way.
- Deepen the patient's self-understanding.
- Promote flexible management of conflict within a framework of personal meaning.

Key Clinical Concepts

- The interpretive process can be conceptualized in terms of repeated cycles of clarification, confrontation, and interpretation.
- *Clarification* entails helping the patient to elaborate his dominant experience, initiating a process of self-observation.
- *Confrontation* calls attention to discrepancies and contradictions in the patient's communications, inviting the patient to observe and think about what she is doing and experiencing.
- Confrontation plays an especially central and complex role in the treatment of BPO patients by supporting reality testing, introducing alternative perspectives, and promoting reflection on an area of conflict.
- *Interpretation proper* begins with the development of a hypothesis about why the patient might experience things as he does, focusing on the anxieties, fears, and wishes motivating defense.
- In the treatment of BPO patients, anxieties motivating defense often have to do primarily with wishes to create or hold on to an idealized relationship or a safe haven that is protected from aggressive attack, and secondarily with depressive anxieties pertaining to guilt, loss, and self-regard.
- In the treatment of NPO patients, motivations for defense often relate to efforts to ward off guilt, to support self-regard, and to militate against fears of object loss.

- A repeated cycle of interpretation (the process of working through) promotes the capacity to contain and contextualize conflictual aspects of experience, corresponding with integrative changes in the patient.

References

Auchincloss AL, Samberg E (eds): Psychoanalytic Terms and Concepts. New Haven, CT, Yale University Press, 2012

Britton R: Naming and containing, in Belief and Imagination. London, Routledge, 1998, pp 19–28

Caligor E, Kernberg OF, Clarkin JF: Handbook of Dynamic Psychotherapy for Higher Level Personality Pathology. Washington, DC, American Psychiatric Publishing, 2007

Caligor E, Diamond D, Yeomans FE, Kernberg OF: The interpretive process in the psychoanalytic psychotherapy of borderline personality pathology. J Am Psychoanal Assoc 57(2):271–301, 2009 19516053

Etchegoyen RH: Fundamentals of Psychoanalytic Technique. London, Karnac Books, 1991

LaFarge L: Interpretation and containment. Int J Psychoanal 81(Part I):67–84, 2000 10816845

Levy ST, Inderbitzin LB: Neutrality, interpretation, and therapeutic intent. J Am Psychoanal Assoc 40(4):989–1011, 1992 1430771

Sandler J, Dare C, Holder H: The Patient and the Analyst, 2nd Edition. Madison, CT, International Universities Press, 1992

Steiner J: Psychic Retreats: Pathological Organizations in Psychotic, Neurotic and Borderline Patients. London, Routledge, 1993

Intervening II

Transference Analysis and Tactics Guiding the Interpretive Process

IN THIS CHAPTER, WE COMPLETE OUR DIS-cussion of the interpretive process. In Part 1, we focus on transference analysis, and in Part 2 we cover tactics that guide interpretive interventions.

Part 1

Transference Analysis

IN OUR DISCUSSION OF THE INTERPRETIVE process in Chapter 10, we described the therapist's task of elaborating and exploring the object relations organizing the patient's experience, making use of the techniques of clarification, confrontation, and interpretation proper. We turn now to the process of transference interpretation, also referred to as *transference analysis* (Auchincloss and Samberg 2012). The process of transference analysis begins with procedures outlined in Chapter 9 for identifying the affectively dominant object relations, now focused on how the affectively dominant object relations are currently enacted in the patient's experience of the therapist and the interactions between them. Next, the therapist applies the techniques outlined in Chapter 10 to explore the patient's experience of the therapist, making use of clarification, confrontation, and interpretation.

We encourage the reader, before proceeding, to quickly revisit Chapter 5, in which we introduce the construct of *transference* and review in detail its variable presentations across the spectrum of severity. Our discussion of transference analysis in this chapter integrates some of the prior material presented in this book for continuity of discussion.

Centrality of Transference Analysis Across the Spectrum of Severity

Borderline Personality Organization

In the treatment of patients with a borderline level of personality organization (BPO), paranoid transferences colored by hostility and characterized by role reversals are universal developments that typically assume affective dominance. Other common developments assuming affective dominance are idealizing transferences that defend against hostility, and acting-out behaviors in response to transference developments. In middle- and low-BPO patients, paranoid transferences predominate, whereas in high-BPO patients, idealizing transferences play a more prominent role. The transference will typically organize the BPO patient's dominant, conscious experience of the therapist and/or the patient's behavior in session and in relation to the treatment frame. As a result, much of the clinical work in transference-focused psychotherapy—extended (TFP-E) with BPO patients tends to focus on the paranoid and idealized object relations organizing the patient's experience of the therapist; these treatments tend to be *transference focused*,[1] and countertransference analysis plays a central role in the clinical process as well. In the treatment of BPO patients, dominant transference themes are often most clearly communicated nonverbally, through the patient's behavior and the countertransference (Kernberg 1980).

Focusing clinical attention on the paranoid and idealized object relations that organize the BPO patient's experience of the therapist has a number of important benefits:

- Clarification and confrontation of the patient's experience in the transference can provide affect containment and support reality testing.
- Focusing on the transference enables the therapist to have a clearer understanding of, and to better manage, developments in the treatment that often lead to acting out or dropping out of treatment.
- The transferences of BPO patients closely mirror difficulties in the patients' interpersonal lives; exploring the transference provides a real-life understanding of problems in a patient's relationships outside the treatment.

Neurotic Personality Organization

As described in Chapter 9, in patients with a neurotic level of personality organization (NPO), affectively dominant object relations may be relatively inaccessible in the transference, and exploration of the patient's world of internal object relations is often not focused on the transference, but rather on interpersonal relationships and subjective states that do not directly involve the therapist. As a result, although transference analysis may play a role, the treatments of NPO patients are generally not transference focused.[2] In this setting, the relationship with the therapist often remains relatively neutral and realistic; for much if not most of the treatment, the therapist may be experienced predominantly as a benign figure who helps the patient observe her behavior and experience (i.e., as aligned with a relatively stable observing ego within the patient).

With NPO patients in TFP-E, transference developments are typically subtle, often socially appropriate, and ego-syntonic (e.g., the familiar defensive NPO transference in which the patient views the therapist as especially skilled or wise, and the patient assumes an attitude that is quietly admiring or appreciative); these developments often fail to assume affec-

---

[1]Transference analysis in the treatments of patients with severe personality disorders is discussed in great detail in *Transference-Focused Therapy for Borderline Personality Disorder: A Clinical Guide* (Yeomans et al. 2015).
[2]Transference analysis in the treatment of this group of patients is discussed in detail in *Handbook of Dynamic Psychotherapy for Higher Level Personality Pathology* (Caligor et al. 2007).

tive dominance. Although the therapist will in his own mind note developments in the transference, it is often the case that focusing excessively or prematurely on the transference in the treatment of NPO patients can function to alienate the patient and will do little to promote the therapeutic process. As a result, it may be preferable to explore affectively dominant object relations in the patient's interpersonal relations if this is where they are more fully expressed and more affectively invested, rather than attempting to force exploration of the transference.

We recommend prioritizing the transference in the treatment of NPO patients in the following situations:

- When the transference is conscious and affectively dominant
- When the transference leads to acting out (e.g., if a patient starts behaving in a hostile fashion toward her boss as an expression of feelings activated in the transference)
- When the transference is negative (e.g., if the patient experiences the therapist as critical or hostile, or treats the therapist in an overtly hostile fashion)
- When the transference is interfering with open communication or exploration (e.g., if the patient coming for help with sexual inhibitions feels unable to speak about her sexual life because her therapist "reminds [me] of my mother")

Empirical Literature on Transference Analysis

Until recently, the results of empirical studies on the impact of transference interpretation on clinical process and change in psychotherapy have been variable and contradictory (Høglend 2014). The variability of findings across studies likely reflects the following, among other factors: the nature of the patients (e.g., severity of pathology, gender), the nature of the treatment (duration, frequency of sessions, level of support), the frequency of transference interpretations (many vs. only a few per session), and the competence with which transference interpretations are introduced (e.g., timing, tact, use of preparatory interventions). Høglend and Gabbard (2012) reviewed the empirical literature on transference work and concluded that a moderate use of transference interpretations has specific, positive effects on long-term functioning in patients treated in dynamic therapy. These effects are mediated by an increase in insight during therapy; they apply in particular to patients with personality disorders. Høglend and Gabbard argue for the positive impact of preparatory interventions prior to transference interpretation—in particular, interventions that affirm the patient's internal situation—in paving the way for effective use of transference interpretation.

In the most elegant studies to date, using a randomized dismantling design, Høglend et al. (2006) found that in a year of weekly therapy, patients with lower-quality object relations (and a higher frequency of personality disorders) had significantly better functional outcome in a treatment arm using transference interpretations delivered at low to moderate frequency (with an average of one such interpretation per session) than in a matched treatment arm that proscribed transference interpretations. In contrast, patients with a higher quality of object relations did better in treatments in which therapists did not make transference interpretations.

In these studies, insight mediated the relationship between transference analysis and change in patients with personality disorders, whereas transference analysis did not lead to insight in patients without significant personality pathology (Johansson et al. 2010). The TFP-E approach to the use of transference interpretation is consistent with these findings; the therapist focuses on material that is affectively dominant, while anticipating that as pathology becomes more severe, affective dominance is increasingly likely to be concentrated in the transference for more of the time. Table 11–1 summarizes the efficacy and quality of transference analysis and countertransference analysis across the spectrum of severity.

Exploratory Interventions and Transference Across the Range of Severity of Personality Pathology

In the seven clinical illustrations that follow, we highlight the process of identifying an affectively dominant object relation and then making use of the interpretive process (as discussed in Chapters 9 and 10) in the process of transference analysis across the range of personality pathology. We focus on common clinical situations and illustrate the differential application of the basic techniques of clarification, confrontation, and interpretation of the transference. We refer back to a number of patients and clinical situations introduced in previous chapters, so we encourage the reader to refer back to the introductory vignettes in Chapters 6, 9, and 10 when reviewing the vignettes that follow.

TABLE 11–1.   Typical transference and countertransference across level of personality organization

Neurotic level of personality organization	Borderline level of personality organization
Transference	
Transference is often not affectively dominant.	Transference is often affectively dominant.
Transference is often not conscious.	Transference is often conscious.
Transference is subtle, gradually developing, and may be ego-syntonic.	Transference is affectively charged, rapidly developing, and ego-dystonic.
Transference is often conveyed in verbal communication.	Transference is often conveyed in nonverbal communication and countertransference.
Excessive attention to transference can tax therapeutic alliance.	Attention to transference can support therapeutic alliance.
Transference analysis is not preferentially associated with positive outcome.	Transference analysis is preferentially associated with positive outcome.
Transference analysis may not be a major source of insight.	Transference analysis is often a major source of insight.
Transference analysis may come across as peculiar, forced, or divorced from patient's concerns.	Transference analysis typically directs clinical attention to dominant issues in the treatment and in patient's life.
Transference analysis may not be a major vehicle of change.	Transference analysis is seen as a major vehicle of change.
Treatment is not consistently transference focused.	Treatment is often transference focused.
Countertransference	
Countertransference is typically not the dominant channel of communication relative to verbal communication.	Countertransference is the dominant and often primary channel of communication.
Countertransference is relatively subtle and easy to overlook.	Countertransference is often extreme, intrusive, and affectively charged.
Countertransference can be contained within the mind of the therapist with reflection.	Countertransference induces pressure for the therapist to act and may be difficult to contain.
Countertransference reflects interaction of the patient's transference and the therapist's transferences to patient.	Countertransference often reflects largely the patient's transference; says more about the patient than therapist.
Utilization of countertransference need not be central to clinical technique.	Utilization and containment of countertransference are central to clinical technique.

Paranoid Transference
Clarification of Therapist-Centered Interpretations

In the treatment of BPO patients, paranoid transferences are common, typically affectively dominant, and frequently highly affectively charged. In this often challenging clinical situation, *therapist-centered interpretations* (Steiner 1994) can be extremely useful interventions.

Clinical Illustration 1: Clarification of Paranoid Transference

We return to Ms. M, the BPO patient diagnosed with borderline personality disorder with prominent paranoid and narcissistic features, who was discussed in the extended clinical illustration in Chapter 6. For a protracted period, Ms. M struggled with the requirement of twice-weekly sessions, the need to begin and end sessions on time, and the inconvenience of her commute to Dr. C's office.

Ms. M came into one session 15 minutes late, visibly agitated, complaining about the traffic and about the "selfish bitch" who had been driving her bus. When Dr. C attempted to clarify what had happened that particular morning, Ms. M fell mute and scowled at Dr. C, communicating clearly in the nonverbal channel that now that she had arrived at the office, all her aggravation and outrage were directly focused on Dr. C. In the face of Ms. M's stony silence, Dr. C made several efforts to clarify what was happening. Ms. M remained visibly angry but said nothing.

Dr. C decided to shift gears, to comment rather than to inquire. "I can see that you are upset and agitated; it seems that the commute to my office was particularly aggravating today." Ms. M responded immediately, "Yes, it was impossible!" Dr. C asked for elaboration: "Can you tell me more?"

Ms. M glared at Dr. C and said, "I've told you over and over—the appointment is too early! I have to wake up at 7:00 to get here and I can't fall asleep at night. Your location sucks. I have to take two buses and I never make the connection. So I missed the second bus, the bitch driver just drove off! I knew I'd be late and you always comment on it and I hate it."

Continuing to use the process of clarification to invite Ms. M to elaborate her experience, Dr. C asked, "Why do you think I comment?" Ms. M responded, "Because you're really a pain in the ass! You don't care about anyone's feelings, just your own convenience. You insist everyone do things your way, because you're in control here. But anyone can see that you're really just selfish and lazy—you're just kidding yourself." Ms. M's hostility was palpable. Her comments left Dr. C feeling simultaneously bullied, defensive, and diminished.[3]

Dr. C proceeded to put into words her own understanding of Ms. M's experience of Dr. C in the moment. Making use of all three channels of communication and her memory of Ms. M's frequent complaints about her mother, Dr. C suggested, "It sounds like I have become yet another person in your life who cares only about herself, abuses power, and bullies others to meet her own needs."

Ms. M enthusiastically corroborated that this was indeed what was happening: "Exactly! Just another selfish bitch." But at this point, Ms. M's tone was more triumphant than paranoid, and she seemed less agitated and guarded. Dr. C opted to further pursue clarification of Ms. M's experience in the transference. She asked, "Can you tell me more about what I do or how I treat you that leaves you feeling bullied or suggests that I'm being selfish or lazy?" Ongoing clarification and elaboration of Ms. M's experience in the transference, putting it into words and sharing it openly with Dr. C, who listened attentively and tried to understand, appeared to help Ms. M feel calmer and more reflective.

Comments: In this vignette, Dr. C can be seen to make three levels of intervention—all, technically speaking, forms of clarification. Dr. C's initial efforts, asking Ms. M to explain what was happening, seemed only to further aggravate the patient, and she remained mute. When Dr. C shifted gears to comment on Ms. M's aggravation rather than inquiring, Ms. M did begin speaking, but her tone remained hostile, although perhaps a bit less paranoid. When Dr. C finally commented on Ms. M's view of Dr. C, the atmosphere in the session began to change.

In the treatment of BPO patients, the process of elaborating and putting words to the patient's experience of the therapist (i.e., identifying and describing the affectively dominant object representation organizing the transference) is often the optimal first step in managing the affectively charged, typically paranoid transferences that emerge in treatment (Caligor et al. 2009). The therapist will link the patient's immediate affective experience (rage, fear, hatred) to more fully elaborated representations (someone who is powerful, abusive, self-serving), an intervention that simultaneously communicates the therapist's capacity to empathize with the patient's situation and provides cognitive containment of affect (Bion 1962, 1959/1967, 1962/1967; Britton 1998; Steiner 1994). An example of such an intervention is this comment of Dr. C's to Ms. M: "It sounds like I have become yet another person in your life who cares only about herself, abuses power, and bullies others to meet her own needs." We refer to interventions of this kind as *therapist-centered interventions*.[4]

---

[3]This countertransference provided Dr. C with a window into Ms. M's dominant self experience in the paranoid transference.

[4]In the psychoanalytic literature, these interventions are described as *therapist-centered interpretations*, a term coined by John Steiner (1994).

Therapist-centered interventions serve the following functions:

- Put words to the patient's experience of the therapist (clarification).
- Stay within the patient's perspective (communicating empathy).
- Avoid confrontation and interpretation (do not incorporate alternative perspectives).
- Provide containment of affect.
- Support reality testing.
- Communicate empathy—that the therapist "gets it."
- Support an observing stance within the patient.
- Pave the way for the patient to "take back projections."

Therapist-centered interpretations (Steiner 1994) provide emotional containment. In a therapist-centered intervention, the therapist focuses on putting words to the patient's dominant, conscious experience of the therapist, without calling it into question and without commenting on the patient's role in the interaction. The therapist adopts the patient's perspective whole cloth, as if it were a concrete reality, without questioning, modifying, commenting, or introducing an alternative perspective. Rather, the therapist simply puts words as much as possible to the patient's exact view of the therapist in the moment, while skirting the issue of subjectivity (e.g., "I have become yet another selfish bully," rather than "You see me as a bully" or "From your perspective, I seem like a bully")— and without in any way challenging the patient or implying the possibility of alternative perspectives. Therapist-centered interventions offer no challenge to the affectively overstimulated patient whose experience may be quite concrete and paranoid; therapist-centered interventions "go with" the patient's dominant experience in the moment.

Putting words to the extreme representations and motives that the patient may attribute to the therapist, and demonstrating the capacity to look at them and evaluate them calmly and neutrally with the patient, may serve a number of functions. Most immediately, therapist-centered interpretations provide cognitive containment of affect and communicate empathy. From a different perspective, such exchanges implicitly communicate that the therapist is able to contain the patient's projections—that the therapist is able to tolerate being seen by the patient as embodying the powerfully negative object representations that she, the patient, feels the need to project. This experience may reduce the patient's anxiety in the moment and may also make projections seem less malignant and not quite as threatening.

In the longer term, the therapist's containing function may perhaps make it easier for the patient to "take back" or to assume responsibility for her projections—that is, to tolerate awareness that what she is experiencing as part of the therapist is also part of herself. Finally, without challenging the patient's experience, therapist-centered interpretations can gently introduce the potential for an external perspective; by describing what the patient sees and feels, the therapist very subtly invites the patient to adopt an observing stance on her experience. Over time, this process should lead the patient to question the absolute veracity of her most extreme attributions, improving her reality testing (unless the patient is psychotic).

Role Reversals

In the paranoid transferences typical of BPO patients, role reversals are common and typically generate confusion. At the same time, working with role reversals in the transference provides a powerful opportunity to increase the patient's self-awareness and may lead to relatively rapid improvement in interpersonal functioning.

Clinical Illustration 2: Confrontation of Role Reversals in Transference Analysis

Mr. G is the 35-year-old patient with narcissistic personality disorder, now in the middle phase of treatment, who was introduced in Clinical Illustration 2 in Chapter 9, as he was complaining about his wife's refusal to help with his car payment (for discussion of phases of treatment, see Chapter 13). Continuing where the illustration left off, Dr. Y was thinking about the affectively dominant object relation, enacted with Mr. G's wife and seemingly emerging in the transference as well: a powerful, hostile figure in relation to a diminished, enraged figure, associated with mutual hostility and frustration.

Dr. Y asked Mr. G for further clarification of the situation with his wife. In response, Mr. G became enraged. He lit into Dr. Y, raising his voice and using a self-righteous and derisive tone: "I can see that you're taking her side, criticizing me! I bet you also feel I should take a stupid job that is beneath me. You're just another stuck-up, condescending twat who thinks she is above me and thinks she knows what's best for me."

Mr. G glowered contemptuously at Dr. Y, who felt flustered, struck by the intensity of Mr. G's hostility and derision, and somewhat shocked by his referring to her as a "twat." She was mindful of what seemed to be escalating agitation on Mr. G's part; it was clear that the object relations that had initially been enacted with respect to Mr. G's wife at the opening of the session were currently affectively dominant in the transference.

Dr. Y gathered her thoughts and reflected on her countertransference. She saw Mr. G's behavior and attitude toward her in the session as offering an up-close view of what must often take place between Mr. G and his wife. At the same time, from the perspective of understanding Mr. G's experience, Dr. Y inferred that the derision and devaluation that she experienced Mr. G to be directing at her must be similar to what *he* experienced when he described her or his wife as critical, condescending, and hostile.

Mr. G went on: "You say we have this contract that I have to be working, but it's bullshit! I know that deep down you're a woman who likes to feel superior to men. Seeing me working as a barista would give you satisfaction. It would make you feel big and make me seem small—you win. It's like that with your charging me a full fee, too—you could charge me less, you don't need the money, but this makes you feel powerful and superior."

Dr. Y restated, "So if I understand correctly, I charge you a full fee because I want to feel powerful and superior, and I want you to take an entry-level job because I would enjoy your sense of humiliation. Is that accurate?" Mr. G corroborated that this was indeed what was happening: "You got it! To me, you're just another controlling, superior therapist-bitch." Though the content of Mr. G's communications remained unchanged, and he continued to speak loudly and employ an accusatory tone, he seemed to relax a bit, and he was less agitated, paranoid, and overtly aggressive.[5]

Over the course of the next several weeks, Mr. G was able to speak about his resentment both at being "forced" to find work and at needing to come to Dr. Y for help. In his mind, these realities placed Dr. Y in a superior position from which she could enjoy devaluing and diminishing him. As these experiences, linked to core narcissistic dynamics, were explored over time, Mr. G gradually seemed less acutely enraged; at moments, he seemed able, fleetingly, to tolerate his feelings of shame and humiliation in relation to his failures, and was less certain that Dr. Y's only motivation was to depreciate and sadistically humiliate him.

In one such moment, during a discussion of Mr. G's resentment, his sense of Dr. Y as dismissive, and his underlying feelings of humiliation, Dr. Y felt that Mr. G seemed somewhat calmer and more self-contained, despite his ongoing hostility and intermittent devaluation. Dr. Y intuited that in his current frame of mind, Mr. G might be able to be sufficiently self-observant to consider the constant and chronic role reversals that characterized the transference; such an intervention could potentially help Mr. G begin to get a handle on his interpersonal difficulties both with his wife and in the workplace, as well as to gain better understanding of his experience with Dr. Y.

Dr. Y suggested, "I'm thinking about how you see me as enjoying placing myself above you and treating you derisively, and how this leaves you feeling dismissed, humiliated, and justifiably angry. I understand that the very fact that I am the doctor, and you come to me for help, brings us to

---

[5]This is an example of how putting the patient's experience into words as part of a process of clarification can provide containment of affect.

that relationship pattern almost automatically. This is something we've been discussing for quite some time now, recognizing the impossible position this puts both of us in. But something else strikes me about our earlier interaction. Would you be interested in hearing my thought?"

Mr. G indicated that he would. Dr. Y continued, "At the same time that you experience me as devaluing and derisive, when you raise your voice and refer to me as a 'twat' or just another superior 'bitch-therapist,' or describe me as a pathetic woman enjoying dominating a man, someone might say that you are behaving in a dismissive and derisive manner toward me—in some sense, humiliating me as a woman. It's as if you are turning the tables, putting me in a vulnerable and devalued position and mocking me. Does what I'm saying make sense?"

Comments: This vignette recapitulates some of the elements discussed in relation to the previous vignette with Ms. M. We would highlight here the role of nonverbal communication and the countertransference in transference analysis, and the need for the therapist to attend to and contain her countertransference, to gather her thoughts and reflect, before reflexively reacting to the patient's projections. This vignette also highlights the observation that if a patient responds with increasing agitation to clarification of his experience outside the transference, it is likely that the transference is becoming affectively dominant and that it has a paranoid flavor. Finally, in this example, the therapist's ability to contain and articulate the patient's projections may prepare the patient to consider that part of what he is attacking in the therapist is also a part of himself.

Nonverbal Communication

The transferences of BPO patients may be expressed predominantly through nonverbal channels—in the patient's behavior in relation to the treatment frame or in nonverbal communications in session. The first step in analyzing the transference is to put words to the patient's actions and to describe the object relations organizing the patient's behavior.

Clinical Illustration 3: Nonverbal Communication and Transference Analysis

We return to Ms. P, the 23-year-old student with a diagnosis of borderline personality disorder and a history of superficial cutting, who was introduced in Clinical Illustration 1 in Chapter 9. She came to treatment with the goals of improving her affect regulation and stabilizing her relationships; she had a history of threatening suicide. Dr. K began by putting into words the object relation organizing the transference, as it had been elaborated during the process of countertransference analysis described in Chapter 12. Dr. K commented, "It sounds like you view me, at least in this moment, as callous and detached, enjoying your powerless position and the possibility of your suffering." Ms. P's response was to verbally agree with Dr. C and to grin slyly.

Dr. K proceeded to confront the dissociation between Ms. P's grin and the verbal content of their communication: "I'm struck by how we are discussing your experience of me as taking pleasure in your suffering, and at the same time you smile." Ms. P again grinned but seemed a bit perplexed, commenting that she wasn't really aware she'd been smiling in response to Dr. K's asking for her thoughts about why she was again grinning. Dr. K commented, "It's as if there is a part of you that enjoys this." Ms. P remained silent.

Dr. K went on: "I wonder if when you mention suicide, there is a part of you that wants to make me uncomfortable or worried about you; it's as if when you raise the possibility of hurting yourself, you are threatening *me*. In the same way you imagine my enjoying your suffering and vulnerability, it's as though a part of you, perhaps largely out of your awareness, enjoys the idea of making me suffer in kind and takes pleasure in highlighting my vulnerability. I wonder if it is that part of you that smiles when we talk about sadism. What are your thoughts?"

Comments: Dr. K began by describing the object relation organizing Ms. P's dominant experience of herself in relation to Dr. K: that of a victim in relation to someone uncaring and detached. Next, Dr. K confronted Ms. P's nonverbal communications—her threat to hurt herself and her grinning in response to his confrontation—as expressions of a dissociated, callous, and sadistic part of Ms. P that she was projecting onto Dr. K in the transference. Finally, Dr. K called attention to the role reversal, in the form of a confrontation. He then offered an early interpretation, addressing potential motives within Ms. P for the role reversal: he suggested that Ms. P enjoyed watching him suffer as retaliation for the suffering that she felt he had induced in her.

Idealized Transferences and Transference Analysis

We have thus far focused on analyzing paranoid transferences. Analysis of idealized transferences, in both their wishful and defensive functions, also plays an essential role in TFP-E with BPO patients. In the treatments of high-BPO patients in particular, idealized transferences may be especially stable, and exploring and interpreting their functions becomes a central task.

Clinical Illustration 4: Confrontation of Splitting and Denial

We return now to Ms. J, the high-BPO patient described in the vignette on interpretation in Clinical Illustration 2 in Chapter 10. Dr. C and Ms. J continued to identify and explore the instability of Ms. J's experience of her boss, Hal, and of her new boyfriend. They noted that she routinely shifted between two polarized, contradictory states in which she either was mistreated and felt incompetent or was highly valued, was taken care of, and felt special. The former was associated with anger and anxiety, and the latter with gratification and relief from anxiety.

Meanwhile, throughout this process, Ms. J maintained a relatively stable, positive (idealized) relationship with Dr. C. The hostility and passive-aggressive power struggles around the frame that had characterized the early treatment phase had entirely disappeared, replaced by a childlike compliance. In her sessions, Ms. J would frequently complain and express hostility, devaluation, and criticism toward her mother, siblings, and girlfriends, as well as her boss and her boyfriend, but never toward Dr. C.

One day, Ms. J came in and said, "I hate everyone! I always get angry at everyone—I am just so angry and frustrated. You are the only person who always treats me well, who never makes me angry. I don't know how you do it. You always take such good care of me."

Dr. C responded with a confrontation: "I've been thinking about that as well. To me, it doesn't entirely make sense. As you point out, you get angry at most people sooner or later and, truthfully, you were angry at me all the time when we first began working together; whenever I raised the issue of your lateness or your drinking or your need to find steady work, you got furious at me. You felt I was controlling you or didn't care about your feelings, or that I sounded just like your parents. But now there seem to be no points of friction between us. Instead, it's as though I can do no wrong."

Ms. J persisted with her idealization, which she was apparently highly motivated to maintain: "What do you mean? It's just that I've found out what a good therapist you are." Dr. C responded, "Perhaps, but it seems extreme—that is, the way you went from taking issue with so much of what I suggested to now agreeing with virtually anything I say. It doesn't entirely make sense and somehow seems unreal."

Ms. J responded, "Well, I can see what you're saying, but it certainly feels real. I have come to see that you're really smart and really know what you're talking about. I'm doing so much better than when I first came."

Persisting in her confrontation of Ms. J's defensive idealization, Dr. C continued: "Well, you certainly are doing better. At the same time, the view of me that you describe seems somewhat exaggerated; it's 'all good,' as if I were a perfect therapist, and of course no one is perfect."

Ms. J responded to this more complete confrontation: "Why *can't* you be perfect? I want you to be perfect!"

Dr. C offered an interpretation: "That's just it. It's as if you need to keep your image of me entirely blemish-free, as if you couldn't tolerate letting in any critical or negative feelings. It feels like a way to protect our relationship, as if you believe that there is absolutely no room for any negative feelings in a positive relationship, that even the smallest disagreement, disappointment, or frustration could lead to the collapse of the whole thing. So to avoid that, you have to keep it totally positive."

Ms. J seemed genuinely perplexed. She said, "Well, what's the problem with that—it feels good, and I'm doing better." Dr. C replied, "Yes, both these things are true—but the problem is that it makes our relationship unreal and superficial. And as you have it set up, it's based on denying parts of your experience or splitting them off, and perhaps risking that they'll bubble up in some of your other relationships."

Comments: In this illustration, Dr. C begins by confronting Ms. J's idealization of her in the transference. In her confrontation, Dr. C reviews the history of the treatment relationship and the friction that characterized the transference early on, recognizing that Ms. J has in the moment split off and is denying these aspects of their current relationship and of their history together. In a series of interventions, Dr. C invites Ms. J to recall the negative side of their relationship, at the same time that Ms. J is immersing herself in an idealized view. Dr. C clearly acknowledges both sides of the split when she reminds Ms. J of the early difficulties while at the same time acknowledging that Ms. J has benefited from the treatment and formed an attachment to her therapist.

These interventions can be considered as a series of confrontations of splitting and denial in the transference, as Dr. C invites Ms. J to join her in cognitively bridging idealized and paranoid sectors of her experience in the transference. In subsequent sessions, Dr. C continued to refrain from making an interpretation proper until Ms. J acknowledged that she could at least appreciate Dr. C's perspective. At that point, Dr. C felt Ms. J might be able to make use of an exploration of the motives driving the idealization that she was clinging to so tenaciously; it was then that Dr. C offered an interpretation, suggesting a way to understand Ms. J's motivation for defensively splitting off all negative affects from the therapeutic relationship.

It is common in the treatment of high-BPO patients for the patient to settle into a relatively stable idealizing transference of the kind illustrated in this vignette. Some patients settle into idealizing transferences midtreatment, once there has been a resolution of the stormy transferences of the opening phase that typically revolve around maintaining the frame. In contrast, other patients may begin treatment with relatively stable idealizing transferences readily in place. Idealized transferences are often relatively comfortable for both patient and therapist, and these may in some ways promote positive developments in the treatment and in the patient;

idealizing transferences may enable the patient to form a positive attachment to the therapist and to the treatment, to adhere to the frame, and often to function better in life overall.

As a result, it can be tempting for therapists to leave idealizing transferences untouched, especially if they do not involve gross distortions or lead to acting out. However, we strongly recommend against allowing idealized transferences to remain unexplored for extended periods of time in the treatments of BPO patients. The positive developments that may accompany idealized transferences are predicated on defensive distortion of the therapeutic relationship, and **they come at a price to the patient.** To leave idealized transferences unaddressed in the treatment is to accept idealization as a viable solution for managing hostility and negative affects, and to leave the patient reliant on splitting to maintain positive attachments. The patient's relationships are relegated to being superficial and brittle, and her sense of self is compromised by a need to split off and reject (or project) all critical and aggressive parts of the self, which are experienced as threatening and potentially destabilizing.

Narcissistic Defenses and Transference Analysis

In the treatment of patients with prominent narcissistic defenses—whether narcissistic personality disorder proper or prominent narcissistic conflicts and defenses in the setting of a different personality disorder—much of the early phase of treatment will often be devoted to analyzing enactment of narcissistic defenses in the transference (Kernberg 2008; see Clinical Illustration 2: "Confrontation of Role Reversals in Transference Analysis" earlier in this chapter, and in Chapter 13, the subsection "Negative Transferences" and the related Clinical Illustration 3: "Containment and Technical Neutrality Around Narcissistic Defenses" for additional discussion of the analysis of narcissistic defenses). The overall approach is similar for these two groups of patients, but narcissistic defenses are far more rigid and far more affectively invested in narcissistic personality disorder than they are in other personality disorders. With both groups of patients, but especially those with narcissistic personality disorder, enactment of narcissistic defenses tends to dominate the transference-countertransference in the early phase of treatment, and analysis of narcissistic transferences is a necessary and often protracted first step in exploring underlying paranoid and depressive anxieties and object relations.

Clinical Illustration 5: Confrontation of Narcissistic Defenses

Ms. H, 40 years old and married, with a diagnosis of narcissistic personality disorder and organized at a middle borderline level, presented after having recently moved out of her home for no apparent reason, abandoning her husband and 10-year-old son, leaving her marriage in crisis. Carefully and stylishly dressed, Ms. H walked into Dr. B's office and settled comfortably in the chair as if she had not a care in the world. She spoke freely about her plans to find an apartment and then began to discuss her interior decorating plans in excessive detail.

As she spoke, Ms. H's attitude toward Dr. B was detached and dismissive. She made virtually no eye contact. The interaction left Dr. B feeling empty, insignificant, and strangely lost in the countertransference. As he sat with Ms. H and listened to her, Dr. B had the thought that Ms. H could go on like this forever, using the therapy hours to deliver monologues about trivial matters and generally turning the therapy into an endless waste of time. Several minutes later Dr. B noted that his mind had been wandering.

Dr. B identified the dominant object relation enacted in the transference as one in which Ms. H played the role of a disinterested, disengaged, dismissive maternal figure, conveyed in her overall attitude, in her body language, and in the countertransference, while Dr. B was cast in the complementary role of someone initially making an effort to connect but being totally cut off and at the same time diminished,[6] someone who ultimately met the patient's withdrawal in kind.

Dr. B decided to address the object relation enacted in the transference-countertransference by focusing on Ms. H's behavior and attitude in the session, and on the contrast between the ongoing crisis in her life and her talking about furnishings in her therapy. "I'm struck by your attitude here today," he began. "You seem relaxed, unconcerned, even detached—speaking about apartment hunting and conveying no sense of urgency with regard to the problems that bring you here."

Ms. H paused for a moment, barely acknowledging that Dr. B had spoken, and then went back to speaking about her new furnishings. Dr. B attempted again to call attention to Ms. H's behavior, this time commenting, "I notice you barely acknowledged my comment, and then you went on speaking about your apartment as if I had not spoken—as if you have no concern about the crisis in your marriage or that you have not seen your son in 2 weeks." Dr. B noted a flicker of irritation before Ms. H returned to her musings about furniture, seemingly without missing a beat. In the countertransference, Dr. B felt frustrated; he also suddenly became worried for Ms. H, who seemed not only dismissive but also bizarrely dis-

---

[6]One could say that Dr. B's initial experience in the countertransference was an identification with the healthier, dependent parts of Ms. H that she projected.

connected, both from Dr. B and from her own circumstances, as she continued to talk about interior decorating.

Dr. B responded to Ms. H's nonverbal communication. "It seems that my comments are irritating to you…an uninvited interruption." Ms. H nodded in agreement and then returned to her musing about furnishings. Dr. B persisted: "You nodded when I suggested my comments are an unwelcome irritation." Ms. H concurred. "Yes. I am here to speak about what is on my mind; but you dismiss my concerns, you do not listen. You seem to have your own agenda."

Rather than defending his position or again attempting to take up the topic of Ms. H's denial of the crisis in her current situation, Dr. B focused on the transference, beginning with a therapist-centered intervention, in an effort to elaborate Ms. H's experience of him at those times he attempted to interject. "I am someone who does not listen, who cares most about my own agenda and dismisses your concerns. Can you tell me more?"

Comments: Dr. B began by confronting Ms. H's denial of her difficulties. For Ms. H, and in general for those with narcissistic defenses, the tendency to deny difficulties functions to avoid awareness of imperfection and vulnerability, and persistent dismissal of the therapist functions to deny all need for help. Dr. B's initial confrontations of the discrepancy between Ms. H's having felt herself in sufficient trouble to warrant needing treatment, on the one hand, and, on the other, her dismissive, superior, and detached attitude in session, had no apparent impact. Ms. H continued to maintain her dismissive attitude in the transference, enacting a defensive object relation of a superior and dismissive self in relation to a devalued therapist—ignored, dismissed, barely a presence outside of whatever the patient might need of him in the moment. This common transference in the treatment of narcissistic patients can be understood in terms of the patient's split-off expectations of how the therapist would view and treat *her* were she to allow herself to become vulnerable or to accept a dependent relation.

Narcissistic transferences tend to be quite stable and concrete, organizing the clinical field and assuming affective dominance in the treatment for extended periods of time. Analysis of narcissistic transference requires both persistence and patience on the part of the therapist; because narcissistic transferences are so highly invested, *repeated* clarification and confrontation of the patient's attitude and behavior in the transference over time are required for the patient to gain perspective on them.

Focusing on the patient's responses to (or dismissal of) the therapist's comments is typically the point of entry into exploration of the transference (Kernberg 2008). It is only as the therapist tactfully but persistently calls attention to what the patient is *doing* (e.g., in the case of Ms. H, ignoring and dismissing) in the transference that more specific object relations (e.g., in the case of Ms. H, that Dr. B had his own agenda that involved dismissing her concerns) and underlying conflicts in relation to dependency, inferiority, envy, and aggression begin to come to light.

Some more grandiose narcissistic patients, such as Ms. M (see Clinical Illustration 1 earlier in this chapter, in the subsection "Paranoid Transference"), remain stably identified with the superior position for extended periods of time, whereas others may oscillate between superior and devalued positions in the transference. In contrast, "thin-skinned," or vulnerable, narcissistic individuals remain stably identified with a devalued, envious self representation in the transference, while the therapist is placed in the superior position; at the same time, the patient will harbor covert feelings of superiority that must be uncovered as part of the process of transference analysis.

Unconscious Conflict in the Transference

In the setting of a neurotic structure, ego-syntonic defensive object relations tend to organize the transference initially, while more conflictual object relations may remain largely unconscious. As repressive defenses become less rigid, and especially as the patient begins to make changes, conflictual object relations may come to assume affective dominance as they color the patient's experience of the therapist.

Clinical Illustration 6: Interpretation of Unconscious Conflict

We return to Ms. S, the 50-year-old married volunteer research assistant functioning at a neurotic level of personality organization, with depressive and dependent features. In the previous vignette of Ms. S (Clinical Illustration 4 in Chapter 9), Dr. C noted to herself that Ms. S was describing two separate object relations: a defensive object relation of an inferior, inadequate self, unworthy of positive attention from someone powerful and superior, and an underlying, highly conflictual object relation of a self able to garner and potentially enjoy the attention and admiration of an attractive and powerful man. Ms. S's initial attitude toward Dr. C in the transference seemed most manifestly to be one of Ms. S somewhat shyly but happily sharing a good feeling. In the countertransference, Dr. C was simultaneously pleased for Ms. S and also vaguely aware of subtle feelings of jealousy in relation to Ms. S's academic successes.

Dr. C. began by describing the two object relations that Ms. S had brought into the session, beginning with the defensive one, and focusing outside the transference: "I hear you describing two very different views of yourself. The first, which is familiar, something we've discussed many times, is a sense of yourself as inadequate, inferior, and unworthy, the subject of condescension from those more fortunate. That view of yourself goes along with feelings of smallness and humiliation." Dr. C paused; Ms. S was attentive but remained silent. Dr. C continued, "But I also hear you introducing a new sense of yourself, one that perhaps is colored with some anxiety. In this view, you are someone enjoying the limelight…pleased about being admired by desirable people. This view is associated with feelings of power and pleasure."

Ms. S immediately looked very uncomfortable and commented, "When you say that, it makes me very anxious." Dr. C inquired about the source of Ms. S's anxiety. The patient responded, "I don't know—first off, it's like I want to shrink down to nothing in my chair, almost literally, like I could disappear. I feel so foolish to think that you see me as wanting to be admired."

Dr. C pointed out Ms. S's retreat to her familiar defensive position, which they had identified and explored repeatedly in previous sessions, and then Dr. C asked for clarification, inquiring of Ms. S why wanting to be admired would have to be viewed as foolish. Ms. S responded, "Because there is nothing admirable about me. I imagine you secretly feeling sorry for me, thinking I am pathetic. Look at who you are and look at me—from your chair, I must sound like a deluded old woman, just pathetic."

Dr. C pointed out that Ms. S's expectations of her response did not sound particularly sympathetic. Ms. S appeared thoughtful, then responded, "No, I guess I don't really see you as sympathetic at this moment. It's funny, I usually do…. I worry you find me contemptible, a foolish old woman."

Dr. C pointed out that as soon as she had called attention to Ms. S's successes, both professional and personal, Ms. S imagined Dr. C to be hostile and contemptuous—as if, Dr. C pointed out, Ms. S's experience of Dr. C as sympathetic was predicated on Ms. S's feelings of inferiority. Ms. S acknowledged that this seemed to be true, that she felt more comfortable being in the inferior position; it felt "right," perhaps because it was familiar.

Dr. C agreed that familiarity was likely part of it, but suggested that there seemed to be more: "It's almost as if you use feelings of inferiority to protect and to ingratiate yourself; as soon as you feel more successful or powerful, you imagine my resenting you, as if I might say to myself, 'Who is she to feel desirable or successful? I am the one with the successful career and the stylish wardrobe. That's my place—how dare she impinge, even in fantasy.'"

Ms. S responded, "Yes, exactly. It's how it was with my mother; she dragged me to watch her shop, or to sit in her office and watch her work. I was happy to admire her; I never thought to want to be admired." Dr. C continued, "And when you start to feel those desires here with me, it leaves you expecting me to respond as you fear your mother would have, with resentment and contempt, wanting to keep you in your place." Ms. S agreed, and Dr. C continued, completing her interpretation: "This experience may have begun with your mother, but your mother is no longer with us. It is not she who leads you to retreat to inferiority. It is a part of you that believes the only way to maintain your attachments is to diminish yourself, make yourself small. It is as if you believe that I would not tolerate your wanting to be my equal, let alone a competitor."

Comments: This vignette illustrates the emergence into consciousness of a conflict that had been stably defended against when Ms. S came to treatment. At this point, the defensive object relation of a humiliated, inferior self is no longer able to fully support repression of underlying pleasurable but highly conflictual strivings to be admired. In essence, the gains Ms. S has made to date, in her treatment and in her life, have functioned to confront her defensive self representation and to call its veracity into question; underlying wishes are being enacted in her changing behavior, and associated anxieties are emerging in the transference.

In her intervention, Dr. C begins with clarification of the familiar, defensive object relation and then describes the more conflictual object relation, repressed until recently, that is beginning to emerge into Ms. S's consciousness. As Dr. C restates what Ms. S has described, putting words to the conflictual object relation in which Ms. S enjoys attention and admiration, the conflict becomes affectively dominant in the transference. In the dominant transference paradigm, Ms. S fears Dr. C's hostility and rejection as a condemning mother and anticipates that she will be condemned for her wishes for admiration, which are viewed as a competitive challenge to Dr. C or to mother (also heard are wishes to be admired by Dr. C, much as Ms. S felt admired by the attractive male scholar). Dr. C's interpretation focuses on Ms. S's anxiety and can be seen, in essence, as implicitly communicating a rather complex meta message, approximating the following: "You assume in a concrete fashion that wanting admiration is the same as making your therapist-mother hate you. However, perhaps your assumption that your wishes automatically constitute a destructive danger is fallacious, and perhaps your anxieties, rather than constituting concrete facts, are beliefs that can be understood as having meaning."

A classical interpretation in the setting of a neurotic conflict has the following structure: defense, anxiety, impulse. Applying this structure to the current situation results in something such as the following: "You seem to retreat to seeing yourself/the two of us in a certain way [*defensive object relation*] to avoid anxiety. It is as if to see it otherwise would endanger/threaten our relationship [*anxiety, fear, or 'danger' motivating the defense*]—as if any possibility of competitive feeling [*underlying conflictual motivation*] would be totally unacceptable." The objective of interpretations structured in this fashion is to help the patient feel less threatened by and better able to tolerate awareness of her conflictual wishes—in this example, wishes to be admired.

Helping the patient tolerate awareness of conflictual motivations is consistent with the overall goal of the interpretive process in a neurotic structure: to promote containment of previously repressed, conflictual motivations within the patient's overall conscious sense of self (see Chapter 10) so that they are contextualized. As long as conflictual motivations and associated object relations remain split off and repressed, the anxieties associated with their expression remain concrete, and the impulses themselves have an all-or-nothing quality (i.e., if a patient is aware of her conflictual motivations, she fears that they will be expressed—and if they are expressed, this automatically will lead to disaster for the patient).

In contrast, if impulses are conscious, contained, and contextualized within an integrated sense of self, they are experienced as thoughts and feelings that are part of a greater whole, and that can be experienced and/ or expressed to a greater or lesser degree. As a result, they need not pose an overwhelming psychological threat (as reflected next in Clinical Illustration 7).

Toward the ending of a successful TFP-E treatment, rather than enactment of individual, conflictual object relations in the transference, the transference may come to reflect enactment of an integrated and realistic experience of the relationship between patient and doctor, an object relation that reflects both the history of their relationship and the patient's personal history, as well as the patient's hopes for herself.

Clinical Illustration 7: Transference Interpretation in the Setting of a Largely Integrated Self Experience

Ms. T is a 45-year-old divorced lawyer with a traumatic developmental history who presented in crisis at the time of her divorce. Now in the advanced phase of treatment, Ms. T shared a dream and then a series of associations.

In her dream, Ms. T was on a fishing boat, looking out and anticipating what she would see on the horizon. In the dream, she had the thought that in the past she would have been sitting in the back where fishing is done, looking at what was behind, at the wake. She associated to having spent the weekend with a childhood friend J, "She is so different from me, she reaches out so freely for help… I'm packing up the old house and found my mother's dishes. We had lunch on them every day as kids, and then I fed *my* kids from them when they were children. Mother never really engaged with us, but she did so well with the traditions, the ceremonial parts of life. I have such a sense of time with J's daughter getting engaged: my father's dementia is progressing, I'm finally building my house to make it a home where someday grandchildren can visit.... there's a sense of time and generations, looking forward rather than coming from where I was. It used to feel so choppy."

Dr. C heard Ms. T describing in her words, associations, and dream an emerging sense of herself as intact and sufficiently secure to manage loss and hope in relation to objects that can be loved and trusted, without having to deny their imperfections or shortcomings.

Dr. C began by describing the object relation organizing Ms. T's verbal communication in the session: "I hear you feeling more secure in yourself and in your ability to build a life that emerges from but is not mired in your past—a newfound optimism and a hope that others can meet you halfway and can help you along." Ms. T began to tear up and responded, "Yes, well, it all started here." Dr. C remained silent, feeling that Ms. T did not need a response to understand that she was listening. After a brief pause, Ms. T went on, "*You* have met me halfway, more than halfway. You focused on my needs when I had no idea that that was a possibility. I've learned here to ask for help and that others can be there for me. It's a new beginning."

Comments: This vignette is from the final months of a successful treatment. The transference no longer represents enactment of conflictual parts of the self in relation to conflictual aspects of the therapist (i.e., enactment of a conflictual object relation), as has been demonstrated in previous vignettes; in the place of component object relations, Ms. T experiences an integrated, whole, and complex self with a history, in relation to a therapist also experienced as an integrated, whole other. This object relation approaches what may be considered a "real" or realistic relationship, developed over time between a patient who has benefited from treatment and a helpful but imperfect therapist.

Part 2

Tactics Guiding the Interpretive Process

WE HAVE DISCUSSED THE INTERPRETIVE process and illustrated how we make use of the different components of that process—clarification, confrontation, and interpretation proper—

both in the transference and outside the transference, with patients with personality pathology at different levels of severity. As we have described the interpretive process, we have also pointed to the impact that different interventions have on the patient, on her capacity to observe her behavior and internal experience, to contain and better regulate her affects, to entertain alternative perspectives, and to contextualize experience in areas of conflict, as well as her capacity to experience the therapist as empathizing with her internal situation and as understanding her.

Clarification, confrontation, and interpretation and their application to analysis of transference are core interventions in TFP-E. Along with countertransference management and managing technical neutrality (discussed in Chapter 12), they constitute the five basic techniques of TFP-E, what the therapist does moment to moment in each therapy session to promote the clinical process.

At this point, we now consider the *tactics* guiding the interpretive process—that is, general principles that the therapist can turn to when it comes to deciding *when* to make a particular intervention and *how* it can best be formulated—with the objective of optimizing the impact of the intervention on the clinical process (Busch 1996; Fenichel 1941; Levy and Inderbitzin 1992; Schafer 1997). Historically, these principles have often been referred to in the psychoanalytic literature as guidelines for therapeutic *tact and timing* (Table 11–2). Some of the tactics of the TFP-E interpretive process have been introduced in earlier chapters preceding this text; this discussion further integrates those concepts.

Initiating Exploratory Interventions From the Patient's Dominant Perspective

Having identified a focus for intervention (see Chapter 9), the therapist begins exploration with clarification, which we have described as a process that involves inquiring about, elaborating, and ultimately putting into words the patient's dominant conscious experience. In this process, the therapist always attempts to first approach the material from within the patient's subjectivity, assuming an *empathic perspective*. The therapist does not add to or comment on the patient's experience but simply elaborates it, as in the following example: "You've described a variety of ways in which your wife is withholding and leaves you feeling frustrated."

TABLE 11–2.   Tactics guiding the interpretive process: therapeutic tact and timing

---

1. Initiate interpretive interventions from the patient's dominant perspective, from within the patient's subjectivity (often described as *assuming an empathic perspective*).

2. Begin with what is most accessible to the patient and move toward material that is less accessible (classically described in the psychoanalytic literature in terms of intervening *from surface to depth*).

3. Begin with defensive object relations and move toward those that are closer to the expression of conflictual motivations (classically described as *addressing defense before impulse*).

4. Begin with dissociative defenses (if present) before taking up repression.

5. Prioritize quality of patient's experience over content.

6. Keep in mind that ego-dystonicity is a prerequisite for interpretation proper.

Moving From Surface to Depth: Beginning With Defensive Object Relations and Moving Toward Those More Conflictual

After the therapist characterizes the patient's dominant conscious experience from an empathic perspective, she then proceeds to make use of confronting interventions to incrementally broaden and deepen the patient's view to include aspects of his experience of which he is not fully aware— that is, that he is defending against. Thus, the therapist begins from the "surface" of the patient's dominant conscious experience and gradually moves toward material that is progressively less accessible to consciousness, either dissociated or repressed. This trajectory is metaphorically described as moving *from surface to depth*.

Defensive object relations are by definition more accessible than those defended against; thus, moving from surface to depth—beginning from the patient's dominant conscious experience and moving toward aspects of experience less accessible in the moment—corresponds with beginning from object relations serving defensive functions and then moving toward those defended against. This approach entails beginning with aspects of experience that are more familiar and acceptable to the patient and moving toward those that are more difficult to tolerate and more threatening, often more closely linked to underlying conflictual motivations or "impulses" and the anxieties associated with their expression. This trajectory is often described as *defense before impulse*. In the foregoing example, we might highlight this as follows:

> You're describing a variety of ways in which your wife is withholding and leaves you feeling frustrated [*clarification of defensive object relations organizing patient's surface experience*], and we've discussed how your view of her at this moment is discrepant with views you've held at other times [*confrontation of instability and dissociation of contradictory representations*]. It seems that no matter how well things are going, this negative view of the two of you always seems to creep in; I seem to recall your having described the same thing happening with your first wife, who was a very different person from Marcia [*confrontation of repetitive nature of relationship patterns*]. It's almost as if you are in some way more comfortable when you see yourself in a relationship with a woman who is withholding and frustrating, as if at some level it makes you anxious to see yourself as having a wife who wants to take good care of you [*interpretation of unconscious anxiety motivating defense*], so you retreat to the negative view.

A more advanced interpretation might address the conflictual motivations associated with the anxiety described, the aspects of experience least accessible, as follows:

> It's almost as if you are in some way more comfortable when you see yourself in a relationship with a woman who is withholding and frustrating, as if at some level it makes you anxious to see yourself as having a wife who wants to take good care of you [*interpretation of anxiety motivating defense*], perhaps for fear it would leave you feeling too dependent on her. (*This more complete interpretation includes a reference to highly conflictual dependency needs.*) So you retreat to the negative view.

In sum, as the therapist sequentially makes use of clarification, confrontation, and finally interpretation proper, she moves from surface to depth and from defense to impulse.

Beginning with Dissociative Defenses Before Addressing Repression

Moving from surface to depth, from material most accessible to the patient to material less available to conscious experience, implies that the therapist typically addresses dissociative defenses before addressing repression. This means focusing first on aspects of the patient's experience that are currently dissociated—not part of his dominant experience in the moment, but that have been fully conscious at other times. Thus, in the example above, the therapist began by addressing dissociative defenses:

> You've described a variety of ways in which your wife is withholding and leaves you feeling frustrated; this seems discrepant with our discussion last week when you were telling me about how generous she is when you really need her to come through.

> You're describing a variety of ways in which your wife is withholding and leaves you feeling frustrated; I'm struck by how these are the exact same words you told me that she used to describe *you* last week, when you had that argument.

Having addressed dissociative defenses, the therapist next focused clinical attention on uncovering and exploring repressed aspects of psychological experience. In the vignette, after reviewing dissociative defenses, the therapist moves on to an interpretation of unconscious conflict, focusing on the anxiety motivating repression of the patient's conflictual dependency needs:

> It's almost as if you are in some way more comfortable when you see yourself in a relationship with a woman who is withholding and frustrating, as if at some level it makes you anxious to see yourself as having a wife who wants to take good care of you, perhaps for fear it would leave you feeling too dependent on her. So you retreat to the negative view.

In sum, from the perspective of *content*, we move from surface to depth and from defense to impulse as we make use of clarification, confrontation, and finally interpretation proper. At the same time, from the perspective of *capacities* within the patient, we begin with interventions that demand less of the patient, focusing on his dominant, conscious, and ego-syntonic experience, and move gradually toward interventions that call on more advanced capacities for affect containment, self-observation, introspection, and greater flexibility of thinking. We conceptualize each intervention as supporting capacities in the patient needed to make use of the interventions that follow.

If the patient is not in a frame of mind to make use of a particular level of intervention, the intervention will be less than helpful—often simply useless and at times temporarily derailing the clinical process (Caligor et al. 2009; Steiner 1994). In this case, the therapist temporarily returns to a more basic level of intervention. As a result, there is typically a back-and-forth quality to the clinical process; the therapist intervenes at levels that progressively stretch the patient's capacities, returning to more basic interventions when need be.

Prioritizing Quality of the Patient's Experience Over Content

It is generally futile to interpret the motivations driving a patient's behavior, thoughts, and feelings if patient and therapist are working from discrepant views of reality, or if the patient's current thinking is extremely concrete or ego-syntonic. Rather, in these settings, the therapist tailors the interventions to target the *quality* of the patient's experience and thinking—the patient's relationship to or *attitude toward* maladaptive behaviors, thoughts, and feelings, rather than their content. The objective here is to help the patient shift from a perspective embedded in rigidly distorted or concretely experienced views of internal and external reality, one in which maladaptive defensive behaviors, beliefs, and feelings are entirely ego-syntonic, and instead move toward greater flexibility in his thinking and the ability to step outside his dominant experience in the moment to consider alternative perspectives.

Concrete Thinking and the Interpretive Process

The following are examples of concrete thinking: A patient is convinced that her therapist dresses with the intention of impressing the patient. When asked what makes her think this is the case, she explains that it is "just a feeling" that somehow seems perfectly true. Another patient knows herself to be a "bad" person—from her perspective, a "fact" about the nature of her fundamental essence that merits no further consideration. Yet another patient explains that because her boyfriend is often late, she knows that he cannot really love her; if he loved her, he would always be on time. None of these patients is psychotic, yet the thinking of each is extremely concrete.

Describing the patient's experience as *concrete* refers to a situation in which the patient *fails to make a clear distinction between internal and external reality*; the patient does not distinguish between what she thinks, feels, and believes and what actually is, or between what she wants to be true and real or what she fears is true and real, and what in fact *is* real. When in this frame of mind, a patient has little or no capacity to see beyond her own experience in the moment; she is unable to entertain alternative perspectives (see also Chapter 2).

Everybody is vulnerable to concrete thinking at moments of stress and in areas of conflict; patients with personality disorders across the BPO spectrum become concrete more frequently and more readily than do those with normal identity formation. In treatment, BPO patients often become concrete in relation to highly affectively charged or conflictual themes, especially in the transference.

In TFP-E, when a patient's thinking is concrete, the therapist's first objective is to help the patient elaborate and describe her experience, while being careful to avoid directly challenging it (Steiner 1994).[7] This process encourages an "observing" perspective by "going with" the patient's view while at the same time subtly introducing space between the patient as observer of her experience and her immediate experience. The therapist's second objective when addressing concrete levels of experience is to supplement clarification with confrontation, while carefully maintaining a neutral position in relation to the veracity of the patient's belief. Here the therapist will call attention to inconsistencies and contradictions in the patient's experience, and will also draw out the logical conclusions of the patient's firmly held beliefs. These sequential interventions help the patient to step out of her immediate experience and invite her to reconsider the absolute veracity of that experience; the therapist gently supports the capacity in the patient to entertain alternative perspectives, while carefully avoiding getting into a debate with the patient.

In sum, when the patient's thinking is concrete or when patient and therapist do not share a common view of reality, the therapist focuses exploration on the concrete *quality* of the patient's thinking before interpreting *content* (i.e., before exploring meanings and motivations that might explain why the patient is experiencing things as she is). In this process, the therapist relies on clarification followed by confrontation, in an effort to open up the patient's perspective while abstaining from interpretation proper until the patient's thinking and experience are more flexible.

---

[7]When the therapist takes this approach in the setting of transference analysis, the process corresponds to *therapist-centered interventions* introduced earlier in this chapter (see the Commentary for Clinical Illustration 1in the subsection "Paranoid Transference.")

Clinical Illustration 8: Working With Concrete Thinking

In a rainstorm, a therapist arrived 5 minutes late to a session with Ms. U, who carried a diagnosis of histrionic personality disorder with borderline features. The therapist apologized for his lateness and explained that several major roads on his way to the office had been closed because of flooding, and he asked if Ms. U could make up the time at the end of the session. Meanwhile, it emerged that the patient understood the therapist's lateness to be confirmation that he did not like her; she was certain that his apology was disingenuous and that he was attempting to hide his true feelings. Ms. U responded to the therapist's apology by explaining that she had been about to leave, and that the wait had been intolerable as she began to realize she'd been right all along that he did not want to treat her.

The therapist was struck by the paranoid and concrete experience of Ms. U; he was tempted to focus on the bad weather and how unreasonable it was not to understand the difficulty of travel in such conditions. However, rather than correcting, confronting, supporting reality testing, or interpreting, the therapist began with clarification, asking Ms. U to elaborate on her experience, while refraining from commenting further. He invited her to tell him more about her experience of him and of his lateness, of her certainty that he didn't like her, and about how his lateness confirmed this understanding. As Ms. U elaborated, the therapist also inquired as to what it was in his behavior up to this point that had convinced her that he didn't want her as a patient. The patient described wondering from the first day they met whether he really wanted to treat her. He had not reduced his fee as her previous therapist had done and as she had assumed he would, although she had said nothing at the time. Also, he was not as warm or supportive as she wanted him to be.

Patient and therapist spent the next several sessions elaborating Ms. U's current and past experience of the therapist as disliking her and not wanting to treat her, and the therapist helped her put the details of that experience into words. He subtly confronted her beliefs by drawing them to their logical conclusion—pointing out, for example, the implication of what she was saying about his charging her a higher fee because he didn't like her, something that would be highly unethical and a violation of the standards of his profession. At the same time, the therapist nonverbally communicated his capacity to comfortably tolerate being seen by Ms. U as hostile, rejecting, and dishonest. Over time and with help from the therapist, the patient became somewhat more flexible in her thinking; she began to notice that what had happened with the therapist was familiar— that over the years, similar experiences in which she had felt despised and rejected but said nothing had led to the demise of a number of her close friendships. This increased level of self-observation and reflectiveness was associated with a subtle but significant shift away from the extremely rigid and concrete quality of her belief that the therapist didn't want to treat her; perhaps she was not as sure of this as she had been. At this point, the therapist felt Ms. U was in a frame of mind in which exploration of potential meanings and motivations behind her idea of his dislike for her could be of use, both to promote further flexibility into her thinking and to begin to deepen her level of self-understanding.

Comments: This vignette illustrates the TFP-E approach to working with concrete thinking. The therapist's initial approach addresses the concrete quality of the patient's experience, rather than the distorted content that she is endorsing. The therapist's initial interventions focus on supporting Ms. U's capacity to observe her experience, a capacity compromised in the setting of her powerful reaction to the therapist's late arrival. To this end, the therapist helps Ms. U elaborate her experience in the transference, encouraging her to think about and put into words her long-standing belief that the therapist is rejecting and disdainful. This process of elaboration can be understood as providing cognitive containment of affect, by linking the patient's affective experience to specific representations of the therapist while at the same time demonstrating nonverbally that the therapist is able to tolerate and contain the patient's hostile projections. In response, over time, Ms.U's thinking becomes somewhat more flexible, and the intensity of her conviction of the therapist's malevolence and dislike for her slowly diminishes. At this point, the therapist's confrontations (e.g., "Is the therapist truly unethical? If yes, why am I remaining in treatment with him?") help Ms. U to reflect on her experience and entertain alternative perspectives. In essence, the therapist's approach aims to help Ms. U observe and reflect on, rather than simply enact, the paranoid object relation organizing her experience. This observing stance helps her shift from a concrete, comprehensive view of the therapist as rejecting and disdainful toward a view that is more flexible and reflective. Finally, as she becomes more reflective, Ms. U is able to step back and to observe herself and her experience not only in the moment, but also across time. Her increasingly reflective stance enables her to view her current experience as part of a pattern, with the possibility of appreciating that the pattern reflects not only a history of maltreatment, but also perhaps a difficulty within herself.

In sum, with the patient who does not share a common view of reality with the therapist or whose experience is markedly concrete, the therapist abstains from interpretation.[8] Rather, the therapist relies on an extended process of clarification ultimately supplemented by confrontation, in which the patient is encouraged to elaborate the details of her experience, and in that process to observe and examine it. Clarification helps the patient to begin to take a step back to observe and think about what she has experienced concretely, supporting reality testing. Confrontation invites the patient to consider her beliefs from an alternative perspective and to reflect on implicit contradictions in her thinking (e.g., "Is the therapist truly unethical? If yes, why am I remaining in treatment with him?"). As the patient becomes somewhat more open in her thinking, it becomes possible, in addition, to confront the repetitive nature of certain relationship patterns, typically across different relationships and in different contexts. In concert, these interventions support the patient's reality testing, her capacity to entertain alternative perspectives, and a dawning appreciation of the internal, subjective (in contrast to concrete) nature of her experience.

Ego-Dystonicity and the Interpretive Process

At those times when patient and therapist *are* working from a shared view of reality and the patient is making a distinction between internal and external reality, the therapist turns his attention to interpretation and to the matter of *ego-dystonicity*. In the treatment of personality pathology, the therapist focuses on behaviors, thoughts, and feelings that are familiar to and accepted by the patient—that is, those that are ego-syntonic. It is only when these habitual thoughts, feelings, and behaviors become ego-*dystonic*, somewhat foreign to or noticeable by the patient, and are associated with anxiety or met with confusion (e.g., see Chapter 10, Clinical Illustration 1 [*continued*], "Interpretation With an NPO Patient," in the subsection "Interpretation and Severity of Pathology") that interpretation is likely to be effective in promoting integrative processes. Toward this end, the therapist will repeatedly call attention to ego-syntonic ways of thinking, feeling, and behaving that are maladaptive or in some way problematic.

The process of repeated clarification and, in particular, confrontation helps patients experience familiar, habitual, and ego-syntonic patterns of behavior, thinking, and feeling as ego-dystonic personality traits. (This

---

[8]For example, the therapist might have interpreted the patient's conviction about her negative attitude toward him as a projection of her own hostility, or as a way to defend against the threatening possibility of a positive relationship developing between the two of them. These interventions would have been accurate, and these themes were fruitfully explored later in the treatment, but at this point, they would have been poorly timed—not compatible with the patient's current mental state and, as a result, useless at best.

process overlaps with the process of addressing concrete thinking, illustrated earlier in Part 2 of this chapter.) As habitual patterns of behaving, thinking, and feeling become ego-dystonic, the object relations embedded in and organizing personality traits become less effective in their defensive functions. At this point, underlying conflicts become accessible not only to interpretation proper, but also to exploration of underlying motivations and personal meanings. Thus, before introducing an interpretation, the therapist looks for evidence that defenses have become ego-dystonic and that underlying anxieties and conflicts are beginning to be accessible to the patient (e.g., see Chapter 10, Clinical Illustration 1 [*continued*], "Interpretation With an NPO Patient").

Clinical Illustration 9: Ego-Dystonicity in an NPO Patient

Ms. N was the young woman with hysterical personality traits and sexual inhibitions who functioned at a neurotic level of personality organization, described previously in Clinical Illustration 1, Chapter 2; and Clinical Illustration 2, Chapter 7. She experienced herself as unattractive to men, even though she was objectively both personally appealing and extremely attractive. Initially, her therapist attempted to make what proved to be premature, albeit accurate, interpretations of underlying dynamics, having to do with guilt in relation to competition and conflictual wishes to be the center of attention, experienced unconsciously by the patient as aggressive transgressions. These interpretations were of interest to the patient, and she felt they rang true, but they appeared to have little if any impact on her sense of herself or on her behavior.

Recognizing that his response to this well-integrated patient had been to assume incorrectly that she could quickly benefit from interpretations of meanings and motivations, the therapist shifted his approach to emphasize more basic interventions. Rather than attempting to promote Ms. N's understanding of her conflicts, he focused instead on supporting her capacity to observe and be aware of the impact of her defensive self representation on her subjective experience. The therapist conceptualized this objective in terms of helping to promote a shift within the patient, away from the rigid, subtly concrete quality of her thinking and experience in relation to sexual conflicts, organized by her defensive self representation ("I am unattractive to men, who are not interested in me; this is a fact, not a feeling, fear, or belief; no man will ever be interested in me; if someone indicates interest, I automatically and out of my conscious awareness disregard it or misinterpret it in order to avoid having to question my defensive perspective").

The therapist focused on the rigidity of Ms. N's view of herself, pointing out that she repeatedly had the same experience regardless of the setting, and he confronted her ego-syntonic denial or dismissal of obvious

indications of interest from a number of men. He helped her articulate the
defensive object relation organizing much of her experience—that of an
unattractive, inferior self in relation to more attractive, happy women or
to kind but disinterested men—and then repeatedly called her attention to
her denial of evidence supporting other views of herself.

With time, Ms. N began to understand what the therapist was seeing
and describing: that she seemed to choose to see herself in a single way,
and that when she began to entertain alternative views of herself, feelings
of anxiety and waves of nonspecific self-criticism quickly followed. While
her defensive view of herself had not yet changed, this view was no longer
concretely held and was becoming ego-dystonic; it was beginning to seem
strange to her that in this aspect of her thinking and experience, she was
so rigid, and that her view seemed to be distorted and constricted. She
wondered what this was about, why it was that she saw herself so differently from the way that others apparently saw her. At this point, both therapist and patient found themselves thinking about the therapist's early
interpretations; the patient felt curious and saw this as an opportunity to
understand something about herself and potentially to expand and modify
her self representation.

Comments: This vignette begins with an illustration of a premature interpretation with an NPO patient. The therapist's interpretations are accurate, but they are superficially accepted by the patient, and they have
little impact. Even though overall, Ms. N is a reflective person, at this
juncture in her treatment and in relation to this core conflict, she is not
able to make use of self-understanding to change her behavior or her feelings about herself. In contrast, when the therapist moves away from interpretation of unconscious motivations and meanings to focus on more
basic interventions, things begin to shift. As the therapist repeatedly confronts the rigidity of Ms. N's experience and the subtle distortions introduced by her defenses, what had been ego-syntonic character traits (e.g.,
Ms. N's reserved behavior in relation to suitable men) and seamless, defensive self representations (e.g., "I am not attractive to men," "I am inferior to other women") are transformed into ego-dystonic ways of
functioning. It is only at this point that Ms. N comes to fully appreciate
the extent to which she is actively doing something, organizing her experience in a particular manner; this insight opens up in her mind the possibility that she might be able to see and do things differently.

The shift in the quality of Ms. N's experience resulting from the therapist's confrontations can be understood in terms of the emergence of a
greater capacity to fully appreciate the symbolic and constructed nature
of her experience in an area of conflict. As Ms. N's defenses become ego-
dystonic and she becomes frustrated by habitual behaviors linked to character defenses, underlying anxieties motivating defensive object relations

became more accessible to consciousness. At this point, interpretation of unconscious meanings and motivations could be effective, promoting integrative processes associated with more flexible and adaptive functioning, including modification of Ms. N's habitual behaviors and ultimately, of her sense of self.

Clinical Illustration 10: Ego-Dystonicity in a BPO Patient

Mr. E, a patient with narcissistic personality disorder organized at a high borderline level, had chronic financial problems. In his work as a midlevel salesman, he routinely went on sprees in which he would take friends out for a night on the town, visiting swank restaurants and high-end bars, and then at the end of the evening expansively pick up the entire tab. When his therapist pointed out that this behavior seemed to run at cross-purposes with the patient's stated goal of improving his financial situation, Mr. E explained that he had no intention of giving up these evenings, that the therapist failed to understand how important they were to him; he said that such events formed the center of his social life and served as a prominent source of self-esteem.

Over time, Mr. E's therapist was able to help the patient flesh out the object relations embedded in his maladaptive behavior: when Mr. E was out on the town, he felt like a king, expansive and able to take generous care of his subjects; however, if he imagined not being able to engage in this behavior, he thought of himself as a wretched pauper—dismissed, isolated, and pitied by all. The patient concurred that this was indeed how he felt. The therapist also pointed out Mr. E's assumption that his friends spent time with him only to the extent that they were able to exploit him financially.

For many months, the patient's sessions focused on this and similar material. Throughout, the therapist maintained an attitude of neutrality, concerned about Mr. E but refraining from being directive; and all the while, the patient insisted that he couldn't agree to relinquish his expansive behavior, regardless of the ramifications.

Several months into this process, Mr. E acknowledged a point of confusion in his view of the therapist that troubled him. The patient explained that he found it difficult to understand how and why the therapist remained patient with him since he, Mr. E, consistently failed to modify his behavior in response to the therapist's comments. But, Mr. E went on to explain, he felt better now because he had come to understand; he now realized that the therapist was simply exploiting him, that the therapist didn't care about the treatment or about the patient, but was happy to just play along, pretend that he cared, and get paid.

At this juncture, the therapist was able to point out that Mr. E was experiencing the same set of expectations of him that they had identified in relation to the patient's friends: that the therapist was interested in the patient only insofar as he could exploit him, and that embedded in this was a view of the therapist as enjoying a feeling of superiority and privately mocking the patient. The therapist went on to comment that this seemed to be the prototype in Mr. E's mind for all relationships—that someone superior, exploiting, and mocking looked down on someone inferior, exploited, and humiliated. It was as if the patient could not imagine a relationship based on anything except one person taking advantage of another, and this view held true even in the protected situation with his therapist.

At this point, Mr. E became pensive and then anxious. He said, "I can see that maybe you aren't just exploiting me, that you enjoy getting paid, but also maybe you want to be of help or to handle things well in here. But I can't truly assimilate that view of you and our relationship; I keep going back to 'you're in it only for the money and to be in a superior position to me.' It's so weird."

The therapist understood Mr. E's comments as reflecting that at least for the moment, his assumptions about the basics of human relations had become ego-dystonic. The therapist saw this as opening the door to the long process of exploring and interpreting the conflicts underlying the patient's split, paranoid view of his interactions with others, with the goal of helping him modify them over time.

Comments: This vignette illustrates confrontation of ego-syntonic, maladaptive narcissistic personality traits. The therapist's initial interventions, calling attention to Mr. E's expansive and extravagant behaviors and attitudes, are met with Mr. E's unwavering investment in maintaining them; Mr. E does not view his behaviors or attitudes as problematic, and his underlying assumption that all relationships are based on exploitation is, from his perspective, neither open to question nor something he is motivated to change. As long as Mr. E is able to sustain his expansive state, anxieties in relation to vulnerability, inferiority, and exploitation are successfully split off from his dominant conscious experience. However, as the therapist repeatedly confronts Mr. E's insistence on spending money and elaborates Mr. E's split view that the world is comprised of magnanimous lords and pitiful paupers, Mr. E's defenses begin to weaken and become ego-dystonic. At this point, anxieties in relation to vulnerability and exploitation can no longer be completely split off from Mr. E's dominant, grandiose, self state; as Mr. E's defenses become less rigid, the underlying conflict is activated in the transference. As Mr. E struggles to maintain his view of the therapist as an exploiter, the therapist understands that Mr. E's grandiosity and splitting are no longer seamless, and underlying anxieties are emerging in the treatment; for the first time there is room to explore and interpret the motivations driving Mr. E's maladaptive behaviors and attitudes.

Key Clinical Concepts

- Analysis of transference makes use of clarification, confrontation, and interpretation to explore the patient's moment-to-moment experience of and behavior in relation to the therapist and the treatment.

- When affectively dominant object relations are enacted in relation to the therapist, the therapist's interventions will be transference focused.

- Treatment of BPO patients tends to be transference focused much of the time, whereas treatment of NPO patients is often focused on other relationships outside the treatment.

- Therapist-centered interpretations focus on articulating the patient's experience of the therapist without introducing any modifications.

- The interpretive process moves from surface to depth and from defense to impulse, focusing first on the patient's dominant experience and then gradually broadening and deepening the patient's view.

- The therapist attends not only to the content of the patient's experience in session, but also to the quality of that experience.

- When the patient's thinking is concrete, the therapist uses clarification and then confrontation to help the patient adopt an observing perspective.

References

Auchincloss AL, Samberg E (eds): Psychoanalytic Terms and Concepts. New Haven, CT, Yale University Press, 2012

Bion WR: Learning From Experience. London, Heinemann, 1962

Bion WR: Attacks on linking (1959), in Second Thoughts. London, Heinemann, 1967, pp 93–109

Bion WR: A theory of thinking (1962), in Second Thoughts. London, Heinemann, 1967, pp 110–119

Britton R: Naming and containing, in Belief and Imagination. London, Routledge, 1998, pp 19–28

Busch F: The ego and its significance in analytic interventions. J Am Psychoanal Assoc 44(4):1073–1099, 1996 8987011

Caligor E, Kernberg OF, Clarkin JF: Handbook of Dynamic Psychotherapy for Higher Level Personality Pathology. Washington, DC, American Psychiatric Publishing, 2007

Caligor E, Diamond D, Yeomans FE, Kernberg OF: The interpretive process in the psychoanalytic psychotherapy of borderline personality pathology. J Am Psychoanal Assoc 57(2):271–301, 2009 19516053

Fenichel O: Problems of Psychoanalytic Technique. New York, Psychoanalytic Quarterly, 1941

Høglend P: Exploration of the patient-therapist relationship in psychotherapy. Am J Psychiatry 171(10):1056–1066, 2014 25017093

Høglend P, Gabbard GO: When is transference work useful in psychodynamic psychotherapy? A review of empirical research, in Psychodynamic Psychotherapy Research: Evidence-Based Practice and Practice-Based Evidence. Edited by Levy A, Ablon JS, Kächele H. New York, Springer, 2012, pp 449–467

Høglend P, Amlo S, Marble A, et al: Analysis of the patient-therapist relationship in dynamic psychotherapy: an experimental study of transference interpretations. Am J Psychiatry 163(10):1739–1746, 2006 17012684

Johansson P, Høglend P, Ulberg R, et al: The mediating role of insight for long-term improvements in psychodynamic therapy. J Consult Clin Psychol 78:438–448, 2010 20515219

Kernberg OF: Internal World and External Reality: Object Relations Theory Applied. New York, Jason Aronson, 1980

Kernberg OF: The destruction of time in pathological narcissism. Int J Psychoanal 89(2):299–312, 2008 18405285

Levy ST, Inderbitzin LB: Neutrality, interpretation, and therapeutic intent. J Am Psychoanal Assoc 40(4):989–1011, 1992 1430771

Schafer R: The Contemporary Kleinians of London. Madison, CT, International Universities Press, 1997

Steiner J: Patient-centered and analyst-centered interpretations: some implications of containment and countertransference. Psychoanal Inq 14:406–422, 1994

Yeomans F, Clarkin JF, Kernberg OF: Transference-Focused Psychotherapy for Borderline Personality Disorder: A Clinical Guide. Washington, DC, American Psychiatric Publishing, 2015

Intervening III

Integrating Supportive and Exploratory Interventions

IN THE PRECEDING TWO CHAPTERS ON
intervention techniques, we discussed clarification, confrontation, and interpretation (Chapter 10) and transference analysis and the tactics guiding intervention (Chapter 11) in transference-focused psychotherapy—extended (TFP-E). We complete our discussion of clinical techniques in this chapter, in which we cover 1) the use of supportive techniques in TFP-E, followed by coverage of exploratory interventions with 2) management of technical neutrality, 3) use of countertransference, and 4) the process of working through. Although exploratory interventions are central to TFP-E, we begin with discussion of supportive interventions because their use may be needed first in the treatment flow, integrated with the exploratory interventions discussed later in this chapter.

Use of Supportive Interventions

In the following discussion, we address the use of supportive interventions in TFP-E, and consider how to integrate the use of supportive techniques into a predominantly exploratory treatment. The supportive interventions most commonly employed in TFP-E are contracting, limit setting, recontracting, providing advice or encouragement, and expressing concern.

Differentiating Between Exploratory and Supportive Interventions

Exploratory, or "expressive," interventions can be conceptualized as those interventions that explore the patient's internal experience and behavior with the objective of increasing his level of self-awareness and self-understanding (Gabbard 2010). In TFP-E, exploratory interventions are made from a position of technical neutrality. Clarification, confrontation, and interpretation proper are exploratory interventions, as detailed in Chapter 10.

In our discussion of the interpretive process (Chapter 10) and its application to transference analysis (Chapter 11), we emphasized that exploratory techniques in TFP-E are conceptualized as serving multiple functions. In addition to promoting self-awareness and self-understanding, exploratory interventions at the same time function to support and help consolidate central psychological capacities that are often vulnerable in patients with personality disorders. We focus in particular on capacities for reality testing, affect containment, self-observation, introspection, reflection, entertaining alternative perspectives, and contextualizing experience. Thus, while maintaining a neutral stance and making use of the interpretive process, the TFP-E therapist intervenes to support psychological capacities often compromised in the patient with a personality disorder.

Although the TFP-E therapist employs the interpretive process to support core psychological capacities in the patient and also to communicate empathy with the patient's experience, the therapist does not *routinely* make use of *conventional* supportive interventions. Examples of these conventional supportive interventions include limit setting, skills training, directly intervening in the patient's life (e.g., helping the patient negotiate with his family or spouse), and providing guidance, advice, praise, or reassurance (Winston et al. 2012). All of these interventions can be classified as supportive, in contrast to the exploratory or expressive interventions that are the mainstay of the TFP-E approach. Use of supportive interventions is characterized by the therapist's deviation from the neutral stance of TFP-E for a particular, temporary, and necessary purpose: to ally with one part of the patient in relation to another, to assume responsibility for intervening on the patient's behalf, or to actively promote particular behaviors in an area in which the patient's functioning is compromised. Table 12–1 shows the role of exploratory and supportive interventions in TFP-E.

TABLE 12–1. **Exploratory and supportive interventions in transference-focused psychotherapy—extended (TFP-E)**

Exploratory interventions: central techniques of TFP-E

Purpose

Explore internal experience and behavior

Increase self-awareness and self-understanding

Support capacities often vulnerable in patients with personality disorders

    Reality testing

    Affect containment

    Self-observation

    Introspection

    Reflection

    Entertaining alternative perspectives

    Contextualizing experience

Stance: technical neutrality

Clarification, confrontation, interpretation

Transference analysis

Countertransference analysis

Working through

Supportive interventions: ancillary techniques of TFP-E

Purpose

Limit destructive and disruptive behavior

Maintain necessary conditions for treatment

Protect therapeutic alliance

Stance: temporarily abandon technical neutrality

    Contracting

    Limit setting

    Recontracting

    Advice, encouragement, concern

Ancillary Role of Supportive Interventions

Despite the central role played by exploratory interventions and the therapist's neutral stance in TFP-E, there are times when the therapist will opt to deviate from neutrality to make use of supportive, or structuring, techniques.[1] Thus, technical neutrality (described in Chapter 5 and later in this chapter, in the section "Managing Technical Neutrality") can be seen as the TFP-E therapist's baseline stance, a stance the therapist deviates from when circumstances indicate but to which the therapist always returns.

The Consultation and Contracting Phase

As discussed in Chapters 8 and 9, in TFP-E, the viability of what is predominantly an exploratory treatment rests upon establishing a frame that provides sufficient structure for the patient with personality pathology to safely and productively engage in treatment. Structured aspects of the treatment are introduced before treatment begins in the form of the treatment contract and treatment goals, and treatment does not formally begin until the contract and goals are in place. This structured framework provides a stable setting within which an unstructured (but systematic) exploratory process can unfold in a relatively controlled and therapeutic fashion. Thus, during the consultation and contracting phase, the therapist is not neutral, but rather assumes a supportive, structuring stance, with the objective of creating a treatment setting in which it becomes possible to maintain technical neutrality.

In the transition from the contracting phase to treatment proper, the therapist shifts her stance and her style of intervention. In the consultation and contracting sessions, the therapist has clear, short-term objectives in each session, and she actively structures the sessions to meet those objectives; when she introduces the necessary conditions for treatment, her stance is directive and to some degree authoritative (i.e., "This is what is needed for this treatment"). In contrast, once treatment begins, the therapist assumes a neutral stance; the therapist waits for the patient's communications and behavior to determine the content of the session, relies on exploratory interventions, and abstains from being directive.

The Start of Treatment

In the ideal case, careful assessment and contracting will create a treatment setting that successfully contains destructive and disruptive behavior. In this ideal situation, from the beginning of treatment through the time treatment ends, the necessary conditions of treatment will be maintained, with the therapist maintaining a neutral stance throughout. However, many cases are less than ideal. It is relatively common, especially in

---

[1]In addition, there are times when driven by countertransference pressures or by inexperience, the therapist will unintentionally abandon neutrality to provide support to or to direct the patient.

the early phase of treatment (see Chapter 13) and with patients who are especially prone to acting out or who have more severe pathology, for the structuring functions of the frame combined with the exploratory interventions of confronting and interpreting to be insufficient to contain all behavior potentially threatening the patient's safety or the viability of the treatment (Yeomans et al. 2015).

When patients persist in destructive or treatment-disrupting behavior, the therapist will abandon neutrality to set limits, structuring the treatment to support behavioral control, as needed. Limit setting is the central nonexploratory technique employed by the TFP-E therapist during the course of treatment. If needed, limit setting will be supplemented by recontracting (see Chapter 8), and in certain circumstances, a meeting with a member of the patient's family or his significant other may be necessary. These interventions are complemented by techniques related to managing technical neutrality.

In the treatment of patients functioning at a borderline level of personality organization (BPO), especially those with prominent borderline, narcissistic, or antisocial features, the need to temporarily deviate from neutrality to introduce a limit is a relatively common development. Especially early in treatment, clinical situations routinely arise that call on the therapist to actively intervene by setting limits in order to protect the patient, the therapist herself, or the viability of the treatment. In contrast, in the treatment of patients organized at a high borderline level and especially patients functioning at a neurotic level of personality organization (NPO), clinical developments calling on the therapist to provide supportive interventions are less common; it is generally possible to maintain the frame, to make use of exploratory interventions, and to maintain a neutral stance with relative consistency.

Limit Setting

Limit setting entails the TFP-E therapist's stepping out of her baseline neutral stance to introduce additional structure, as needed to maintain the treatment frame and the necessary conditions for treatment. When limit setting is employed in TFP-E, it is most frequently directed toward 1) ensuring that the boundaries established by the treatment contract are maintained; 2) controlling destructive acting out, both in and outside sessions; and 3) limiting secondary gain (see also the next subsection, "Managing Secondary Gain"). The TFP-E therapist is selective with regard to limit setting, doing so only when clinically necessary to protect the viability of the treatment or the safety of the patient and others, and by introducing the minimal degree of structure needed.

Central to the TFP-E model is the observation that the objective of limit setting in response to acting-out behavior goes beyond securing behavioral control; *limit setting* is the process of containing the patient's habitual forms of acting out that leads to activation and elaboration in the treatment of the object relations organizing maladaptive behaviors and associated personality traits. These object relations then become the focus of exploration in the therapy.

In sum, in the face of destructive or disruptive acting out, the TFP-E therapist's goal is to explore the object relations being acted out or enacted as they relate to the patient's core conflicts and defenses, and in particular as they are played out in the transference. To achieve this goal, it is typically necessary to contain destructive behavior; at those times when confrontation and interpretation prove insufficient to provide behavioral control, the therapist will make use of limit setting.

Clinical Illustration 1: Limit Setting Around the Treatment Frame and Contract

Ms. Q is a 28-year-old visual artist functioning at a high borderline level, with prominent histrionic and dependent traits. For several years prior to beginning treatment, she had been drinking moderately, with good control, but she reported a prior history of binge drinking with serious sequelae during and after college. In the contracting phase, she and her therapist agreed that she would limit her drinking to one or two glasses of wine or beer two or three times weekly during the treatment. If she found herself drinking in excess of this restriction, she would immediately bring up her behavior as the priority issue at the beginning of her next therapy session.

Six months into what had been a relatively smooth and seemingly productive opening phase, Ms. Q came into a Friday morning session 10 minutes late, poorly groomed and with bloodshot eyes. She apologized for her lateness and then launched into a description of the "super-fun" evening she'd had the previous night; she had discovered a new club and met a new group of established young artists who, she had no doubt, would foster her professional development.

As Dr. K asked for more specifics about the evening [*clarification*], it emerged that Ms. Q had been out until 4:00 A.M. and had then slept very poorly. Dr. K asked about Ms. Q's alcohol consumption over the course of the evening. Ms. Q casually commented that it had been a long evening and she had "a fair amount to drink." Dr. K inquired specifically if her drinking represented a violation of their agreement, to which Ms. Q responded, "Yes, I guess so, but not a big deal—it won't happen again."

Over the course of the session, Dr. K shared his concerns, focusing on Ms. Q's failure to directly bring up the drinking as a problem at the beginning of the session, as they had agreed, as well as her minimizing its significance when he inquired. He reminded her of their initial discussion about her history of drinking and the problems it had caused her, and also commented that anything more than very limited consumption of alcohol was incompatible with the kind of treatment she was pursuing.

Ms. Q ultimately acknowledged the significance of her behavior and assured Dr. K that it would not happen again. Dr. K shared his concern that Ms. Q's behavior reflected a wavering commitment to the treatment. He reminded her of recent gains she had made and pointed out that her behavior the previous evening seemed to be part of a long-standing pattern of making gains and then undoing them by turning to alcohol and/or destructive relationships that undermined her stability and personal and professional growth. Ms. Q nodded in agreement, saying that up until then, she hadn't thought about the evening in these terms; it had simply felt "so exciting."

The following session focused on Ms. Q's perception of Dr. K as weak and conventional, unable to appreciate the exciting, risk-taking, and creative parts of Ms. Q that were necessary for her artwork. Together they came to understand Ms. Q's recent drinking as a rebellion against constraints and as an expression of her freedom, but in a form that was destructive and that distanced her from the helpful view she held of Dr. K, and from the more controlled parts of herself that had forged a positive, somewhat idealized relation with him. They agreed that they were touching on important conflicts closely tied to her presenting complaints and best explored in the setting of ongoing control of her drinking, as they had originally agreed.

The following Monday morning, Ms. Q again arrived late to her session, again with bloodshot eyes. Dr. K wondered to himself whether she was mildly intoxicated. When he inquired, she said that she was thinking clearly, but with a grin, she acknowledged having spent the evening with the same group of artists and having gone on "quite a bender." After briefly exploring Ms. Q's attitude toward her behavior—and especially her pleasure in casting Dr. K as weak and conventional, while she felt superior and part of an exciting "darker side"—Dr. K returned to a discussion of the treatment contract. He shared with Ms. Q that he understood her behavior as an active effort to abort her treatment; no doubt, there was a part of her—the part that came to sessions and engaged in honest discourse with him—that was committed to the treatment, but there seemed to be another part, connected to her "darker side," that was making continuation of the treatment impossible, perhaps stimulated by recent gains she had seemed to be making.

Ms. Q asked Dr. K, "Are you kicking me out?" Dr. K replied that he thought they should consider the best way to proceed, but that it would be foolhardy and potentially destructive to continue under the present conditions. From his perspective, Dr. K explained, Ms. Q's recent behavior was destructive and perilous, threatening to disrupt her treatment and potentially endangering her life. He pointed out that they had already spoken about it at length but that she seemed unable or unwilling to change her behavior; it seemed she had put him in the position of having to step out of his usual role to revisit the treatment contract and to institute new limits on her drinking in an effort to preserve the treatment.

Dr. K went on to suggest that Ms. Q abstain from drinking entirely and return to Alcoholics Anonymous. If she felt unwilling to do these things, they could consider switching to a once-weekly, behaviorally oriented treatment, focusing on her drinking and associated destructive behaviors. The session then ended, and Ms. Q walked out after having expressed resentment at Dr. K's "inflexibility and conventionality." Dr. K was left unclear as to what was likely to transpire, and somewhat concerned that Ms. Q would return to the active alcohol abuse that had characterized her college and postcollege years.

Ms. Q came to her next session on time, seemingly clearheaded. She resentfully told Dr. K that she had been complaining about him to her parents and sister, sharing with them that he insisted on her not drinking, when everyone in the arts used recreational drugs and alcohol. To her surprise, her parents had supported Dr. K's position; they reminded Ms. Q in painful detail of the price she had paid for her drinking in the past, and of the family history of alcoholism (noting her father was a "sober alcoholic"). Ms. Q then begrudgingly told Dr. K that she would comply with the new arrangements.

Dr. K shared his hesitation based on concern that her attitude revealed very mixed feelings and a wavering commitment to the treatment. They would continue to assess whether, at this point in her life, Ms. Q was sufficiently motivated to get a grip on the more destructive aspects of her personality. If she proved unable to adhere to their new agreement, they would have to interrupt the treatment and consider alternative options.

Comments: In this example, Dr. K dealt with the first contract violation with clarification, confrontation, and ultimately interpretation of the object relations organizing the patient's behavior, while maintaining a neutral stance. He reviewed the contract, reminding Ms. Q of both the rationale for and the necessity of their agreement, while maintaining technical neutrality.

After the second contract violation, Dr. K again alluded to the conflict within Ms. Q and the dangers of her behavior, but opted at this point to deviate from a neutral stance in order to set a limit—in essence, saying that treatment could not rationally continue under the present conditions, and suggesting a new contractual arrangement of attendance at Alcoholics Anonymous and total sobriety. At that point, it was up to Ms. Q to decide whether she was interested in continuing the treatment under the newly introduced conditions. She was free to refuse, but in that case, the treatment would be discontinued in its current form.

Clinical Illustration 2: Limit Setting Around Acting-Out Behavior Inside Sessions

Ms. D, a 34-year-old homemaker functioning at a middle borderline level, with both borderline and narcissistic personality traits, had a history of anger outbursts, especially in relation to her husband and children when they did not do as she wanted. In the first months of treatment, she was frequently hostile and derisive toward Dr. Z.

In one session, Ms. D started to raise her voice, insulting Dr. Z and yelling at her, cutting her off when she attempted to speak and leaving the therapist distracted by concerns about disturbing other clinicians in adjacent offices. Ms. D continued to escalate her behavior, intermittently getting out of her chair and moving around the office. Her repeated interruptions made it impossible for Dr. Z to explore what might be happening between them; when Dr. Z attempted to comment on Ms. D's behavior, Ms. D spoke over her until Dr. Z fell silent. Meanwhile, it was clear that Ms. D was obtaining a great deal of satisfaction from her own behavior.

Dr. Z started to feel that she couldn't think clearly because of Ms. D's nonstop barrage of insults and complaints, along with her moving around the office. Dr. Z firmly interrupted Ms. D to introduce a limit: "I am going to have to ask you to lower your voice and take your seat so that we can discuss what is happening here."

Ms. D responded, "Discuss, discuss! I can do whatever I want here. I am here to express my feelings, to tell you 'whatever comes to mind,' and what comes to mind is that I can shout if I so choose!"

Dr. Z responded by concurring that Ms. D was free to share her feelings, and indeed Dr. Z was very interested in hearing what Ms. D had to say, but raising her voice in that way precluded their working productively together. The doctor explained that she was asking Ms. D to modify her behavior because she found it difficult to think when Ms. D was yelling and pacing; also, the noise was disruptive to other clinicians in the office suite, which was not acceptable.

Ms. D again began to shout derisively. She insisted, "It's my therapy hour, I'm paying for it, and I'm free to do whatever I want here!"

Dr. Z responded that in fact that was not true. She went on to say that if Ms. D was unable to control her behavior, Dr. Z would have to ask her to leave the session to collect herself. She added that she thought that what Ms. D was playing out with her today was important, and if she could sit down and lower her voice, they might be able to learn something valuable. Dr. Z stated that simply unloading hostility and disrupting the office was not productive in terms of Ms. D's therapy, but taking a look at and trying to understand her behavior was important, and was closely linked to the difficulties in her home life that had brought her to treatment in the first place.

Clinical Illustration 3: Limit Setting Around Acting-Out Behavior Outside Sessions

Mr. X, a 55-year-old man functioning at a high borderline level, with masochistic and narcissistic features, had a history of severe hypertension treated with a combination of three different medications. He had a long history of poor compliance with his medications, leading to several emergency room visits for hypertensive crises. As part of his treatment contract with Dr. Y, Mr. X had agreed to take his medications as prescribed, to see his internist's nurse monthly for blood pressure monitoring, and to arrange for her to contact Dr. Y to keep her abreast of Mr. X's medical management.

A year into the treatment, Dr. Y noticed that things had started to feel empty in Mr. X's sessions, and at the same time, Dr. Y realized that she had not heard from Mr. X's medical team for several months. Dr. Y commented on the lack of communication and asked Mr. X what was going on with his medication and follow-up. Mr. X responded that he had been busy and unable to get to the doctor, but that "everything is fine."

Dr. Y was alarmed, concerned about the possibility that Mr. X's blood pressure was or would become dangerously out of control. She recognized that her anxiety was distracting her from thinking clearly and neutrally about the object relations organizing Mr. X's behavior. Dr. Y then inquired specifically about medication compliance, and Mr. X glibly acknowledged that he had been "missing a few doses here and there."

Dr. Y commented on how destructive Mr. X's behavior was and wondered if it explained the empty quality that they had noted in recent sessions; it seemed the real action in the treatment was being played out in Mr. X's failure to care for himself, while concealing his actions from Dr. Y. Dr. Y commented that it would be important to understand what was motivating Mr. X's behavior, but first it was necessary to ensure his safety. She reminded Mr. X that his behavior represented a violation of their treatment contract, given that compliance with his blood pressure management was a necessary condition for his treatment; there was no point in treating his personality pathology if he was at the same time putting his long-term health and even his life in danger. Dr. Y told Mr. X that he would need to have his blood pressure checked before attending his next therapy appointment, and that he should bring a note from his doctor to the therapy appointment as documentation of his blood pressure and his medication compliance.

Comments on Ms. D and Mr. X: The vignette with Ms. D illustrates limit setting to manage in-session acting-out behavior (frequently referred to as "acting in"). The vignette with Mr. X illustrates limit setting in relation to destructive acting out outside the therapy hour and a contract violation. In TFP-E, patients may turn to acting out as a way to express the pathogenic object relations activated in the treatment and in the transference, without being fully conscious of or reflecting on them. In this setting, the first step toward productive exploration is behavioral control, to the extent needed to ensure that the patient is out of acute danger, the therapist is able to think clearly without undue distraction, and the behavioral boundaries established in the treatment contract are maintained.

The therapist can infer that Ms. D was enjoying acting on her hostility and disrupting Dr. Z's ability to think and her office mates' ability to work in a professional environment. Central goals for the treatment were to help Ms. D take responsibility for the sense of omnipotence and sadistic pleasure that she derived from her behavior, to appreciate the negative impact of such behavior on herself and her relationships, and to understand the complex motivations organizing both her destructive rage and her refusal to take responsibility for it. In the session we describe, Dr. Z's initial efforts to comment on or explore Ms. D's behavior were futile. At the same time, Dr. Z felt strongly that allowing Ms. D to simply vent in session as she was doing would be counterproductive and would represent a destructive transference-countertransference enactment of a hostile, bullying, entitled patient and a weak, cowed, ineffective therapist. In Dr. Z's judgment, setting limits in relation to the acting-out behavior was the necessary first step toward helping Ms. D better manage her hostility.

Mr. X, on the other hand, was endangering himself and violating his treatment contract, necessitating limit setting and at the same time creating an opportunity to clarify and explore the object relations organizing his chronic poor compliance and self-destructive behavior: a defiant, sadistic self, happy to hurt himself in return for the pleasure of tormenting a helpless, panicked, and frustrated authority.

Clinical Illustration 4: Limit Setting Around Secondary Gain Threatening Viability of Treatment

Mr. U, 20 years old, was in treatment for failure to work in school. Carrying a diagnosis of narcissistic personality disorder, he had a long history of truancy and of failing to study or to hand in assignments, and was currently on academic probation. He spent much of his time holed up in his dorm room, either sleeping or listening to music. His parents were totally exasperated and agreed to pay for his therapy, which allowed the patient to protect a small inheritance he had received from his grandfather.

Dr. P had met with Mr. U and his family before treatment began, and had explained his policy of charging for missed sessions unless the patient contacted him 24 hours in advance. Mr. U frequently missed sessions. In exploring his behavior, it became clear that behind Mr. U's habitual explanation of "lacking motivation" was a long-standing and highly gratifying pattern of frustrating those in positions of authority: his parents, his teachers, and now Dr. P. It also emerged that Mr. U derived particular pleasure from his parents' frustration at paying for sessions that Mr. U failed to attend.

Although discussions of this kind were perhaps illuminating, they did nothing to modify Mr. U's behavior. It became clear to Dr. P that the gratification Mr. U derived from wasting his parents' money, frustrating them in the process, was contributing to his poor attendance, seemingly overriding whatever motivation he had to make productive use of the therapy.

Dr. P explained his concern to Mr. U and suggested that they set up a meeting with Mr. U and his parents to discuss the problem and ideas to remedy it. In that meeting, Dr. P explained to Mr. U's parents that the arrangement for the payment and their eagerness to see their son do better were perversely working against the treatment by motivating Mr. U to skip sessions freely and to waste time when he was in session. Dr. P went on to explore with Mr. U and his parents what alternative arrangements could be made. Dr. P suggested that perhaps they could agree that Mr. U would find a job that would enable him to pay on his own for any sessions he missed.

Mr. U's parents were concerned that this was not realistic, given Mr. U's difficulty even in getting his schoolwork done; they questioned his ability to work both at a job and in school. After much discussion, it was agreed that Mr. U would use funds from his inheritance to pay for any missed appointments, and that his parents would continue to pay for sessions that he attended. Dr. P made clear that this was only a first step, and if Mr. U continued to routinely miss sessions and to waste time when he did attend, they would be forced to reconsider the viability of the treatment.

Comments: This clinical illustration portrays a patient's motivations for both primary and secondary gain. *Primary gain* refers to the basic motivation for a symptom or maladaptive behavior. In this case, Mr. U's grandiosity (his need to feel above all constraints and demands, which he experienced as a humiliation) was motivating him to miss sessions. These dynamics made it difficult for him to actively participate in treatment, just as they made it difficult for him to participate fully in his education.

Secondary gain refers to additional benefits that accrue to symptoms and maladaptive behaviors and that tend to reinforce them. In this case, Mr. U's pleasure at frustrating his parents and wasting their money provided secondary gain. Dr. P ultimately found it necessary to deviate from neutrality to meet with Mr. U's family, to set limits with Mr. U, and to work with the family to arrange for alternative ways to pay for missed sessions.

Managing Secondary Gain

Many patients with personality disorders experience themselves as unable to control or modify maladaptive behaviors (e.g., Mr. U maintained that he was simply unable to consistently attend his therapy sessions—that to do so was impossible). In contrast, TFP-E is predicated on the clinical observation that patients with personality disorders are typically less behaviorally constrained by their personality pathology than they and/or their loved ones may imagine; we find that many patients with personality disorders presenting with "intractable" destructive behaviors are able to modify these behaviors within a number of months of beginning treatment. This is especially true if secondary gains that have reinforced maladaptive behaviors can be removed or contained.

Secondary gain comes in many forms. Often, secondary gain is financial—for example, a patient who receives social benefits for psychiatric disability when he is unable to work, or a patient who remains financially dependent on his family. Another form of secondary gain is illustrated by the patient who uses the fact that he is "working on it in therapy" to avoid having to address his real-life problems or destructive behavior. Other forms of secondary gain involve the control and torture of others that can result from destructive and suicidal behavior (e.g., the patient whose wife, family, or therapist must walk on eggshells for fear of provoking him and stimulating his self-destructive behavior; the patient who leaves an anxiety-inducing message for her therapist or boyfriend in which she says she is suicidal).

In general, management of secondary gain requires contracting and limit setting, ideally before treatment begins but not uncommonly during treatment as well, as in the case of Mr. U. The TFP-E treatment frame and contract are designed to eliminate many potential sources of secondary gain. In particular, as part of the contracting phase, the therapist makes clear 1) that she is "out of the loop" of the patient's self-destructive behavior, and rather that these behaviors are the domain of emergency or crisis services; and 2) that she does not accept into treatment a patient who rejects the expectation that he will engage in productive, structured activity outside the treatment (see Chapter 8, "Essential Treatment Contracting," sections "General Principles: Introducing Specific Parameters Into the Treatment Contract" and "Contracting Around Specific Behaviors, Adjunctive Treatments, and Medication"). In addition, the therapist may opt to introduce specific arrangements during the contracting phase, tailored to the individual patient and his situation, to reduce the impact of secondary gains on the clinical process (see Chapter 8).

In many cases, as illustrated by Mr. U, the need for special arrangements in relation to secondary gain may become apparent only after treatment has begun. Often, it becomes necessary to set limits and, if need be, to recontract around sources of secondary gain. In those cases where it is not possible to adequately control secondary gain (e.g., if Mr. U's parents had insisted on continuing to pay for all his sessions), the viability of the treatment should be called into question. It is often best in such situations to openly discuss with the patient, and his family if appropriate, the prospect of interrupting TFP-E to switch to basic clinical management or some other form of "maintenance" treatment.

Use of Exploratory Interventions

In the following discussion, we further address the exploratory interventions of managing technical neutrality, utilizing countertransference, and the process of working through.

Managing Technical Neutrality

As we have emphasized, the TFP-E therapist's baseline stance is one of technical neutrality, in which she observes and comments on, rather than taking sides or participating in, the patient's internal conflicts (Auchincloss and Samberg 2012). However, technical neutrality is not a stance that the therapist adheres to rigidly, and she does not do so blindly. When the therapist assumes a directive stance in the face of a contract violation or behavior that is acutely dangerous or that threatens the viability of the treatment, she is temporality deviating from neutrality.

The therapist will always first attempt to address a clinical situation from a neutral position, making use of clarification, confrontation, and interpretation of the object relations and conflicts organizing the patient's experience and behavior. However, there will be times in any treatment when the therapist decides to deviate from neutrality to secure behavioral control or perhaps to provide practical or emotional support. After deviating from neutrality, the therapist will explore the patient's experience of the deviation, and in that process reestablish her neutral stance.

Deviating From and Reinstating Neutrality

In TFP-E, when the therapist deviates from technical neutrality, she *temporarily* assumes a supportive stance. When the therapist decides to deviate to provide limits on destructive behavior to maintain the frame, she begins by reviewing with the patient the events leading up to her decision. As part of this process, the therapist shares with the patient her thinking in choosing to deviate, making clear that she is responding to a clinical necessity created by the patient. The therapist then introduces a limit in an effort to help the patient attain behavioral control.

TABLE 12–2. Tips for deviating from and reinstating neutrality

Deviating from neutrality to set limits

1. Attempt to intervene from a neutral position.
2. If necessary to deviate, explain reason for deviation.
3. Announce deviation and introduce a limit-setting intervention.

Reinstating neutrality

1. Wait until crisis has passed and patient is more reflective.
2. Review the deviation and reasons for deviating.
3. Review patient's experience of the deviation.
4. Explore object relations organizing the transference and enacted in the deviation.

Once the crisis is past and the patient is more reflective, the therapist reviews the deviation and the therapist's reasons for having deviated. She then reviews the patient's experience of the deviation and links the deviation to the object relations enacted in the therapist's modifying her stance and her taking a directive position in relation to the patient. The final stage in the process of reinstating neutrality entails exploring and elaborating the object relations embedded in and concealed by the patient's behavior and the therapist's response. This process often leads to a deeper understanding of previously split-off aspects of the transference. Table 12–2 provides tips for deviating from and reinstating neutrality.

Clinical Illustration 5: Deviating From and Reinstating Neutrality

In a Friday afternoon session, Ms. W, a single mother diagnosed with borderline personality disorder, told her therapist that she was going out of town for the weekend. She mentioned in passing her plan to leave her 6-year-old daughter with Ms. W's boyfriend. Dr. P pointed out to the patient that Ms. W had repeatedly complained about the boyfriend, who was known to abuse cocaine, as someone irresponsible and unreliable. Dr. P then asked Ms. W about her thoughts and feelings in relation to leaving her daughter in this man's hands. Ms. W shrugged, acknowledging Dr. P's words, but as if to communicate "this is not my problem."

Maintaining a neutral stance, Dr. P called attention to Ms. W's apparent nonchalance in relation to endangering her child, but her attitude remained bland, and she demonstrated no apparent intention to modify her plans. Dr. P reminded Ms. W that one of her treatment goals was to be a good mother and not to repeat the mistakes made by her own mother, who had abused substances and neglected her children.

Ms. W's attitude remained bland. She appeared free of all anxiety, while Dr. P noted that he was feeling afraid for the child and in some way responsible for protecting her. Making use of this countertransference, Dr. P ventured an interpretation, pointing out that it seemed Ms. W was handing off to him the part of herself that anxiously wanted to be a good mother, while in her behavior she was identifying with the part of herself that would callously neglect the child, as her own mother had neglected her. The patient was dismissive, responding that whatever the risk the weekend might pose to her child, it was hers to manage as she wished.

Comments: This vignette illustrates that **neutrality does not imply passivity.** Confronting a patient with her denial of reality, as Dr. P did in pointing out the obvious dangers to which Ms. W was exposing her daughter, is consistent with maintaining a technically neutral stance. Similarly, reminding Ms. W of her treatment goals is also consistent with technical neutrality. Both interventions represent confrontations of aspects of reality that the patient is denying or dissociating in the service of engaging in destructive acting out without the encumbrance of experiencing anxiety or conflict.

Clinical Illustration 5 *(continued)*: Deviating From Neutrality

Ms. W's session was coming to an end, and the weekend was nearly upon them. Up to this point, Dr. P had maintained a neutral stance, but at this juncture, he decided to become directive and set a limit, fully aware that to do so represented a deviation from his usual, neutral stance. Dr. P said, "You have told me that you are leaving your daughter in a situation that we both understand to be unsafe, yet you do not seem concerned about the danger you are exposing her to. While it is not my customary role to tell you what to do, in light of all you have told me, you leave me no choice but to suggest that you change your plans, either by leaving your daughter with your mother or by canceling your trip." Ms. W grumbled but conceded that she would call her mother.

Clinical Illustration 5 *(continued)*: Reinstating Neutrality

Ms. W came to her Monday session to announce, with irritation directed toward Dr. P, that she had canceled her weekend away. When Dr. P commented on her irritation, Ms. W responded by recounting that her boyfriend had overdosed over the weekend and had been taken to an emergency room. Dr. P remained silent. After a pause, Ms. W spontaneously acknowledged that it was "probably a good thing" that she had not left her daughter with her boyfriend.

At this point, Dr. P felt he could reinstate neutrality. He pointed out to Ms. W that in asking her to change her plans, he had stepped out of his usual role of helping her to make her own choices while abstaining from advising or telling her what to do. He commented that he had done so because he felt she had left him no alternative; she had been knowingly exposing her child to danger and did not seem concerned.

They went on to explore Ms. W's thoughts and feelings about what had happened in the last session and over the weekend. Two things emerged clearly: First, as Dr. P had interpreted, Ms. W had externalized and enacted her conflict about being a good mother. Second, a new perspective emerged, previously unexplored in the treatment, in which Ms. W was in some sense testing Dr. P to see what kind of mother *he* was. Would he protect Ms. W and her child from her destructive acting out, or would he be callous and neglectful, allowing her to engage in destructive behavior, as had her own mother? At this level of understanding, Ms. W was identified with a dependent and vulnerable, anxious child self, projected also into her daughter.

Comments: This example is rather compressed in time, and the dynamics involved were quickly clear. There are other situations, however, in which it takes much longer, sometimes weeks, to explore and work through the events leading up to a deviation from neutrality, along with the patient's experience of the therapist's behavior. These moments in treatment, typically highly emotionally charged, often prove in retrospect to be especially meaningful to the patient, and may be intermittently revisited through the course of the therapy as part of the process of working through. They typically convey central aspects of the transference that have not been sufficiently addressed before the deviation—in this case, Ms. W's wish for an ideal mother who would protect her and her child from harm and neglect.

Flexible Implementation of Technical Neutrality

Maintaining a stance of concerned neutrality is a cornerstone of the technique of TFP-E, first promoting activation of conflictual object relations in the treatment, and next enabling therapist and patient to explore, rather than simply to enact, the object relations organizing the clinical process. The therapist's overall objective, however, is not to blindly maintain a neutral stance, but rather to be aware of the occasions when she is intervening from a position of neutrality and when she is deviating from neutrality—and to have an understanding of why she would choose to maintain or to deviate from neutrality in any given clinical situation. This understanding entails the therapist's measured consideration (either in advance or, if this is not possible, after the fact) of whether her choice is being driven by her best clinical judgment, reflecting what she deems best for the overall trajectory of the treatment, or is being driven by countertransference pressures.

In sum, rather than a monolithic and rigid description of the therapist's position, technical neutrality is a conceptual framework within which therapists can organize their interventions and their understanding of how psychodynamic therapy works in order to promote integrative processes in patients.

Deviations from neutrality typically emerge from some combination of the therapist's response to the patient's behavior or life circumstances, countertransference pressures, and clinical judgment. As we have described, deviations from neutrality represent most commonly the therapist's best efforts to protect the treatment from the patient's destructive or disruptive behavior; at these times, setting limits on the patient's behavior becomes the highest priority, superseding other goals and principles of technique.

Countertransference pressures can also play a role in deviations from neutrality, at times guiding the therapist to introduce needed limits, and at other times leading her to make unnecessary deviations from neutrality (this can be considered a form of "countertransference acting out"; see the subsection "Failures of Containment" and related clinical illustrations later in this chapter). In addition, there are a variety of nonurgent situations in which the therapist may feel that maintaining a neutral stance would appear to cause undue or unnecessary strain on the therapeutic alliance, risk verging on unprofessional behavior, or neglect other priorities that in the moment supersede general clinical principles (see the following Clinical Illustration 6).

Although we have focused primarily on deviations from neutrality related to limit setting, in the course of a psychotherapy in which the patient develops a deep and trusting relationship with the therapist, it is only natural that situations will arise in which the patient asks for direct help from the therapist, often in a very appropriate and reasonable fashion, or in which the therapist may feel the patient requires help that she is in a privileged position to provide. When the therapist chooses to respond to these clinical developments by providing advice or a direct expression of concern, she is making use of supportive interventions not routinely employed in TFP-E, but that in her clinical judgment represent the best choice in the clinical moment. These decisions are based on clinical experience and judgment, along with an understanding of the individual patient.

Commonly encountered examples include responding to a patient's direct request for a medical or psychiatric referral for the patient or a family member, requests for advice about how to manage a critical situation with a child, and implicit or explicit requests for an expression of sympathy around a significant loss. Also relatively common (and challenging) are situations in which the patient's parenting is problematic in a manner that the patient may not appreciate, drawing the therapist temporarily into being instructive or into recommending consultation with another professional who can help with parenting skills.

Although as a rule the TFP-E therapist explores rather than directly responds to requests or a perceived need for advice and support, there are times when responding in a professionally responsible or socially appropriate fashion is called for. The therapist who rigidly adheres to prescribed rules of conduct can leave the patient with the not-unreasonable impression that the doctor is socially off, or even professionally irresponsible. If the therapist's actions stand out as a break in "business as usual," the deviation can be acknowledged and explored, following the procedure outline above.

Clinical Illustration 6: Flexible Implementation of Technical Neutrality

Mr. A, a 55-year-old patient with obsessive traits, organized at a neurotic level, had been in treatment for a year when his wife was diagnosed with a rare form of breast cancer. An expert in treating this kind of cancer worked at the same institution with which his therapist, Dr. M, was affiliated. Mr. A explained that he had been unable to get his wife an appointment in a timely fashion and asked if Dr. M could make a call on his behalf. Dr. M did in fact have a relationship with the oncologist and arranged for the patient's wife to be seen the following day.

Mr. A began his next session by expressing how deeply grateful he was. Dr. M asked Mr. A if he had other feelings about what had happened. Mr. A acknowledged having had the thought that Dr. M "must really care"—and also explained that he was aware that this made him somehow uncomfortable. This led to fruitful exploration of Mr. A's deep-seated conflicts around wanting and at the same time fearing to settle into a dependent relationship, conflicts that had been intensified in the setting of his current anxieties about his wife's health.

Comments: In this vignette, the patient is psychologically quite healthy; he easily tolerated and worked through his complex response to Dr. M's actions. When a therapist is treating a patient with more severe pathology, however, the choice to step out of role to provide direct support often leads to more complex and at times extreme reactions; identifying, exploring, and working through the object relations activated and enacted by the therapist's actions becomes an integral part of the clinical process.

The specific nature of the object relations activated will vary depending on the severity of the patient's personality pathology and the nature of his core conflicts. For example, a patient with paranoid personality disorder might experience the therapist's efforts as a ploy to gain control over the patient or to earn his indebtedness; a narcissistic patient might experience the therapist's behavior as an indication of his own specialness, or perhaps of the therapist's efforts to show up or depreciate the patient; and a histrionic patient might experience the therapist's efforts as an expression of the therapist's secret love for the patient.

Regardless of the specific nature of the patient's reaction, the therapist will work with the patient to explore in depth the object relations enacted. This process can be painstaking and slow, sometimes taking months and often returned to at different times during the treatment; nonetheless, it often leads to a more complete or deeper understanding of the object relations organizing the transference.

Utilizing Countertransference

The therapist's capacity to contain her countertransference determines whether countertransference can help the therapist better understand the patient's inner world and deepen the clinical process—or whether it limits the therapist's ability to understand and empathize with the patient or leads to countertransference acting out (Kernberg 2004). The therapist's capacity to contain the patient's affects in the countertransference not only provides a more complete understanding of the patient, but can at times be a therapeutic intervention in and of itself. Conversely, failures of containment rob the therapist of an important therapeutic tool and are the most common cause of unnecessary deviations from technical neutrality.

Containment

In TFP-E, countertransference serves as a central channel of communication, and in the treatment of patients with more severe personality pathology, it is often the most direct access the therapist has to what is going on in the treatment. The therapist's ability to make use of her countertransference rests on her ability to do the following:

1. Allow the patient to affect her internally.
2. Reflect on, rather than react to or deny, her own internal responses.

3. Identify, in her own imagination, the internal object relations enacted in the countertransference.
4. Use her internal experience to deepen her understanding of the patient's internal situation and of the object relations currently active in the treatment.

We refer to this process as the therapist's *containing* the countertransference (Bion 1962, 1959/1967, 1962/1967; Britton 1998; Joseph 1987/1988; Ogden 1993).

In the most general sense, *containment* refers to the capacity of thought to modify psychological content, especially highly affectively charged content. *Containment* implies the capacity to be open to fully experiencing an emotional experience without being controlled by that experience or having to turn immediately to action; containment calls on the therapist to be self-aware, responsive, reflective, and restrained. It is the process of containment that enables the therapist to make use of the countertransference as a source of information about the object relations currently being enacted in the treatment, and to empathize at any given moment with all parts of the patient and with all sides of any given conflict. Containment may lead to interpretation but need not necessarily do so (Lafarge 2000; Ogden 1993; Schafer 1997).

The containing therapist needs to have the emotional freedom to respond internally to the patient, along with the restraint to delay acting on these responses until she has had an opportunity to reflect on them. Another way to say this is that the containing therapist is internally responsive but not interpersonally reactive, replacing action and reaction with self-observation and reflection. In this sense, containment of countertransference is the opposite of countertransference acting out; the former involves reflection and promotes understanding, whereas the latter avoids awareness and eschews understanding. Over the course of treatment, patients with personality disorder hopefully traverse this gradient. In TFP-E, patients move away from expressing internal states through action and symptoms that avoid awareness; instead, they move toward containment of underlying affects and object relations, managing them through self-awareness and reflection, facilitating enhanced behavioral control and resolution of symptoms.

To demonstrate containment, in Video 7, "Therapeutic Neutrality," Dr. Yeomans works with a male college dropout with a severe personality disorder whose primary treatment goal is to complete college. The patient precipitously announces his plan to drop out of school and to leave treatment. The patient explains that he feels compelled to leave in order to escape the pressure that he feels as a result of the treatment, and he complains that Dr. Yeomans is pressuring him to be in school. In his response, Dr. Yeomans maintains a neutral stance, despite his wish in the countertransference to encourage the patient to stick with both the treatment and school. He reminds the patient that it is his treatment goal to complete college, his wish for himself rather than something Dr. Yeomans is imposing on the patient. Dr. Yeomans goes on to suggest that the pressure the patient feels reflects his own internal conflict, rather than any external demands that are being placed upon him. This vignette illustrates how the therapist's ability to maintain a neutral stance enables the patient to come to appreciate the internal nature of his difficulties, rather than to simply externalize his conflicts, and the central role of countertransference containment in that process. This vignette also highlights the central role played by the treatment goals in TFP-E, and how they can help to anchor the treatment, especially during times of crisis.

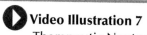

Video Illustration 7
Therapeutic Neutrality (3:20)

Working With Countertransference: The Process of Containment

Working with countertransference is a complex and challenging process that can be thought of as taking place in several steps (as listed in the previous subsection, "Containment"), although in practice, the steps may be superimposed on one another. In psychotherapy, containment of countertransference always follows an interaction between therapist and patient in which the patient affects the therapist internally, stimulating affects and activating representations of self and others in the therapist's internal world.

The first step in working with countertransference is for the therapist to allow herself to be both open to and fully aware of the feelings—sometimes very uncomfortable ones, and at other times barely perceptible—that underlie her emotional reaction to the patient or the clinical situation. Thus, the therapist both allows the patient to move her internally and allows herself to be aware of what is being stimulated within her. In the second step, she tolerates what is being stirred up internally, abstaining from reflexively turning to action or denial to alleviate discomfort.

We can return to our example of Ms. W and Dr. P, in which Dr. P ultimately asked Ms. W to change her weekend plans, which illustrates how

Dr. P worked with his countertransference. Early in the session, as Ms. W casually let him in on her weekend plans, Dr. P became aware of his feelings of anxiety in relation to Ms. W's child. He also noted that his experience contrasted with the attitude that Ms. W conveyed. Dr. P consciously registered and tolerated these feelings without immediately doing something to alleviate them. He neither resorted to action nor reflexively deviated from neutrality. Instead, Dr. P opened himself up to Ms. W's projections, paying attention to his internal responses to her behavior and communications.

To conclude the second step, after allowing herself to respond internally to the patient, the containing therapist moves into the position of observer of her internal experience and to reflect on that experience. From this vantage point as a third party, progressing into the third step, the therapist identifies and observes the object relation activated in her own mind in response to her interactions with the patient. It is this process of *triangulation* that enables the therapist to use the countertransference to further her understanding of the object relations currently dominant in the treatment. In the fourth and final step, the containing therapist uses her experience to make inferences about the internal object relations being activated in the patient and enacted in transference. In this process, she will ask herself to what degree her responses emerge from the patient's attitude and behavior and to what degree her own conflicts and attitudes shape her response.

Returning to our example, Dr. P inferred that Ms. W was projecting into him the protective, maternal parts of herself, as well as the vulnerable, anxious, and childlike parts, while she consciously identified with a callous maternal object in relation to a neglected child. Dr. P's use of his countertransference enabled him to identify and empathize with Ms. W's *entire* emotional situation, including the vulnerable and anxious aspects of her experience that she was defensively splitting off and projecting in the moment. Dr. P's use of his countertransference also enabled him to formulate an intervention; specifically, he called Ms. W's attention to the dissociation and projection of her anxious maternal self (and ultimately of her vulnerable, dependent-child self that longed for an ideal mother) by suggesting that Ms. W was handing off to him the part of herself that wanted to be a good mother but feared she was inadequate, while identifying with the part of herself that would neglect the child as her own mother had done.

Before turning to another clinical illustration, we want to emphasize that containment need not necessarily lead to a verbal intervention. Sometimes the act of containment is in and of itself the most effective intervention that a therapist can offer in the moment. As the therapist contains the object relations enacted in the transference-countertransference, she is also in some way modifying the internal experience initially stimulated within her by the patient. In our immediately previous example, after accepting Ms. W's projections, Dr. P used his reflective capacities to feel less anxious and afraid than he had initially. In essence, his internal processing of his countertransference enabled him to modify, within himself, an initial experience of anxiety and helplessness close in quality to that of his patient's dissociated experience, transforming it into an experience that was better integrated and less affectively charged, as well as less threatening.

Clinical Illustration 7: Working With Countertransference

Ms. O was a 45-year-old divorced, professional, childless woman with narcissistic and histrionic features organized at a very high borderline level. She began a session by speaking at some length about her wonderful weekend with her new boyfriend, focusing on the great sex and the great fun she had enjoyed, the colorful people, the beautiful homes. As the session progressed, Ms. O became more and more excited. Her tone became shrill; she spoke and laughed loudly as she told humorous stories in an extremely animated fashion.

Initially, Dr. T (several years younger than her patient) was swept up in Ms. O's mood, feeling excited herself and wanting to laugh along with her patient. (This is an example of *concordant identification* in the countertransference; see Chapter 5.) However, as Dr. T continued to sit with Ms. O, she started to feel diminished and demoralized; she found herself thinking about things Ms. O had that she herself would never have. (This is an example of *complementary identification* in the countertransference; see Chapter 5.)

Reflecting on her own responses to her patient's verbal and nonverbal communications, Dr. T identified an object relation of an excited person who "has it all" and an excluded and inferior person who feels envious. Thinking about it further, Dr. T was struck by how exaggeratedly diminished she had been feeling. She remembered the envy Ms. O had felt in the past toward Dr. T, whom Ms. O knew was married and had children. As Dr. T reflected on what was being enacted in the session and why, she found herself feeling calmer in the face of Ms. O's manic style, and she was able to empathize with the painful feelings underlying her patient's excitement.

As the session went on, Ms. O, too, began to calm somewhat and became more self-reflective.[2] Meanwhile, Dr. T's ability to contain her countertransference enabled her to empathize with Ms. O's entire emotional situation, including the inferior, devalued sense of self she was defending

---

[2]This is an example of the impact on the patient of the therapist's containment of the patient's projections, even in the absence of verbal interaction between them.

against and projecting into Dr. T; at the same time, Dr. T's equanimity seemed to help Ms. O become less agitated and more reflective.

Failures of Containment

Though generally undesirable, failure to contain countertransference pressures may not be entirely avoidable in TFP-E, even when the therapist is experienced. Treating patients with personality disorders, and in particular those with more severe pathology, can stir up strong and often very uncomfortable feelings in the therapist. At times, the therapist will act in response to these feelings, sometimes despite active efforts not to do so, engaging in various forms of countertransference acting out by turning in some way to action to relieve uncomfortable emotional states activated within the therapist by the patient or by the clinical situation.

Thus, even though countertransferences in the treatment of patients with more severe personality disorders tend to be relatively easy to identify, they are often difficult to contain, leaving the therapist at risk for engaging in some form of countertransference acting out (Joseph 1987/1988; Pick 1985). Common forms of such acting out in this setting include emotional withdrawal from the patient or, conversely, being drawn into a dialogue, inadvertently communicating hostility, behaving seductively, unnecessarily setting limits, or inappropriately tolerating contract violations.

In contrast to the relatively extreme, acute countertransference reactions often encountered when treating patients who function at a borderline level of personality organization, chronic forms of these reactions are frequently expressed in the therapist's maintaining a particular attitude toward or feeling about a patient over time. Chronic countertransferences that are especially likely to be overlooked may be activated by patients whom a therapist views as in some way special—for example, as particularly needy, vulnerable, or desirable—or, in the setting of more severe pathology, perhaps particularly fragile, brittle, or unstable. Chronic countertransference reactions may go unnoticed by the therapist for extended periods of time. Consultation with a supervisor or trusted colleague is the most effective way to diagnose chronic countertransference reactions.

Clinical Illustration 7 *(continued)*: Acute and Chronic Countertransference in Failures of Containment

In the previous clinical illustration, Ms. O, the 45-year-old divorced woman, stimulated feelings first of excitement and then of diminishment in Dr. T. Let's now consider what might have happened if Dr. T had failed to contain her responses to her patient:

Acute Countertransference. One possibility is that Dr. T might have joined Ms. O in her manic excitement, identifying with Ms. O's conscious, expansive self representation. In this scenario, patient and therapist would have enacted a defensive object relation of an expansive patient and an idealized therapist engaged in an exciting dialogue, supporting Ms. O's defensive efforts to deny the painful, diminished self representation that she was splitting off.

Acute Countertransference. In another possible scenario, Dr. T might have gotten lost in her own feelings of envy, inferiority, and demoralization, allowing this experience to interfere with her capacity to reflect on how and why she felt the way she did in relation to Ms. O. As in the previous scenario, this countertransference could leave Dr. T with a blind spot, unable to empathize with Ms. O's underlying feelings of envy and inferiority. In addition, feelings of demoralization might lead Dr. T to withdraw from Ms. O, a common countertransference reaction in the treatment of patients with narcissistic conflicts.

Chronic Countertransference. The case of Ms. O can also illustrate the therapist's failure to contain chronic countertransference reactions. At this point, we add that Ms. O was extremely successful professionally, maintaining a high-profile and highly influential position. Further, she was physically very attractive and always dressed in extremely elegant clothing. Dr. T had great admiration for the things Ms. O had accomplished, as well as for how attractively she presented herself. It was only after Ms. O had been in treatment for almost a year that Dr. T became fully aware of the subtle way in which her admiration for Ms. O had limited her capacity to fully empathize with the parts of Ms. O that felt small and diminished, left out, and sad.

Comments: In the first two examples, Dr. T's possible failure to contain her acute countertransference in response to Ms. O's grandiose defenses might have led Dr. T either to feel diminished and demoralized or to be drawn into joining Ms. O in her grandiose excitement. Either of these reactions on the part of Dr. T, if unexamined and uncontained, would have interfered with the doctor's ability to appreciate and help Ms. O with the painful feelings of inferiority and envy that were hidden beneath her more grandiose self-presentation and were closely tied to her presenting complaints.

In the third example, portraying Dr. T's chronic, unexamined countertransferential admiration of Ms. O, Dr. T's implicit attitude toward Ms. O covertly supported Ms. O's defenses by enacting in the countertransference an object relation that was both familiar to and ego-syntonic for patient and therapist alike; this is often the case in chronic countertransferences that go unnoticed and are therefore uncontained. Ms. O needed to feel special and, defensively, to leave Dr. T feeling vaguely diminished; Dr. T was chronically admiring of people like Ms. O, whom she saw as more colorful and dynamic than she. Although Dr. T's attitude toward Ms. O had been fully conscious, because it was familiar and ego-syntonic, she had failed to fully acknowledge her countertransference or to explore it, leaving her vulnerable to unwittingly colluding with Ms. O's defenses for an extended period of time.

As another example, in Clinical Illustration 5 (continued below), we return to Ms. W, the patient diagnosed with borderline personality disorder who has a young daughter and substance-abusing boyfriend, introduced earlier in this chapter (in the subsection "Deviating From and Reinstating Neutrality").

Clinical Illustration 5 *(continued)*: Countertransference Acting Out in Failure of Containment

As the treatment proceeded over a number of months, Dr. P recognized that he was becoming increasingly anxious about the safety of Ms. W's child. Even though Dr. P tried reminding himself that in the end, Ms. W always seemed to protect her child from danger, he often found himself preoccupied on weekends about the child's safety. As time passed, Dr. P found himself increasingly unable to contain his feelings, eagerly looking forward over the weekend to Monday, when he would see Ms. W and his anxieties would be allayed. In this setting, the patient had successfully offloaded her anxiety about her daughter into Dr. P in the countertransference.

Over a weekend when Dr. P was feeling especially worn out and burdened by personal difficulties, he found himself particularly uncomfortable and preoccupied about Ms. W. Impulsively, on Sunday morning, he called Ms. W at home to check on the safety of her child. When Ms. W failed to pick up the phone, Dr. P left a voice mail communicating his anxiety and asking Ms. W to call him back. Ms. W did not return his call. Over the course of the day, Dr. P came to feel that his behavior had been driven largely by his countertransferential need to unburden himself; he recognized that if he felt it clinically indicated to introduce a safety net for the child, there were ways that he could strategically go about doing so.

When Ms. W came to her next session, she was silent. Dr. P inquired about her reaction to his call. Ms. W responded that she had experienced Dr. P's call as both intrusive and disappointing. She questioned why, if he really didn't think her a fit mother, he didn't involve Child Protective Services.

Comments: This vignette illustrates the potentially overwhelming intensity of affective experience (typically paranoid—anxiety, panic, fear, helplessness) that may be stimulated in the countertransference by middle- and low-BPO patients, as well as the extreme difficulty that therapists may encounter in containing these feelings. In contrast to Dr. T in Clinical Illustration 7, who may not have been fully aware of her countertransference to Ms. O, Dr. P was fully cognizant of what he was feeling, and also knew that it was being actively induced in him by Ms. W. Even so, at a time of vulnerability, Dr. P found himself unable to contain his countertransferential anxiety. In the moment, he felt compelled to act, somewhat impulsively, in an effort to alleviate the extremely uncomfortable feelings that Ms. W had engendered in him.

In retrospect, Dr. P was able to see that the clinical situation had activated for him the experience of being a dependent child in relation to a dangerously unreliable mother-patient; he found himself clinging to Ms. W in the countertransference for reassurance of her daughter's safety, rather than containing and using the object relations activated in the countertransference to inform his understanding of what was going on within Ms. W. This object relation, Dr. P came to understand over time, was an unbearably painful conflict between a powerful pressure within Ms. W to identify with her own mother, enacting the role of neglectful mother while projecting into her daughter her neglected child-self, in conflict with a desperate wish that an idealized therapist-mother could protect both her and her child from this unpleasant and potentially dangerous outcome.

Countertransference Pressures and Deviations From Neutrality

In our discussion earlier in this chapter of deviations from neutrality, we focused on situations in which the therapist makes a more or less measured determination of how to proceed before abandoning neutrality to set a limit or to offer support. In the discussion of utilizing, containing, or failing to contain countertransference, clearly there are times when therapists may deviate from neutrality, becoming directive, supportive, or participating in defensive enactments in a less reflective manner, in response to countertransference pressures. In this setting, the therapist turns to action to relieve uncomfortable emotional states activated within her by the patient or by the clinical situation.

Although generally undesirable, resorting to action in response to countertransference pressures may not be entirely unavoidable in TFP-E, even among experienced TFP-E therapists. Treating patients with severe personality disorders invariably stirs up very strong and often very uncomfortable feelings in therapists; when therapists treat patients with personality disorders, if the therapists truly open themselves up, they are exposed in the countertransference to affects commensurate with the level of internal integration or lack thereof that is characteristic of the patient's experience in the moment. As a result, therapists treating patients with severe personality pathology will experience poorly integrated affects—foreign, extremely painful, and often frightening to the therapist—that mirror the patient's internal experience. These feelings can be extremely difficult, at times perhaps impossible, to consistently contain, and not infrequently lead to subtle or not-so-subtle forms of countertransference acting out. As was the case with Dr. P, who called Ms. W on a weekend, this can be the case even at times when therapists are fully aware of the pressures they are under, and sometimes despite their active efforts not to act on them.

In sum, unnecessary deviations from technical neutrality in TFP-E on the part of a relatively experienced therapist typically result from poorly contained countertransference. In more extreme situations, the therapist may flagrantly act out, as in the case of Dr. P. In more subtle cases, the therapist may fail to see the entire situation from a neutral position, leaving herself vulnerable to unwittingly participating in defensive enactments, as illustrated by Dr. T's chronic countertransference in relation to Ms. O.

In situations such as Dr. P's phone call, when failure to contain countertransference leads to unnecessary deviations from technical neutrality, the deviation is handled after the fact in a fashion similar to the management of planned deviations outlined earlier in this chapter, in the subsection "Deviating From and Reinstating Neutrality." The therapist will begin by pointing out that what he did involved stepping out of his usual role, acknowledge that it was in error if he believes it was, and then explore with the patient how she experienced the therapist and his behavior.

For example, in their session after the phone call, Dr. P began by acknowledging to Ms. W that he had been in error to call her over the weekend, and that in retrospect he should have waited until their next session to discuss his concerns. Dr. P then turned the focus back to Ms. W, exploring her experience of him in relation to the call; on the one hand, she saw Dr. P as critically condemning her as an unfit parent, and on the other hand, she saw him as neglecting her by not raising the question of whether she indeed needed additional social support to help with parenting. In a subsequent session, Ms. W revealed yet another, hidden experience of Dr. P's call and of his acknowledgment of his error—that these actions signified that he "really cared." All of these transferences were fruitfully explored and understood in terms of a dyad of a critical, condemning mother and a "bad," shamed, and deservedly neglected child, along with dissociated wishes to be part of an idealized mother-child relationship.

Countertransference Disclosure

Our discussion of working with countertransference would be incomplete without a careful comment on the approach to countertransference disclosure in TFP-E. *Countertransference disclosure* refers to the therapist openly sharing, and perhaps exploring with the patient, her own personal and idiosyncratic emotional reaction to the patient and to the clinical situation.[3] In TFP-E, the therapist generally does not make use of countertransference disclosure; although the therapist actively uses the countertransference, she does not for the most part directly convey or communicate her countertransferential thoughts and feelings to the patient.

Instead, as illustrated in this chapter, in TFP-E, the therapist attempts to use her countertransference to inform interventions that focus on the *patient's* experience of the relationship, an approach that is consistent with an object relational frame of reference. Thus, while recognizing the inevitable contribution and participation of both parties in any interaction, in TFP-E, the therapist attempts to focus exploration on the patient's internal experience while maintaining a relatively restrained stance that as much as possible contains countertransference and minimizes the therapist's active interpersonal participation in developments in the transference.[4]

It is our experience that within the frame of reference of TFP-E, one that focuses on the patient's internal world from a technically neutral position, countertransference disclosure carries the risk of calling too much attention to the therapist's experience in a way that can be confusing to the patient with personality disorder or, conversely, may serve as a welcome distraction from the patient's thinking about himself. As a result, in our earlier example describing Ms. W's plans to leave her daughter with

---

[3]For example, the therapist will freely share her confusion in response to what the patient is saying or doing, in the service of confronting denial or offering a confrontation. For example, the therapist might say, *"I'm confused*; you just told me X, now you are telling me Y. They seem to contradict one another" or *"I am having difficulty following* the events you are describing; you are providing a lot of information but it doesn't seem to add up. Do you understand why I am having difficulty?"

a substance-abusing boyfriend, Dr. P abstained from sharing his personal anxiety with Ms. W. He did not say, "You are making me anxious about the safety of your child." Rather, he commented on her denial of the reality that the situation was clearly unsafe. Although the distinction between these two possible stances may be subtle, it is important. In TFP-E, Dr. P would neither share his discomfort as a venue for deepening Ms. W's understanding of herself and her world, nor assume the position of an expert telling Ms. W what to do (unless he was forced to deviate from neutrality); rather, he would use his discomfort to ask himself, "Why am I uncomfortable? Would a normal or average person find this to be a dangerous and anxiety-provoking situation?" He would then use his internal dialogue to confront the patient's denial of an evident reality—the danger to her child—that part of her must have fully appreciated but that she chose to ignore.[5] Similarly, after Dr. P acted on his countertransference to call Ms. W on a weekend, the therapist subsequently apologized to Ms. W for having made an error and then turned the focus back onto Ms. W's experience; he abstained from delving into his own anxieties or the personal reasons for his vulnerability that weekend.

Working Through and Therapeutic Change

We complete our three chapters on techniques employed by the TFP-E therapist with this discussion of the process of working through. (As a reminder, we began our description of exploratory techniques used by the TFP-E therapist in Chapters 10 and 11, in which we discussed the interpretive process and its application to analysis of transference.) In this chapter, we have covered supportive techniques, focusing on limit setting,

---

[4]This approach is quite different from that assumed in a variety of contemporary psychodynamic approaches, many of which often make use of countertransference disclosure. For example, for therapists working within a relational framework, a focus on the intersubjective field and countertransference disclosure are integral components of the treatment (Auchincloss and Samberg 2012). Therapists using mentalization-based therapy focus on enhancing mentalization in the patient, and in this frame of reference, countertransference disclosure is used as a way to model and stimulate a process of mentalization between patient and therapist (Bateman and Fonagy 2006).

[5]If the patient were truly unable to appreciate that she was endangering her child, the therapist would need to shift gears to provide ongoing supportive interventions, such as recommending that the patient participate in parenting classes or parental supervision, either in conjunction with or instead of TFP-E.

and expanded our discussion of exploratory techniques to include managing technical neutrality and utilizing countertransference. In combination, the techniques of interpretation, transference analysis, managing technical neutrality, utilizing countertransference, and parsimonious use of supportive interventions function to support in the moment, and help to promote over time, capacities for affect containment, self-awareness, reflection, contextualization of experience, and self-understanding in the patient with personality pathology.

However, no single intervention, even when leading to new and meaningful levels of self-awareness or self-understanding, can result in material change in personality functioning. Rather, the effectiveness of TFP-E in promoting long-term change in personality functioning, be it assessed at the level of maladaptive behaviors and symptoms or at the level of personality organization, depends on the *repetitive* and *progressive* application of core techniques. We refer to this process as *working through*.

Working through can be defined as the repeated enactment, exploration, and interpretation over time, and in an emotionally meaningful fashion, of conflictual object relations and associated conflicts (Auchincloss and Samberg 2012). In this process, it is necessary to enact and interpret core conflicts from a variety of perspectives and in a variety of contexts. In the treatment of personality disorders, the process of working through involves repeated identification of repetitive, maladaptive behaviors and symptoms (personality traits) as they are activated in the treatment and in the patient's daily life, followed by exploration of the defensive and impulsive object relations organizing these traits, and ultimately by elaboration and interpretation of underlying conflicts.

In TFP-E, it is the process of working through that provides the link between self-awareness or self-understanding and therapeutic change. Working through constitutes the major task of the middle phase of TFP-E (for further discussion, see Chapter 13). In fact, the bulk of TFP-E therapeutic work involves the process of working through; once core conflicts and associated object relations have been identified, they are repeatedly enacted and explored throughout the course of the treatment, allowing the therapist to make use of clarification, confrontation, and interpretation. What the therapist sees, then, are the repetitive enactment and progressive interpretation of clusters of core conflictual object relations that organize chronic behaviors and subjective experiences (i.e., personality traits). These object relations are explored as they are expressed in different contexts both inside and outside the treatment, and as they can be viewed from different perspectives.

Typically, the therapist first sees the working through of narcissistic and/or paranoid conflicts associated with a particular cluster of conflictual object relations; this process then clears a path for focusing clinical attention on the working through of associated depressive conflicts and anxieties. Over time, the process of interpreting a particular conflict, which may initially take place over the course of weeks or even months, becomes more efficient, as patient and therapist become familiar with defensive object relations and underlying conflicts. In more advanced stages of working through, it becomes possible to complete an entire interpretive cycle within a single session—or even to complete it several times within a session, often in different contexts or from different perspectives.

In sum, it is the process of working through that we believe leads to personality change in TFP-E. Working through provides the patient with a progressively deeper and more comprehensive understanding of the conflicts addressed by a particular cluster of defenses, and ultimately increases his capacity to contain and flexibly manage conflictual object relations. Essential to the concept of working through is the exploration of conflictual object relations and core conflicts as they are enacted 1) *repeatedly over time*, with the patient becoming progressively better able to observe and reflect and to move through the cycle of identification, exploration, and interpretation with increasing efficiency and flexibility, and with decreasing need for the therapist's participation; 2) in *different contexts*, with the patient having the opportunity to view core conflicts as they are activated and can be observed in a variety of settings, including both in important domains of functioning and in the transference; 3) with *progressive deepening*, as patient and therapist acquire a more complete understanding of core conflicts, anxieties, and defenses, ultimately linking them to developmental antecedents; and 4) with elaboration of the *multiple functions served by personality traits* in relation to core conflicts.

Clinical Illustration 8: Working Through in the Treatment of an NPO Patient

Mr. R presented at the insistence of his wife, who complained of his excessive passivity; even worse, from her perspective, whenever she called out Mr. R on his behavior, his response was to become submissive and conciliatory, asking her to tell him what he could do to improve. She found this infuriating.

In his therapy, Mr. R's passivity and submissiveness were identified early on as characteristic of his functioning not only in his marriage, but also at his work, where he failed to ask for a raise or promotion; with his teenage children, with whom he was consistently the "good cop" while leaving all limit setting and disciplining to his wife; and in his relationship with his parents. Mr. R's passive submission was also subtly evident in the way he comported himself in therapy sessions and in his interactions with Dr. L.

Initial exploration and interpretation focused first on helping Mr. R to be more aware of his behavior. Clarification of Mr. R's behavior and experience enabled Dr. L and Mr. R to characterize and elaborate an ego-syntonic object relation of an ingratiating and accommodating, childlike self in relation to a dominant, superior, somewhat feared authority figure, associated with feelings of wanting to be loved and accepted. Dr. L and Mr. R focused on this defensive object relation and on Mr. R's passive-submissive behavior, exploring how these were enacted in a variety of contexts, and attending to ways in which, in many settings, Mr. R's behavior was maladaptive. [*This is an example of clarification and confrontation.*]

Over time, Mr. R's passivity became increasingly ego-dystonic. At this point, Dr. L was able to help Mr. R uncover and explore anxieties motivating the defensive object relation, having to do with fears of being rejected or criticized if he were to be assertive. [*This was the early phase of interpretation.*] With time, Mr. R became increasingly familiar with and understanding of this part of himself as it was activated in a variety of contexts. In his sessions, he would describe his defensive behaviors as he noticed them in his day-to-day life, and he was able to link them to underlying anxieties, often with limited intervention from his therapist. Now, when Mr. R found himself wanting to assume a passive or submissive stance, he was able to catch himself, to identify the temptation to enact the familiar defensive object relation, and to recognize his underlying anxieties. In this setting, Mr. R found himself able, with considerable effort, to be somewhat more assertive with his wife.

At this point, Dr. L invited Mr. R to consider how they might make sense of his persistently fearful expectation that being assertive would lead him to be rejected and criticized. Focusing on Mr. R's defenses, fears, and fantasies, Dr. L was able to help Mr. R become aware of deep-seated fears in relation to the expression of aggressive motivations, still largely unconscious, organized as wishes to lash out or to aggressively criticize and demean those around him. [*This interaction marked a deeper level of interpretation.*] These wishes were highly conflictual, quite horrifying to Mr. R, and entirely discrepant with his dominant sense of self; they could be characterized in terms of a hostile, demeaning attacker in relation to a devalued and enraged victim.[6] This object relation was linked to fears of residing in a world infiltrated with mutual hostility and mistrust.

As a result of the process of repeated clarification, confrontation, and interpretation, Mr. R came to see how defenses in relation to this conflict, along with underlying anxieties and impulses, impacted—and to some degree, organized—his relationship not only with his wife, but also and in different ways with his children, his parents, and his boss. Dr. L also pointed out that Mr. R's accommodating and somewhat submissive behavior in the therapy seemed similarly designed to ward off the possibility of mutual hostility in the therapeutic relationship.

---

[6]At times Mr. R seemed more closely identified with the attacker, and at other times with the attacked.

As Mr. R was able to work through these predominantly paranoid anxieties and conflicts in relation to the expression of aggression, he became more tolerant of his own aggressive wishes and feelings. Now, when he found himself becoming passive or submissive, he experienced himself as "slipping back into old bad habits," and was curious about his motivations for doing so. In this context, Mr. R came to see that at times, he resorted to passivity in relation to his wife not simply as a defense against the expression of hostility, but also as a covert (passive-aggressive) way to express hostility.

As Mr. R became increasingly able to tolerate awareness of the aggressive motivations lurking behind his habitual passivity and submissiveness, he was confronted with the painful awareness of intermittent wishes to sadistically criticize or lash out at his wife, children, and others whom he cared for; these wishes were linked to feelings of guilt and concern. At the same time, he expressed anxiety that if he were to be more assertive or less accommodating in relation to Dr. L, he would seem ungrateful.

Working through these depressive anxieties, and ultimately linking them to long-standing power struggles with his mother during childhood, enabled Mr. R to be more consistently and comfortably assertive in his marriage as well as with his children and parents and, to a lesser degree, at work. He discovered that when he felt his wife was being excessively critical or demanding, he could now "push back" rather than submit, or even respond in kind; with a grin, he reported to Dr. L that he sometimes found himself becoming—and even enjoying being—"a bit nasty" toward her during disagreements. Mr. R's wife, who was relatively comfortable with measured expressions of aggression, welcomed his newfound assertiveness, which she experienced as his being appropriately masculine. In the countertransference, Dr. L noticed that he felt a new respect and admiration for Mr. R and his accomplishments, very much in contrast to his initial experience in the transference-countertransference that had been laced with a subtle form of contempt, a complementary identification in the countertransference.

Comments: This vignette describes in condensed form the process and impact of Mr. R working through the conflicts underlying and organizing his passive-submissive behavior. Preliminary interventions focused on the behavior itself, helping Mr. R to become more aware of habitual responses to conflict as they were played out in a variety of settings, and ultimately helping him to no longer experience his passivity as ego-syntonic; the defensive object relation organizing his behavior and experience could then be characterized. As Mr. R became more aware of the defensive nature of his behaviors and the anxieties motivating them, he became better able to effortfully modify his behavior. This development can be understood as a form of cognitive, or cortical, control of automatic behaviors, and a clear marker of clinical improvement. However, because the deeper conflicts motivating Mr. R's passivity remained unresolved, he initially had to exert significant, conscious effort to override his habitual behaviors.

As a result of Mr. R's practice in being more assertive in a variety of settings, over time, it became somewhat easier for him to override his automatic predisposition to assume a passive stance. As he became better able to be assertive, he began to gain access to the hostile and sadistic motivations underlying and motivating his passivity. In this setting, Dr. L helped Mr. R first to understand—and next, to tolerate—emotional awareness of these conflictual motivations.

Dr. L and Mr. R repeatedly explored Mr. R's hostile and sadistic wishes as they manifested over time, in the setting of different relationships and to some degree in the transference as well. This process of working through enabled Mr. R to better contain his conflictual impulses within his dominant self experience, so that they came to feel like a part of himself, somewhat challenging but manageable, rather than as totally unacceptable and threatening impulses that needed to be entirely split off from his self experience and buried. This process of containment on Mr. R's part entailed exploring and repeatedly interpreting the various anxieties, both paranoid and depressive, that motivated his defenses.

Ultimately, Mr. R became able to comfortably assert himself, to tolerate conflict, and to express hostility, and even to enjoy a measured expression of his sadism within the context of a loving relationship. Although Mr. R maintained a relatively neutral relation toward Dr. L, and Dr. L for the most part did not view the transference as affectively dominant, the therapist did notice a shift in his countertransference over time. Initially, Dr. L had been somewhat put off by Mr. R's self-presentation of a grown man assuming a childlike, passive-submissive stance and wanting only to be loved (a complementary countertransference that Dr. L was able to contain). By the latter phases of the treatment, Dr. L noted that his emotional reaction to Mr. R had quietly evolved, so that he now viewed Mr. R with quiet admiration and respect; Dr. L noted as well some mildly competitive feelings toward a worthy equal and potential rival.

Key Clinical Concepts

- TFP-E relies predominantly on exploratory techniques.
- The TFP-E therapist also makes use of supportive, or structuring, techniques—if they are needed to maintain the treatment frame and to manage destructive and disruptive behavior.
- Contracting, limit setting, and recontracting are the major supportive interventions employed by the TFP-E therapist.

- When the TFP-E therapist uses supportive techniques, she is deviating from technical neutrality, and when the crisis resolves, she reinstates neutrality.
- The process of containment—allowing oneself to be emotionally open and reflective without turning to action—enables the therapist to make use of his countertransference.
- Failures of containment can lead to unnecessary deviations from neutrality.
- Working through entails enacting, exploring, and interpreting a particular conflict repeatedly over time and in a variety of contexts.
- The process of working through promotes the integrative changes that are the goals of TFP-E.

References

Auchincloss AL, Samberg E (eds): Psychoanalytic Terms and Concepts. New Haven, CT, Yale University Press, 2012

Bateman A, Fonagy P: Mentalization-Based Treatment for Borderline Personality Disorder. New York, Oxford University Press, 2006

Bion WR: Learning From Experience. London, Heinemann, 1962

Bion WR: Attacks on linking (1959), in Second Thoughts. London, Heinemann, 1967, pp 93–109

Bion WR: A theory of thinking (1962), in Second Thoughts. London, Heinemann, 1967, pp 110–119

Britton R: Naming and containing, in Belief and Imagination. London, Routledge, 1998, pp 19–28

Gabbard GO: Long-Term Psychodynamic Psychotherapy: A Basic Text, 2nd Edition. Washington, DC, American Psychiatric Publishing, 2010

Joseph B: Projective identification, some clinical aspects (1987), in Melanie Klein Today, Vol 1. Edited by Spillius EB. London, Routledge, 1988, pp 138–150

Kernberg OF: Acute and chronic countertransference reactions, in Aggressivity, Narcissism, and Self-Destructiveness in the Psychotherapeutic Relationship. New Haven, CT, Yale University Press, 2004, pp 167–191

Lafarge L: Interpretation and containment. Int J Psychoanal 81 (Pt 1):67–84, 2000 10816845

Ogden TH: Projective Identification and Psychotherapeutic Technique (1982). Northvale, NJ, Jason Aronson, 1993

Pick IB: Working through in the countertransference. Int J Psychoanal 66 (Pt 2):157–166, 1985 4019040

Schafer R: The Contemporary Kleinians of London. Madison, CT, International Universities Press, 1997

Winston A, Rosenthal RN, Pinsker H: Learning Supportive Therapy: An Illustrated Guide. Washington, DC, American Psychiatric Publishing, 2012

Yeomans F, Clarkin JF, Kernberg OF: Transference-Focused Psychotherapy for Borderline Personality Disorder: A Clinical Guide. Washington, DC, American Psychiatric Publishing, 2015

Section VI

Phases of Treatment and Trajectories of Change

A DYNAMIC PSYCHOTHERAPY CAN BE thought of as having an *early phase*, a *middle phase*, and an *advanced phase of treatment*. Although these three phases are not clearly demarcated and gradually flow from one to the next, there are characteristic features of each phase that can be used to conceptualize the flow of treatment. Understanding the central tasks that define each phase, as well as the clinical issues that characterize it, can help the therapist anticipate and identify expected clinical developments over the course of the treatment, and will also help identify those times when the treatment process is stagnating.

In Section VI, we discuss the three phases of treatment in TFP-E and the clinical issues that commonly arise in each phase of treatment. While the tasks of each phase are the same across the range of severity of personality pathology, the clinical issues that emerge in each phase, as well as their relative centrality to the clinical process, are variable depending on the severity of personality pathology.

497

13

Early, Middle, and Advanced Phases of Treatment

focused psychotherapy—extended (TFP-E) will have an opening phase, a middle phase, and an advanced phase with an ending, or termination. In this chapter, we discuss the three phases of TFP-E, focusing on the central tasks of each treatment phase. We consider the impact of level of personality organization on the overall trajectory of treatment and on the clinical issues that characterize each phase of treatment. In addition, we introduce markers of change that signal the patient's readiness for the next phase of treatment.

Early Treatment Phase

The early treatment phase of TFP-E can be as short as a few months and as long as 6 months, depending on the nature of the patient's personality pathology and affinity for working in exploratory treatment, as well as the therapist's skill. Treatment formally begins only after assessment and contracting have been completed. By the time the patient enters the opening phase, therapist and patient will have established treatment goals and agreed upon a frame for the treatment; the therapist will have clearly explained the patient's tasks and role in the treatment, as well as those of the therapist; and the therapist will have had the opportunity to demonstrate his interest, concern, and expertise, laying the groundwork for development of the therapeutic alliance.

The following are the major tasks of the early phase of treatment:

- Stabilizing the treatment frame
- Supporting ongoing development and stabilization of the therapeutic alliance
- Exploring initial anxieties stimulated by the treatment setting
- Minimizing risk of the patient's dropping out of treatment before she has the opportunity to become fully engaged

These tasks are overlapping and mutually reinforcing, and in concert they function to bring into the treatment the core object relations organizing the patient's daily experience and presenting problems. By the end of the early phase, the core object relations that repetitively organize the patient's experience inside and outside the treatment hours will have been identified, and will be familiar to both patient and therapist.

Stabilizing the Treatment Frame

Stabilizing the treatment frame and securing the necessary conditions for treatment are top priorities in the opening phase of TFP-E. A viable treatment frame is necessary to do exploratory work and at the same time functions to bring pathogenic object relations into the treatment (see Chapter 8). Patients at a neurotic level of personality organization (NPO) and some at the top of the high range of borderline level of personality organization (BPO) typically have little difficulty working within the treatment frame as agreed upon in the contracting phase. For these individuals, any difficulties with attendance, scheduling, payment, or arriving and ending on time—difficulties often present in the early phase of treatment—tend to be minimally disruptive and can often be relatively easily understood as an expression of anxieties activated by starting treatment.

In contrast, many patients functioning at a middle or low borderline level have initial difficulty maintaining the necessary conditions of treatment agreed upon during contracting. When this is the case, stabilizing the frame is a priority issue and becomes a focus of clinical attention. Over time, the structure and limits provided by the treatment contract and the therapist's attention to maintaining the treatment frame, combined with a treatment contract that minimizes secondary gain, help the patient settle into treatment while relinquishing habitual and destructive acting-out behaviors outside the treatment. As the patient's behavior outside the treatment settles down, things in the treatment tend to "heat up," as object relations that had driven acting-out behaviors in the past are now enacted in the transference.

Clinical Illustration 1: Addressing Employment and Attendance in the Treatment Frame

Mr. W, organized at a middle borderline level, with passive-aggressive and narcissistic features, deeply resented being told what to do; he quietly rebelled by dragging his heels in relation to any demand placed on him. This had been highly disruptive in his interpersonal life and had left him chronically unemployed. Although one of his treatment goals was to find a job, when his therapist, Dr. L, made employment a condition of treatment, Mr. W expressed great outrage and resentment. He delayed for many months, making half-baked efforts to find steady employment. This same patient routinely missed morning sessions, oversleeping after having spent a wild night out on the town.

It was not until 6 months into the treatment, after much discussion of the frame and the viability of the treatment, that Mr. W was both working and consistently attending his sessions. These changes were the result of constant attention to the frame on Dr. L's part; the therapist consistently called attention to deviations from the frame and set limits as needed. As Dr. L called attention to his patient's failure to find employment or to consistently attend sessions, he reminded Mr. W of their treatment contract. Dr. L emphasized that employment, along with consistent and timely attendance at his sessions, was a necessary condition for treatment; only if both these conditions were met could the treatment be successful.

Interventions of this kind, focusing on the integrity of the treatment frame as a reality-based condition for successful treatment, laid the groundwork for pointing out the contradiction between Mr. W's wish to be in treatment as a way to make gains in life, on the one hand, and his choice not to meet the necessary conditions of treatment, on the other. At the same time, Dr. L helped Mr. W explore the object relations enacted in the transference: a struggle between a powerful, controlling, and devaluing figure and a helpless, resentful, and diminished one, with Mr. W consciously identified with the diminished figure but enacting the controlling, devaluing figure in his behavior. These object relations organized the chronic maladaptive behaviors that had brought Mr. W to treatment, and that were now being activated in relation to negotiations around the frame.

Clinical Illustration 2: Limit Setting Around Self-Harm and Secondary Gain

Ms. Y, organized at a middle borderline level with prominent sadomasochistic and borderline features, had a history of chronic depression and of superficial cutting as a way of managing anxiety and distress. In previous treatments with other therapists, as Ms. Y had become engaged in treatment, her cutting had escalated in frequency and severity. The cutting quickly became the focus of these treatments, engaging her former therapists in evaluating her lacerations, and ultimately leading to disruption of the treatment and/or hospitalization.

As part of her TFP-E treatment contract, Ms. Y had agreed that if she had an impulse to cut, she would abstain from acting on her impulse and speak about it in the following session, or if she were unable or unmotivated to abstain, she would obtain medical clearance and a note from her nurse practitioner or other clinician before attending her next session. (See the discussion on contracting in Chapter 8 for further discussion of secondary gain and the rationale for this sort of structuring of the treatment.)

As anticipated, in the early months of treatment, Ms. Y's cutting initially escalated. In response, Dr. M consistently set limits while reducing secondary gain by deferring their next appointment until Ms. Y had visited her nurse practitioner. In this setting, the cutting gradually resolved.

Simultaneously, Ms. Y developed an overtly paranoid transference. She experienced Dr. M as coldly depriving, having robbed her of her sole source of comfort and self-soothing. Elaboration of the object relation underlying this self state led to the description of Dr. M as a sadist devoid of compassion, someone who wanted only to dominate the patient, while Ms. Y had the role of a suffering, helpless victim who had nowhere to turn, no source of relief—"like an animal whose skin has been peeled off." Further exploration of this object relation as it organized the transference initiated a process of understanding the motivations that drove Ms. Y's self-destructive behaviors.

In sum, establishing a relatively stable frame for the treatment is a central task in the early months of TFP-E. In the treatment of patients organized at a borderline level, especially those with severe personality disorders, managing challenges to the treatment frame typically becomes a major focus of intervention in the early phase of treatment. As the therapist sets limits and the contract reduces secondary gain, a patient's destructive behaviors tend to resolve. Ultimately, habitual acting-out behaviors are transformed into object relations enacted in the treatment and in the transference, where they can be identified and explored.

In the treatments of patients with higher level personality pathology, deviations from the treatment frame generally are not overtly destructive and do not threaten the viability of the treatment. Across the range of severity of personality pathology, clinical attention to patients' difficulties in maintaining the frame will lead to identification of anxieties activated by the treatment and in the transference.

Supporting the Development of a Therapeutic Alliance

The second major task of the early phase of treatment is to foster the development and gradual consolidation of a therapeutic alliance (Bender 2005). The relationship among an early therapeutic alliance, treatment dropout, and treatment outcome is one of the most robust findings in psychotherapy research (Crits-Christoph et al. 2013; Horvath and Bedi 2002). Thus, while establishing a stable frame for the treatment is perhaps the highest priority in the opening phase, developing a therapeutic alliance is a close second. As the alliance is strengthened during the opening phase of treatment, the patient's wish to maintain the relationship with the therapist becomes a central motivator for adhering to the treatment contract for patients who have difficulty doing so, and the alliance reduces the likelihood of early dropout for patients across the spectrum of severity.

In TFP-E, alliance building is accomplished through attending to shared *goals*, the specific *tasks* of the participants in their work together, and the therapist's attitude toward the patient and her difficulties, supporting the development of a *bond* between them. These approaches to alliance building are adopted in many forms of treatment and are not limited to a specific frame of reference or approach to therapeutic technique. What is specific to TFP-E is that at the same time that the therapist focuses on goals, tasks, and the bond, he also actively addresses *negative transferences* to support the development of a therapeutic alliance. The TFP-E therapist directs attention to negative transferences early, actively, and consistently. In sum, in TFP-E, the therapeutic alliance is built on the combined impact of 1) the therapist's steady interest and concern, accepting and nonjudgmental attitude, and empathic listening and effort to understand (see also Chapter 5 discussion of the alliance, therapeutic attitude, and the therapist's stance); and 2) an exploration of the negative transference.[1]

---

[1]The therapist's attention to negative transference in the opening phase is supported by the work of Levy et al. 2015.

The foundation for the developing treatment alliance is in place even before the opening phase begins (Hilsenroth and Cromer 2007). As we describe in Chapter 7, patient and therapist begin to establish a relationship in their initial meetings during the assessment. In these initial sessions, the therapist lays the groundwork for the development of a therapeutic alliance by maintaining an open, curious, and nonjudgmental stance, and by demonstrating concern for and interest in knowing the patient. The alliance is further fostered toward the conclusion of the assessment phase as the therapist shares his diagnostic impression, helping the patient make sense of her difficulties, and then helps the patient identify treatment goals and select among available treatment options.

In the contracting phase, as part of introducing the frame, the therapist explains in detail how the therapy will proceed and outlines the specific tasks and roles of patient and therapist. Each of these interventions, focusing on goals, tasks, and the bond between patient and therapist (Bordin 1979), contributes to the developing alliance and to the patient's experience of the therapist as knowledgeable, professional, caring, and able to offer useful help.

Differences Across the Range of Severity

Patients organized at a neurotic level typically develop and solidify a therapeutic alliance with relative ease during the early months of treatment in response to the therapist's interest, concern, and attention to early anxieties stimulated by the treatment setting (Caligor et al. 2007; see also Chapter 5 for additional discussion and citations). With this population of patients, the alliance is typically established relatively easily and naturally in early contacts between patient and therapist, and develops relatively smoothly through the initial phase of treatment. The developing alliance deepens as the therapist helps the patient identify the anxieties stimulated in the patient by beginning treatment and links them to early, often preconscious negative transferences.

In contrast to NPO patients, BPO patients typically have difficulty developing a stable therapeutic alliance (Yeomans et al. 2015; see also Chapter 4 for additional discussion and citations). With BPO patients, the initial alliance is often tenuous and unstable; it is inevitably vulnerable to disruption by emerging paranoid transferences, and often fluctuates over the course of a session or from one session to the next.

With BPO patients, the alliance tends to gradually deepen and stabilize through the entire first half of the treatment, but it is often punctuated by temporary ruptures introduced by emerging negative transferences. From this perspective, we can operationalize the therapeutic alliance as the conditions under which the patient establishes a positive bond with the therapist that can survive negative and erotic transferences and associated affects, and under which the therapist maintains a reciprocal positive bond despite the impact of countertransference. In the opening phase with BPO patients, the developing alliance requires consistent attention.

As a rule, as a patient's personality pathology becomes more severe, and as aggression and splitting become more prominent and extreme, the development of an alliance becomes increasingly challenging. However, even quite disturbed and aggressive patients with personality disorders, if motivated for treatment, may be able to establish a rudimentary alliance during the opening phase; conversely, as exemplified in Clinical Illustration 3 (which follows), some patients, although relatively well integrated, may experience a fair amount of difficulty in establishing an alliance. High-BPO patients, for the most part, have less difficulty than patients with severe personality disorders, and patients with narcissistic personality disorder and those with antisocial traits have the greatest difficulty of all. Individuals with antisocial personality disorder proper are by definition incapable of forming an alliance (Patrick 2007).

Negative Transferences

Paranoid Transferences. We can generalize by observing that across the spectrum of severity, early activation of *concretely experienced* paranoid transferences poses a challenge to the developing alliance. When paranoid transferences are concrete, the patient is unable to entertain alternative perspectives that might contextualize her current experience in relation to other, more neutral or positive experiences of the therapist. In this setting, the therapist's attitude of respect and concern, so helpful in alliance building for many healthier patients—or even for the same patient at other times—may have little impact on the paranoid patient, who may experience anything the therapist says or does, regardless of content or intention, as an attack or as further evidence of the therapist's malevolence or untrustworthiness.

In the treatment of BPO patients, the predictable emergence of paranoid transferences in the early phase of treatment calls for active and persistent intervention. The therapist's task in each session is to address any negative transference that may be in evidence, empathizing with, elaborating, and exploring the object relations coloring the patient's view of the therapist and of her self experience in session. Exploring paranoid transference can bolster a faltering alliance in the moment, and over time facilitates the gradual development and consolidation of an alliance that reflects more reality-based aspects of the relationship.

Narcissistic Transferences. Patients with narcissistic personality disorder, as well as those with other personality disorders with extremely rigid narcissistic defenses, present particular challenges to alliance building during the opening phase. These individuals may present an attitude toward the treatment that is implicitly, and sometimes explicitly, rejecting of the therapist's efforts to be of help. The patient's attitude in these circumstances is often driven by painful feelings of envy, conscious or unconscious, that create a psychological situation in which it becomes intolerable for the patient to acknowledge the therapist's expertise or potential contributions. To avoid such misery, narcissistic patients commonly cast the therapist in the role of audience to the patient's independent process of self-exploration, or openly devalue the therapist. Insofar as the patient does not acknowledge the therapist as an autonomous, contributing presence, an alliance cannot develop. With this group of patients, therefore, the opening phase may be prolonged while the treatment focuses on confrontation of these narcissistic transferences. We refer the reader to Chapters 5 and 11 for additional clinical illustrations of management of negative transferences.

Clinical Illustration 3: Containment and Technical Neutrality Around Narcissistic Defenses

Ms. F, a married professional woman, functioning on the border between high BPO and NPO, with prominent narcissistic and masochistic conflicts and character defenses, sought treatment for depression. Several years earlier, one of her young-adult children had been diagnosed with a debilitating chronic illness. Ms. F experienced the diagnosis and its chronicity as a blow that she had been unable to cope with or recover from, and she described suffering profound sadness and envy whenever she heard from friends or colleagues about their own healthy children.

Ms. F's relationships were long lasting and stable, but she had a tendency to be critical and to assume a morally superior stance when others didn't do what she thought correct or when they seemed to "get away with things"; in the face of disagreement, she had a tendency to "get stuck," ruminating on perceived wrongs, and in her mind insisting that the other admit to personal failings.

From the earliest sessions with Dr. A, Ms. F made it clear that she had little faith in the medical profession. She came to treatment angry and mistrustful, ready to criticize Dr. A for the smallest shortcoming, and demonstrating little expectation that Dr. A would understand or help her. Deep down, Ms. F experienced beginning treatment as putting herself in the hands of someone who had all the things that she did not, and who shared none of her heartache, although this was not something she spoke about directly with Dr. A. Instead, Ms. F fell back on her propensity to be critical and morally superior, accusing Dr. A of being thoughtless in his comments, or insufficiently caring or attentive, or charging too much money. Throughout the week, she would ruminate on his transgressions.

Nevertheless, Ms. F continued to attend all scheduled sessions, arriving on time, but often wondered out loud, "What am I doing here?" In the countertransference, Dr. A felt constantly second-guessed, criticized, and devalued. He found himself thinking that perhaps he could not help this patient and wondered whether he might be relieved if Ms. F were to leave the treatment.

In this setting, Dr. A focused on promoting an alliance. He contained his countertransference and whenever possible shared with Ms. F his understanding of her experience of him as potentially uncaring, unsympathetic, incompetent, and unable to empathize with her pain. For example, he would say to her, "I see that my comment reinforced your view of me as loose-lipped, insufficiently caring, and inattentive." Dr. A offered such interventions from a position of technical neutrality, after absorbing— rather than reacting to—Ms. F's criticisms. Dr. A made an effort not to get sucked into debate about his failings, he did not retaliate or respond in kind, and he also abstained from reassuring Ms. F that "everything will be fine." Rather, Dr. A withstood her devaluation and hostility, and contained it; Dr. A communicated concern while retaining a respectful, noncritical, yet self-respecting attitude.

As Dr. A was able to manage his countertransference, and then to stand back and observe and reflect on the object relations being enacted in the treatment, he came to understand Ms. F's criticism and devaluation as defensive. In his mind, he imagined an object relation in which Dr. A was fortunate, superior, and triumphant, while Ms. F was defeated, envious, and resentful. This object relation was colored by feelings of mistrust and resentment, and deeply buried underneath them were unsatisfied longings to be taken care of. (Dr. A made these inferences about Ms. F's dynamics less on the basis of what she told him and more on his understanding of the countertransference and his prior clinical experience with narcissistic defenses and conflicts in relation to dependency.) In sessions, Dr. A began to gently call attention, at times with humor, to Ms. F's critical and devaluing, often scathing behavior toward him; at the same time, he remained mindful of the unconscious subtext of Ms. F's experience, in which she hid her frustrated longings to be cared for.

Dr. A began by reminding Ms. F that she had come to him for help with her sadness. If Ms. F really felt that Dr. A could not possibly understand or help her, she might do better to choose another therapist. However, if she held out some hope that she could benefit from the treatment, as seemed evidenced by her continued attendance and participation, it would make sense to try to understand why she treated Dr. A in the way she did, and to explore how this might relate to the problems that had brought her to treatment.

Dr. A held his ground. Over time he noted a gradual shift in the atmosphere in the sessions. Although Ms. F remained quick to criticize and to suspect Dr. A of either incompetence or inconsiderateness, there was an underlying sense of mutual warmth between them, of a developing collaborative relationship, and of deepening trust on the part of Ms. F that alternated and at times seemed to coexist with her hostility and devaluation. This shift heralded an emerging therapeutic alliance; for the first time, Ms. F spoke openly about the discrepancies she imagined between her life situation and that of Dr. A's privileged position, and how painful it was in that setting to come to him for help. This opened the door to a process of identifying and exploring unconscious expectations, linked to Ms. F's core conflicts and presenting problems; it was then possible to understand Ms. F's unconscious belief that Dr. A secretly enjoyed her sadness, using it in his own mind to reassure himself of his good fortune and superiority.

Exploring Early Anxieties Stimulated in Treatment and Fostering Open Communication

The third major task of the opening phase of TFP-E is to identify and explore initial anxieties stimulated in the treatment, often enacted in negative transferences and/or manifesting as difficulty in communicating openly and freely in session. The relatively intimate and unstructured nature of the therapeutic setting and the patient's vulnerable position in that setting, as well as the invitation to the patient to take the lead in session and to speak openly and freely, tend to stimulate anxiety. Most patients initially find it difficult to share their inner, private thoughts and feelings, and the therapist pays careful attention to the patient's response. Some patients cannot think what to say; others may structure or prepare their communications before they come to session; some fill the space with trivial communications; and still others act out outside the treatment hours in lieu of communicating in them. Some respond to their difficulty by asking the therapist to direct them, some wait in silence until the therapist takes the lead, and others act as if the therapist is not there.

Regardless of the specifics of the patient's responses, early interventions in TFP-E focus on exploring the behaviors and anxieties stimulated by the treatment setting, the therapeutic relationship, and the invitation to communicate openly about inner thoughts and feelings. The therapist's attention to and tactful exploration of anxieties stimulated in the treatment gradually free the patient to communicate more openly with the therapist, while supporting the developing alliance. At the same time, the process of identifying and elaborating early anxieties initiates the exploratory process that characterizes the treatment as a whole; exploring initial anxieties stimulated by the treatment setting helps bring into focus internal object relations linked to core conflicts, while promoting self-observation and reflection.

Clinical Illustration 4: Using Clarification and Interpretation to Address Anxieties

Mr. V, an NPO patient with avoidant and depressive personality traits, frequently found himself feeling anxious in his sessions. As his therapist asked for clarification, Mr. V, a highly introverted person, was ultimately able to share his sense that he didn't know what to speak about, that he was somehow "doing it wrong," and that he was ill-suited for a dynamic therapy.

Dr. Y suggested, "It sounds like part of the problem is that you expect that I will not understand how challenging it is for you to begin in this therapy, as if you anticipate that I will be impatient or even critical of you." As Dr. Y helped her patient become more fully aware of the anxieties stimulated by beginning treatment, Mr. V was able to reflect on them and to some degree distance himself from them, better distinguishing between his therapist in the transference (demanding, critical) and the therapist in her role (empathic, patient, helpful).

Mr. V began to relax as he came to view his anxieties as worries rather than as facts, and as aspects of his experience that were of interest, to be observed and understood in collaboration with Dr. Y. He was able to settle more comfortably into the treatment while developing greater trust in Dr. Y's interest and concern.

Minimizing the Risk of the Patient's Dropping Out of Treatment

Before the alliance has had time to develop—and often precipitated by early anxieties and negative transferences, premature dropout from treatment is common in psychotherapy. Early dropout is especially common in the treatment of BPO patients. Thus, minimizing the risk of dropout is an overriding task of the early phase of TFP-E. Central tactics employed to minimize risk have already been covered in earlier sections in this chapter in which we address stabilizing the treatment frame, supporting the alliance, and exploring initial anxieties simulated by the treatment setting. Individually and in concert, addressing these tasks reduces the risk of dropout, even in patients with severe and/or narcissistic pathology where the rate of dropout is especially high.

Struggles in relation to the frame or spotty attendance are most often the point of entry with the patient at acute and high risk of dropping out. With a patient at high risk for dropout during the early phase, the therapist may feel tempted to attempt to "hold" the patient by adopting a supportive stance and being accommodating and flexible in relation to the patient's demands and behavior (e.g., "I can only meet once a week," when an agreement had been made during contracting to meet twice weekly, or the patient consistently misses sessions while asking the therapist to be flexible "just for now"). However, in most circumstances, the most effective way to retain the patient at risk for dropping out is to combine many of the tasks discussed earlier in this chapter—to acknowledge the patient's difficulties while maintaining the frame rather than bending it, and then to identify and explore the anxieties activated in relation to the setting, in the process supporting the therapeutic alliance.

Clinical Illustration 5: Maintaining the Treatment Frame With a Patient At Risk of Dropping Out

The patient is a 25-year-old female graduate student organized at a middle borderline level with prominent narcissistic traits. Six weeks into her therapy and a week before an upcoming holiday break during which the patient planned to be out of town, the patient left a voice mail for her therapist announcing that she would have to cancel her Monday and Wednesday sessions, the last remaining sessions before the holiday interruption. In her voice mail the patient explained that she had procrastinated over the weekend and now needed to cancel her sessions to make time to work on a crucial term paper. She added that "if needed" she could conduct the sessions on the phone. When she received the patient's message the therapist felt overtly devalued; at the same time, the therapist noted her own temptation to be flexible, fearing that the patient was "hanging on by a thread" and would likely drop out if she did not accommodate the patient with phone sessions. In contrast, the therapist's supervision group suggested that the therapist hold her ground.

The therapist called the patient, making sure to speak with her directly, and after several attempts got her on the phone. During their conversation, the therapist emphasized that she understood the importance of the patient's academic deadlines; at the same time, the positive outcome of the treatment rested on their maintaining a regular schedule, especially before a break. In response to the therapist's call, the patient agreed to come in. In the following session the therapist was able to put into words the patient's view that coming to her sessions when she had academic work to do was a devaluation of the importance of her academic work, as if to say that it was inconsequential relative to the therapeutic work and demands of the therapist; conversely, canceling the appointments was a statement that her academic work was more important than that of the therapist. Putting words to this experience of needing to fend off devaluation in the transference helped the patient to put her sense of injury into perspective, supporting a weak alliance and enabling the patient to begin to settle in more comfortably into the treatment.

Markers of Change and Transition to the Middle Phase

As the treatment transitions from the early phase to the middle phase, the treatment frame will have been firmly established, a developing therapeutic alliance will be in place, and patient and therapist will have explored initial anxieties stimulated by the treatment setting. In this process, core object relations that organize the patient's moment-to-moment experience and presenting problems will have been identified and explored. The patient will have come to appreciate that repetitive enactment of these object relations constrains her, introducing rigidity into her experience and behavior. These developments ready the patient to continue into the middle phase, where conflicts motivating enactment of these pathogenic object relations will be explored and ultimately worked through, the latter being the central task of the middle phase of treatment.

By the end of the early phase of treatment, the NPO patient will have become familiar with the defensive object relations that consistently and stably organize her experience and behavior in areas of conflict. These object relations will have been linked to the maladaptive traits and repetitive thoughts and feelings that brought the patient to treatment. Through repeated cycles of clarification and confrontation, the patient will have come to question familiar rationalizations about her own personality traits and maladaptive behaviors. These changes correspond with an increased capacity for self-observation and introspection in areas of conflict, and with early decreases in personality rigidity as maladaptive traits and defenses become ego-dystonic.

In the treatment of BPO patients, the structure of the treatment frame, supported by limit setting if need be, may lead to significant behavioral change during the early phase of treatment. By the end of the early phase, BPO patients, for the most part, will have relinquished habitual destructive acting-out behaviors and will be engaged in full-time, structured activity. By the time of transition to the middle phase, the BPO patient is familiar with core conflictual object relations through their impact on her experiences in the transference and through awareness of how these relations are enacted interpersonally. The BPO patient will have developed at least a rudimentary awareness of identifications with both sides of pathogenic object relations—at moments viewing herself as aggressor as well as victim in the paranoid dyad, reflecting an increased capacity for self-observation and an ability to entertain alternative perspectives in areas of conflict.

These developments often lead to some degree of stabilization of the patient's interpersonal relationships, even as the transference may become more affectively charged. As the BPO patient transitions to the middle phase, she is more aware of the instability of her experience and can identify shifts between idealized and paranoid perspectives, reflecting increased ego-dystonicity of splitting-based defenses and an early capacity to reflect on internal states—that is, to mentalize—at times of relative calm.

Middle Treatment Phase

The middle phase of TFP-E typically lasts from 1 to 3 years. The central task of the middle phase is to explore and work through the object relations defining core conflicts, with the aim of promoting integrative processes within the patient. This task is an application of the strategies of treatment described in Chapter 6, and it makes use of the techniques and tactics elaborated in Chapters 10–12. Because this material has already been extensively described and illustrated in earlier chapters, here we emphasize typical clinical developments.

As a result of the work of the opening phase of treatment, the patient entering the middle phase has a developing appreciation of the nature of many of the core object relations that organize her experience. The overarching task of the middle phase is to link these object relations to underlying paranoid and depressive anxieties and to work through related conflicts, promoting integrative processes within the patient. This work rests on the foundation built in the early phase, including a stable treatment frame, a therapeutic alliance, and a developing capacity within the patient to observe and reflect on her behavior and internal experience. Working through in the middle phase leads to gradual shifts in the quality of the object relations organizing the patient's experience. In BPO patients, working through leads to the gradual integration of paranoid and idealized object relations—the process of identity consolidation. In NPO patients, working through leads to containment of conflictual object relations within dominant self experience—the process of decreasing personality rigidity and deepening affective experience.

The following are the major tasks of working through in the middle phase of treatment:

- Repeatedly exploring and interpreting core conflicts (i.e., the process of working through)
- Exploring the paranoid and depressive anxieties interfering with integrative processes
- Focusing on the treatment goals
- Working through the developmental antecedents of conflictual object relations
- Working through negative therapeutic reactions if they emerge

Working Through

The process of working through begins in the middle phase of treatment, continues into the termination phase, and ultimately is completed by the patient, working independently of the therapist after treatment ends. However, the bulk of working through takes place during the middle phase of treatment. In the treatment of BPO patients, the transference is often a major focus of working through; at the same time, the therapist will make sure to ground exploratory work in reality by simultaneously calling attention to parallel enactments in the patient's current interpersonal life. In the treatment of NPO patients, working through is typically focused outside the transference, although with most patients there are opportunities for the therapist to point out parallel enactments, even if subtle, in the treatment setting and in relation to the therapist. (See Chapter 12 for additional discussion of working through.)

In the TFP-E approach, it is the process of working through that provides the link between self-exploration and therapeutic change; working through leads to integrative changes corresponding with enhanced capacity for perspective taking and contextualization of experience in areas of conflict, flexible and adaptive functioning, and symptomatic improvement. Across the spectrum of severity, the process of repeatedly activating, enacting, and exploring a given conflict will lead to the containment of conflictual object relations while promoting a more complete level of self-awareness and, ultimately, a more emotionally meaningful level of self-understanding.

In the BPO patient, the repetitive process of working through strengthens the capacity for "top-down" management of maladaptive behaviors, supports the capacity for affect containment, and leads to the gradual integration of paranoid and idealized sectors of experience. In the NPO patient, the process of repeatedly activating, enacting, and interpreting a given conflict facilitates the increasing capacity to tolerate awareness of, and to symbolically manage, conflictual aspects of experience, reducing anxiety and introducing greater flexibility into personality functioning.

Working through rests on the therapist's capacity to contain the paranoid and depressive anxieties activated in the treatment setting and in the transference-countertransference; this process, in turn, promotes and supports the patient's developing capacity to contain the anxieties and mental states associated with activation of conflictual object relations. In this process, the patient will come to appreciate the role of her identifications with both halves of any particular object relation, as well as the ways in which activation of a particular internal object relation or conflict defends against others. It is also during the process of working through that the therapist is able to most effectively link current difficulties to the past. In this setting, folding in a link to the past can promote further containment and symbolic management of conflictual object relations; current experience is enriched as the patient develops a new and deeper appreciation of the role of her developmental past in her current experience. Ultimately, the patient will come to take responsibility for previously repressed and dissociated aspects of herself and of her internal objects, past and present.

Gradual Shifts in the Quality of Object Relations Across the Spectrum of Severity

The object relations that emerge early in treatment of NPO patients are predominantly defensive, relatively realistic, and well integrated. In contrast, as the patient moves through the middle phase, the object relations explored in the treatment may more directly represent conflictual motivations and associated anxieties; this progression occurs as the NPO patient gains greater access to her inner life and becomes more tolerant of awareness of unacceptable, warded-off parts of her inner world. The patient's capacity to tolerate awareness of a broader range of psychological experience in the middle phase is supported by the tolerant and accepting attitude of the containing therapist, as conflictual object relations are enacted in the treatment and explored.

In the treatment of BPO patients, object relations enacted early in the middle phase are by definition split, to a greater or lesser degree, depending on the severity of the patient's pathology and the conflicts currently activated. Through the course of the middle phase, the therapist can expect to see evidence of an uneven but overall progressive shift toward integration and resolution of splitting in the BPO patient. At the level of the macroprocess (i.e., over months and years of treatment), as the patient moves through the middle phase, object relations become less widely split, increasingly complex, and better affectively modulated. In the microprocess (i.e., over the course of a session or several sessions), the patient can be seen to oscillate between better-integrated self states associated with stable reflective capacities, on the one hand, and more poorly integrated self states and a lack of reflectiveness, on the other.

As the patient moves through the middle phase into the advanced phase of treatment, periods of integration become more frequent and more prolonged and are punctuated by more or less transient regressions to split states. In this process, the patient becomes better able to step back, observe, and reflect on her experience even in areas of conflict, enhancing her capacity for containment of affect and facilitating further integration. Throughout, the shift from splitting toward integration, reflected in the patient's developing capacity to tolerate more complex affective states and to appreciate a broader range of psychological experience, is supported by the therapist's ability to contain the patient's projections and highly charged affect states.

Exploring Paranoid and Depressive Anxieties Interfering With Integrative Processes

The topic of phases of treatment raises the question of whether there is a particular order in which therapists typically encounter or explore the patient's conflicts, and also whether these differ among patients at different levels of personality organization. The answers to these questions are complex. There is tremendous variation from patient to patient regarding the order in which conflicts unfold in treatment, and depending on which conflicts are most threatening to the patient.

As described in Chapter 3, conflicts can be divided into those associated with paranoid anxieties and those associated with depressive anxieties. A paranoid orientation implies that threatening aspects of the patient's internal world are split off from dominant self experience and projected. As a result, the patient feels herself to be in danger in relation to an object perceived as in some way threatening. Responsibility is located externally, and the dominant affects are anxiety and fear. In contrast, a depressive orientation implies the capacity to contain conflictual motivations and emotional states rather than project them; the patient fears not for herself but for her objects, who are seen to be in danger as a result of the patient's own aggressive and self-serving motivations. The dominant affects associated with depressive anxiety are guilt and loss, often in conjunction with wishes to make reparations.

Paranoid anxieties are associated with more or less polarized images of self and other. In the setting of a paranoid orientation, these anxieties can be articulated as follows (using first-person "I" for simplicity, as if the patient were able to express the underlying conflicts): "The person whom I fear and loathe is entirely separate from the person whom I love and trust; if I feel hateful, envious, or competitive, it is because the object of my hostility is entirely worthy of being hated or defeated." (Note that there is no conflict as long as the patient maintains separation between the two sets of object relations—the loving and the hateful.)

Depressive anxieties, on the other hand, are associated with relatively well-integrated, or ambivalent, experiences of self and other (using first-person "I" for simplicity, as above): "The person toward whom I am potentially destructive is also someone I love and trust; I am someone who is both loving and destructive, as is my object." (Note that conflict is inevitable in this setting.)

Working through paranoid anxieties and moving toward a more predominantly depressive orientation enhances the patient's capacity to sustain an increasingly deep, stable, and complex image of herself and her objects (Steiner 1996). Because depressive anxieties are most fully experienced in relation to whole, ambivalent objects (Klein 1935/1975; Steiner 1993), addressing paranoid anxieties in therapy before depressive anxieties facilitates the working through of both sets of anxieties.

The strategy of addressing paranoid before depressive anxieties applies both to the microprocess within a given session and to the macroprocess over months and even years of treatment. On a macro level, as paranoid anxieties are worked through during the middle phase, depressive anxieties gradually become a more consistent focus in treatment. On a micro level, once the patient's core paranoid and depressive anxieties and the associated object relations have been identified and explored in treatment, the patient will tend to oscillate between paranoid and depressive dynamics, as part of the process of working through. Thus, while the overall trajectory of the treatment is to more solidly establish a depressive level of functioning in areas of conflict, during the middle phase, moment to moment and session to session, patients will typically oscillate between depressive and paranoid orientations.

Paranoid and Depressive Conflicts Across Levels of Personality Organization

All patients will grapple with both paranoid and depressive anxieties during the course of treatment, and all shift toward increasing centrality of depressive over paranoid anxieties over the course of treatment (Steiner

1993). In the middle phase, the process of working through invariably entails tracking how one set of anxieties can defend against the other, beginning with what is affectively dominant. Respecting the unique makeup of each patient, we note that there are general differences in the typical dynamics encountered with NPO, high-BPO, and low-BPO patients; these differences are not hard and fast. Understanding these general distinctions can enable the therapist to anticipate how dynamics are likely to unfold in the middle phase.

Neurotic Level of Personality Organization. As discussed in Chapter 3, in the setting of NPO, dominant conflicts are depressive. Thus, the TFP-E therapist of an NPO patient who is entering the middle phase of treatment can anticipate that the focus of much of the work ahead will involve exploring and working through depressive anxieties. To review in brief, NPO patients suffer from an inability to assimilate aspects of the self, tied to conflictual motivations, that are viewed as unacceptable. Awareness of conflictual motivations stimulates anxieties—typically, depressive anxiety, but also at times paranoid anxiety. The therapist observes the patient grappling with *depressive* conflicts and anxieties to the degree that the patient is in an integrated world of "whole" objects (representations of self and other are well integrated, neither all good nor all bad) and is taking responsibility for (as opposed to projecting or denying) her impulses (Hinshelwood 1991; Joseph 1987/1988). In a neurotic structure, when paranoid anxieties emerge, they can often be seen as defensive retreats from depressive anxieties. As the patient moves through the middle phase and develops greater capacity to take responsibility for conflictual motivations, tolerates depressive anxieties, and ultimately works through them, paranoid concerns tend to fade.

Clinical Illustration 6: Working Through Depressive Conflicts and Anxieties

Ms. I, a graduate student organized at a neurotic level, experienced conflicts in relation to competitive aggression; she was chronically fearful of being undermined or humiliated by her middle-aged female mentor. As this object relation was explored in the early middle phase of her therapy, the patient acknowledged that she secretly viewed her mentor with quiet contempt, seeing her as older, less attractive, and less capable than she. As Ms. I attended to and reflected on her attitude, she came to feel self-critical and, ultimately, remorseful; her mentor had in fact been generous and helpful, whereas Ms. I had reciprocated with covert hostility and devaluation.

In this example, Ms. I's fears of being undermined and humiliated represented a defensive role reversal within a hostile and competitive object relation—a sort of paranoid retreat from, and projection of, her own hostility and devaluation—all in the service of protecting her from taking responsibility for her aggression and from painful feelings of guilt and remorse. As Ms. I became increasingly able to take responsibility for her competitive aggression and worked through her conflicts in relation to wishes to triumph over other women, she became more comfortable with her mentor. Ms. I found it easy to treat her mentor with respect and to experience gratitude for the mentorship she provided, while also accepting the areas in which her mentor fell short. She came to accept her own competitive side, working hard to succeed and quietly enjoying her triumphs without needing to undermine, or to fear, her competitors.

Another NPO patient, more deeply conflicted and more aggressive than Ms. I, might respond to similar conflicts by activating splitting-based defenses. For example, such a patient might demonize her mentor, becoming enraged while seeing her mentor as untrustworthy and ruthless, single-mindedly needing to triumph over all potential rivals; or the patient might entirely devalue her mentor, seeing her as pathetic and inept, incompetent and totally lacking in any useful expertise, with the patient feeling deprived, resentful, and hostile (see also the discussion of "splitting of the depressive position" in Chapter 3, Clinical Illustration "Dynamic Relationship Between Paranoid and Depressive Orientations in a Patient Organized at a Neurotic Level"). For such patients, interpretation and working through of splitting as a way to obviate depressive anxieties is the first task of the middle phase, opening up the possibility of helping the patient tolerate and work through depressive anxieties as she moves through the middle phase, so as to facilitate her becoming more comfortable with and better able to manage her competitive aggression.

Borderline Level of Personality Organization.   As they enter the middle phase of treatment, BPO patients, in whom splitting-based defenses predominate, struggle primarily with paranoid anxieties. The major task of the middle phase, from a dynamic perspective, is to help the patient relinquish splitting, which entails the patient's development of the capacity to contain first paranoid and then—at more advanced phases of personality integration—depressive anxieties. These developments constitute a gradual process of integration that subsumes the middle phase in the treatment of BPO patients. During this process, shifts toward integration reflect the patient's capacity, in the moment, to contain the paranoid and depressive anxieties that drive splitting, whereas shifts toward less-well-integrated self states reflect a defensive retreat from those anxieties. Tracking these oscillations and exploring the anxieties that drive them characterize the process of working through in the middle phase of the treatment of BPO patients.

Initially, in the early middle phase, as a result of focused clinical attention on splitting and on paranoid and idealized object relations, the patient comes to appreciate how paranoid and idealized object relations mutually defend against one another, and she begins to cognitively bridge the two sectors. Exploring the paranoid anxieties that motivate splitting, while helping the patient to test reality and contain these anxieties, promotes further integration. Repeated confrontation of splitting, followed by exploring and working through the underlying paranoid anxieties, allows for moments of greater integration of idealized and paranoid object relations. By the midpoint of the middle phase, moments of partial integration have become more frequent and more sustained as splitting becomes less pervasive and less extreme.

Moments of integration expose the BPO patient to the experience of a more or less integrated self, vulnerable to and/or directing conflictual impulses toward a more or less integrated vulnerable object—that is, to depressive anxieties. This development represents a major turning point in the treatment of BPO patients; initially, depressive anxieties are poorly tolerated, triggering a defensive return to splitting to avoid depressive as well as paranoid anxieties. During the second half of the middle phase, therapeutic work comes to focus on tracking the patient's oscillation between better-integrated and less-well-integrated split states, each defending against the other, and exploring the depressive and paranoid anxieties that drive splitting, as the patient has the opportunity to work through both sets of anxieties. As integration proceeds, with the patient tolerating more complete and protracted periods of integration, splitting comes to defend predominantly against depressive anxieties. Finally, as these anxieties are explored, worked through, and at least partially contained, the patient is able to consolidate an integrated sense of self.

We have outlined in broad strokes the dynamic shifts that characterize the middle phase of treatment with BPO patients. There are, in addition, important differences between midphase developments in the treatment of low- and middle-BPO patients and midphase developments in the treatment of high-BPO patients. In the more severe groups, the early middle phase is dominated by paranoid object relations, often highly affectively charged and concretely experienced, which are enacted and explored in the transference and in the patient's interpersonal life. Clinical focus on the transference, in particular, provides an opportunity for needed affect containment (see Chapter 6, Part 3, section "Patients Along the Borderline Spectrum of Personality Organization," subsection "Strategy 2"; and

Chapter 11, Clinical Illustration 1: "Clarification of Paranoid Transference") and facilitates confrontation of role reversals within a paranoid object relation.

For some patients, many months of exploring paranoid object relations may be necessary before idealized object relations and transferences become accessible. Once both idealized and paranoid sectors are available, the therapist begins to confront their mutual dissociation and proceeds as outlined above. What is distinctive about the more severe personality disorders is the predominance of paranoid object relations relative to idealized experiences, such that initial interventions focus predominantly on paranoid object relations and the relatively long duration of the middle phase. Depressive anxieties tend to emerge relatively late, after paranoid anxieties are explored and to some degree worked through, allowing moments of integration to become accessible to the patient.

In contrast, idealized object relations often dominate the experience of high-BPO patients as they enter the middle phase. Idealization allows the patient to at least partially gratify dependency needs in the setting of failure of identity consolidation, while warding off enactment of dissociated paranoid object relations. After initial difficulties that often emerge in relation to the contract are resolved in the opening phase, high-BPO patients may fall into relatively stable idealization of the therapist, often mirroring the patient's relations with significant others. In contrast to what is typically seen in the low-BPO patient, depressive anxieties often play a central role from quite early on with high-BPO patients; exploration of motivations for splitting leads to the relatively quick emergence of depressive as well as paranoid anxieties, as the high-BPO patient often comes to treatment already benefiting from moments of partial integration. As these anxieties are explored, worked through, and contained, the therapist sees identity consolidation and the resolution of splitting, reflected in the patient's capacity—in the transference and in the patient's interpersonal and intimate life—to tolerate vulnerability without idealization, and to take responsibility for aggression toward complex objects.

Clinical Illustration 7: Working Through Paranoid Transference

Mr. J, a middle-BPO patient with borderline, narcissistic, and paranoid features, presented with painful feelings of self-loathing and problems at work due to hostile outbursts during which he became quite paranoid. The patient entered the middle phase with a paranoid transference in which he experienced the therapist, Dr. H, as he did his boss: as a powerful and dangerous enemy. The only evidence of an idealized side of the split was Mr. J's seemingly contradictory choice to continue in treatment, despite his hostility toward and mistrust of Dr. H.

During the early phase, Dr. H worked with Mr. J first to articulate Mr. J's paranoid experience of the therapist, and next to tolerate awareness of Mr. J's quite flagrant and hostile attacks on the therapist, by calling attention to constant and rapid role reversals within a paranoid dyad. During this period, Dr. H made great efforts to contain Mr. J's hostility, while noting to himself the apparent absence of an alliance.

Many months later, with the therapy well into the middle phase, Dr. H become aware that Mr. J had stopped complaining about his job; sessions were no longer punctuated by paranoid outbursts focusing on his rage at his boss, who had placed him on probation, and at his coworkers, who he felt bullied and devalued him. When Dr. H inquired about what had been happening at work, Mr. J explained, to the therapist's surprise, that he was no longer on probation. In response to Dr. H's commenting on Mr. J's not having raised in session that his status at work had improved, Mr. J responded that he had not thought it was worth mentioning.

As therapist and patient clarified the specifics of what had been happening at Mr. J's workplace, Dr. H noted what appeared to be the emergence within the patient of a view of himself as potentially able to succeed, coupled with reluctance to bring this into the treatment. The emerging, positive view of himself entertained by Mr. J was linked in his mind to the experience of being under the protection of Dr. H, a man who "knew how to make it." The therapist called attention to the discrepant views that the patient had held of him over time: first a dangerous enemy, and now at times a powerful, healing savior. Dr. H also pointed to Mr. J's reluctance to share the positive side of his experience, and suggested that perhaps Mr. J was motivated to sequester the positive because it seemed fragile; it could be too easily destroyed when, at any moment, the powerful, healing therapist might turn on him to become, once again, an enemy [*this is an example of paranoid anxiety*].

Only after many months during which Dr. H tracked the oscillation between Mr. J's paranoid transferences and brief moments of idealization, highlighting that both were extreme and distorted and pointing out how each defended against the other, did Mr. J begin to have moments of more integrated experience. This shift was heralded by the patient's acknowledgment that after a session in which he had been especially hostile toward the therapist, he'd found himself feeling regretful for having bullied him so aggressively.

Focusing on Treatment Goals

As discussed in Chapter 9, the TFP-E therapist remains mindful of the treatment goals and of related developments (or lack of them) in the patient's daily life. It is easy to become lost in moment-to-moment issues, be they in the clinical process or in the patient's daily life. However, while exploring acute developments, the therapist attempts to maintain awareness, in each session and throughout the treatment, of the difficulties that brought the patient to treatment and of the longer-term treatment goals. As conflictual object relations are enacted in the treatment and the patient's core conflicts come into focus during the middle phase, the therapist will be asking himself, "What is the relationship between the object relations currently being explored and the treatment goals?" Similarly, when a session seems unfocused or confusing, the therapist will contemplate, "How does this material relate to or fail to relate to (i.e., represent avoidance of) the treatment goals?" And while focusing on a particular development in the patient's life, be it an acute crisis or a more chronic issue, the therapist will at the same time consider how this development relates to the problems that brought the patient to treatment in the first place.

Neurotic Level of Personality Organization

TFP-E with NPO patients is oriented toward reducing personality rigidity in circumscribed areas of functioning, defined by presenting complaints and treatment goals. With this objective in mind, as core conflicts are worked through in the middle phase, the NPO patient's therapist will preferentially focus on the relationship between the active conflict and the patient's presenting complaints and treatment goals. Typically (and very much in contrast to what is seen with BPO patients), NPO patients naturally share significant developments in their lives as part of open communication and free associations, and they tend to keep the treatment goals in mind. In addition (and also in contrast to what occurs with BPO patients), typically these developments can be easily linked to presenting problems and treatment goals. If, however, the content of the sessions becomes dissociated from treatment goals, with the patient focusing instead on other issues, the therapist will share this observation with the patient and explore possible motivations for diverting attention away from the problems that brought the patient to treatment.

With NPO patients, the therapist may initially explore a given conflict without necessarily making links to treatment goals or presenting problems. However, as the conflict comes into focus, the therapist routinely considers how it relates to the patient's presenting complaints and treatment goals, folding these considerations into the process of interpretation and working through. The therapist does not do this by raising the issue of the treatment goals out of the blue or by arbitrarily forcing the issue.

Rather, as a conflict comes into focus, the therapist watches for situations in which links to treatment goals present themselves in a natural and meaningful way; that is, the therapist waits for opportunities but does not create them. In fact, sometimes it is less that the therapist chooses to focus on or to pursue certain issues, and more that he chooses to pursue other issues less actively.

Thus, with NPO patients, it is during the process of working through that the treatment goals play an especially central role. Patients have dominant conflicts that may affect many areas of functioning. Some areas of functioning will be very powerfully and obviously affected by a given conflict, whereas others will be much more subtly affected. During the middle phase of TFP-E, the therapist focuses on the patient's core conflicts as they pertain to those areas of impairment that are of greatest concern to the patient and most disruptive of her functioning. The technical objective is to be open to all aspects of the patient's communications, while at the same time streamlining interventions to address specific treatment goals.

Discussion of focusing on treatment goals raises the question of the extent to which the therapist can expect to see improvement in the NPO patient's areas of functioning *outside* the domains defined by the treatment goals. Improvement, and in some cases highly significant improvement, is typically seen in a variety of areas of functioning as part of a ripple effect. This is especially likely when various functional difficulties are viewed as manifestations of the same core conflicts. Paradoxically, our clinical experience suggests that focusing more consistently on a *specific* domain of functioning (in contrast to promoting a more unstructured process) not only leads to greater improvement in that particular domain, but also may increase the likelihood that improvements generalize to *other* domains as well. As a rule, the less severe the patient's personality rigidity, the more likely it is that therapeutic benefits will be seen in areas of functioning not specifically targeted during the treatment, whereas with greater personality rigidity, benefits may be more localized. The fact that the treatment has not ameliorated or possibly even addressed all of the patient's difficulties is a reality that will be confronted and worked through during the termination phase of every TFP-E treatment.

Clinical Illustration 8: Therapeutic Focus on Treatment Goals

Mr. O, a 46-year-old physician's assistant, organized at a neurotic level and diagnosed with depressive personality disorder with obsessive-compulsive features, came to treatment feeling like "a loser"; he described being unable to assert himself or to actively pursue leadership positions in his workplace and the monetary success he desired. This patient had other areas of difficulty apart from self-esteem and professional advancement: He was perfectly happy to maintain a caring and respectful but somewhat constrained relationship with his wife, who, it seemed, was also content in the marriage. Although the marriage lacked sexual passion, Mr. O did not view this as a problem. In addition, he was struggling, with some degree of distress, with the demands of caring for his elderly parents. Although any or all of these areas of difficulty could have been given priority in the treatment, Mr. O was troubled primarily by experiencing himself as a loser in his professional role; this is what had brought him to treatment, and his identified goal was to improve his functioning and self experience at work.

As the patient's conflicts came into focus, his therapist, Dr. T, emphasized links between the object relations being enacted and Mr. O's inhibitions in relation to power, authority, and money, but paid less attention to Mr. O's inhibitions in relation to sexuality and intimacy. For example, as Mr. O's anxieties about his competition came into focus, Dr. T suggested that perhaps one way to understand his holding himself back at work was that doing so helped him avoid finding himself in a position of power, where he might fear losing control and attacking people who were less powerful or more vulnerable than himself.

Similarly, when Mr. O responded to personal successes by feeling anxious or guilty, Dr. T again emphasized the link to the patient's inhibitions in relation to success in the workplace. Though the therapist commented on the links between Mr. O's conflicts and his emotionally restrained and sexually inhibited relation with his wife, these links were not emphasized in the process of working through. In sum, as a particular conflict came into focus, Dr. T emphasized how this related to the patient's inhibitions with regard to pursuing professional and financial advancement, and paid less attention to exploring how these same conflicts left him inhibited in other areas as well.

Borderline Level of Personality Organization

As emphasized in Chapter 9, when working with BPO patients, the TFP-E therapist needs to maintain active awareness of and attention to the treatment goals if the treatment is to stay on course. Because BPO patients may be entirely "in the moment," and are often unable to consistently maintain a big-picture view that incorporates goals and longer-term objectives, it falls to the TFP-E therapist to bridge dissociated aspects of the patient's experience, keeping in mind in every session the treatment goals and the patient's daily functioning. There is always a risk during the middle phase that the therapist and patient will get lost in the moment-to-moment clinical process, losing sight of the connection between the process and the treatment goals or, alternatively, between the treatment and important developments in the patient's life. In the worst-case scenario, the outcome is that the treatment seems to be going fine but the patient's functioning remains unchanged.

To avoid this pitfall—relatively common in unstructured psychodynamic treatments of patients with personality disorders—the therapist's mind must serve as a bridge among dissociated areas of the patient's functioning, the therapy, and the therapeutic goals, while the therapist helps the patient develop a more integrated perspective on her experience and behavior. With this objective, throughout the middle phase, the therapist will consider in each session how the contents of the session and the patient's life outside the treatment relate to (or fail to relate to) one another and to the treatment goals.

In TFP-E, at those times when the relationship between the clinical process and the treatment goals is unclear, or the therapist has only a vague understanding of the BPO patient's recent functioning, the therapist will be active in tactfully but consistently pointing out that the patient appears to be splitting off the treatment from her life and related treatment goals. This approach ensures that the treatment remains anchored in the reality of the patient's presenting problems and daily functioning, while the therapist initiates exploration of dissociative defenses. This exploration may involve active inquiry on the part of the therapist, to whom it falls to bring in relevant issues that the patient does not hold in mind. In contrast to the approach with NPO patients (in which the therapist can wait to see what comes to the patient's mind, so to speak), with BPO patients, the therapist takes a far more active approach in bringing material into the session, with the treatment goals as a central vehicle for doing so. The following are examples of therapists' inquiries:

> You mentioned that you've been doing a lot of partying, which we know means not keeping up with your schoolwork. How does this fit with your treatment goal of completing your degree this academic year?

> One of your goals here is to complete your degree, yet you've said nothing about your studies for a number of weeks.

> We've been talking a lot about how you sometimes undermine your treatment and undermine me. I'm wondering how this relates to the problems in your marriage that brought you here.

In sum, in the treatment of BPO patients, from the opening sessions and throughout the middle phase, the therapist's ability to maintain awareness of the treatment goals and to keep abreast of developments in the patient's life serves the essential function of bridging the dissociative processes introduced into the treatment by the patient's defenses (see Chapter 9 for additional discussion of focusing on treatment goals with BPO patients). This integrative function on the part of the therapist requires constant effort to avoid colluding with the patient's defenses, as well as consistent interventions to call the patient's attention to the impact of her defenses on the clinical process.

Clinical Illustration 9: Focusing on Goals Brings Splitting and Denial Into the Treatment

Organized at a middle borderline level, with passive-aggressive, narcissistic, and dependent features, Ms. Z presented with the complaint of frequently losing her temper with her 6-year-old daughter. The patient acknowledged having at times attempted to "frighten her into behaving." Ms. Z denied any physical contact during these episodes ("I just want to make her feel scared so she'll listen"). The patient was aware that her behavior was destructive, and she dealt with her discomfort after the fact by being lenient with the child while trying not to think about her own behavior.

Ms. Z reported occasional outbursts with her husband as well, but these were less frequent, and he seemed able to manage them without much distress. He would respond by forcefully insisting that his wife calm down, and she was able to respond positively to his limit setting. Ms. Z sought treatment when she noticed that her daughter seemed not to want to spend time with her. At the same time, the daughter began having difficulty at school.

In the early months of this patient's treatment, she spoke nonreflectively about a variety of topics: how her day had gone, struggles with her girlfriends, a recent flirtation, and her disappointment in not having a career. The therapist, Dr. E, noted to herself that Ms. Z's discourse did not appear to be directed toward any specific objective, and that Ms. Z demonstrated no apparent interest in what the therapist might have to say.

It seemed to Dr. E that the dominant issue was Ms. Z's failure to speak about matters of consequence, while shutting out the therapist. Dr. E chose to comment on this observation, sharing with the patient her impression that although Ms. Z was speaking of a number of issues, it was unclear what any of them had to do with the difficulties that had brought her to treatment.

Ms. Z responded by essentially ignoring Dr. E's comment and returning to her monologue. When the therapist pointed this out to the patient, Ms. Z acknowledged that she preferred to pretend in her mind that Dr. E was not present. What emerged was that the patient didn't want to think about the therapist's reactions to her, and especially any reactions to what she had said about her treatment of her daughter during the consultation. This exchange led to fruitful discussion of Ms. Z's reliance on denial and rationalization to support her preference not to think about her behavior with her child, and the fact that this coping style came at the price of perpetuating her destructive behavior.

Several months later, in the early middle phase of Ms. Z's treatment, she became preoccupied with wanting acknowledgment from Dr. E. She described wanting to feel special to the therapist; she had wishes that the therapist would demonstrate this by making special arrangements and accommodations for her. This transference, in which Ms. Z wanted to be a special child who was taken care of by a patient, devoted therapist, was the focus of seemingly fruitful exploration in the treatment.

However, at a certain point, Dr. E realized that recent sessions, focusing on the transference, had seemingly become detached from the patient's daily functioning. Dr. E became aware that Ms. Z had said virtually nothing in recent weeks about what was going on in her daily life or, in particular, in her interactions with her daughter. When she called Ms. Z's attention to these omissions, Ms. Z responded that her behavior at home had remained problematic, and "as usual" she had not wanted to think or talk about it in her sessions. Dr. E pointed out that while the patient had been talking about her wish for an idealized relationship with the therapist, this feeling had become dissociated from the opposite and far more urgent issue at home, in which Ms. Z was enacting with her daughter a hostile, paranoid object relation of a withholding, frustrating, controlling child in relation to a powerless, frustrated, enraged caretaker. Notably, the patient identified with both roles.

Working Through Developmental Antecedents of Conflictual Object Relations

In Chapter 10, when we introduced the process of interpretation, we commented that in TFP-E, the therapist does not emphasize interpretations that link current conflicts to the patient's early history. Instead, the therapist focuses on conflictual object relations as they are enacted in the here and now, both in the patient's current life and in the treatment. However, as core conflicts are worked through in the middle and advanced phases of treatment, it often becomes helpful to link the object relations that are being worked through in the here and now to important figures and experiences from the patient's developmental history. Whereas premature interpretation of the role of the past generally leads to intellectualized discussions with limited therapeutic benefit, or to the patient's externalization of responsibility for her difficulties, well-timed interpretations that link the patient's early history to object relations that are alive in the treatment can provide additional depth and meaning to the process of working through.

In the treatment of BPO patients, this process begins only after the patient has attained some degree of identity consolidation—typically in the later middle phase and during the transition to the advanced phase of treatment. At this point, making links between internal object relations and the patient's developmental history becomes useful, as representations of self and of significant objects from the past become relatively well integrated, coherent, and realistic, and are viewed by the patient from a relatively complex perspective. (See Chapter 6, Part 3, section "Patients Along the Borderline Spectrum of Personality Organization," and the case of Ms. M discussed throughout.)

In the treatment of NPO patients, references to the patient's developmental history routinely become part of the process of working through in the middle phase. As core conflicts are elaborated and are being worked through, links to the patient's past tend to emerge organically and spontaneously in the patient's associations, as her experience becomes more flexible in areas of conflict. (See Chapter 6, Part 3, section "Patients Along the Neurotic Spectrum of Personality Organization," and the case of Ms. S discussed throughout.) At this point, the patient tends to move smoothly between present and past experiences as she deepens her understanding of how both express her internal world.

Commentary on the Role of Working With Dreams

In the process of working through or at any point in treatment, patients may bring up their dreams. Exploration of a patient's dreams has an important place in the history of psychoanalysis. Initially, psychoanalytic "cure" was thought to result from uncovering repressed, unconscious mental contents; and, for Freud (1900/1964), dream analysis was considered the "royal road to a knowledge of the unconscious activities of the mind" (p. 609). In the TFP-E approach, the perspective on working with dreams is more measured and is considered according to the treatment goals and level of personality organization.

Borderline Level of Personality Organization.   As we have emphasized throughout this book, with BPO patients, the therapist focuses preferentially on promoting first self-observation, then self-awareness, and finally self-reflection, before exploring unconscious dynamics with the objective of deepening self-understanding. As a result, through much of the early and middle phases of treatment of BPO patients, the utility of dream analysis is limited relative to the utility of focusing on the impact of dissociative defenses on the patient's behavior, conscious thoughts, and feelings. In the early and middle phases of treatment, if a BPO patient chooses to present a dream in session, the therapist typically should focus on the manifest content of the dream and on the action of the patient's sharing the dream (i.e., considering why the patient is telling about this dream now).

Neurotic Level of Personality Organization. With the NPO patient who is able to freely associate and for whom repression-based defenses predominate, understanding unconscious dynamics plays a more central role in treatment (see Chapter 10, section "Interpretation Proper," and also later within that section, Clinical Illustration 1 (*continued*): "Interpretation With an NPO Patient"), and helping the patient become aware of repressed aspects of experience is a part of this process.

However, even with NPO patients, the therapist's interest is less on bringing repressed aspects of experience to consciousness per se and more on helping the patient develop the flexibility to tolerate full emotional awareness of these parts of herself. As a result, dream analysis typically does not play a central role in TFP-E even with NPO patients. When patients describe dreams, the overall approach for the therapist is to listen to the patient's associations to the dream, to consider her account of recent events that may have triggered the dream, and to observe her attitude in telling the dream. Typically, a central theme will emerge in these communications, much as occurs generally in free associations with NPO patients in the middle phase. The therapist will consider how this theme may relate to affectively dominant object relations in the session, and to conflicts currently active in the treatment and in the patient's life.

Working Through Negative Therapeutic Reactions

The term *negative therapeutic reaction* describes the situation in which a patient makes a therapeutic gain and then reacts by becoming more symptomatic, anxious, or depressed, or by undoing the gains made (Auchincloss and Samberg 2012; Sandler et al. 1992; Tindle 2006). Although negative therapeutic reactions can occur in any phase of treatment, they are most common in the middle phase of personality disorder treatment, as the patient begins to develop a realistic sense of the help provided by the therapist and the treatment.

In patients with higher level personality pathology, the dynamics of the negative therapeutic reaction often relate to depressive anxieties, such as the patient's guilt, either conscious or unconscious, about receiving help and/or making gains. It is common for patients to feel undeserving of the therapist's help, or to worry that whatever gains made will in some way take place at the expense of others or will "leave behind" people whom the patient cares about. Negative therapeutic reactions of this kind, reflecting depressive anxieties, will be worked through—for some patients, many times—over the course of the middle phase, and will be reworked as part of the process of ending the therapy.

In contrast, negative therapeutic reactions in BPO patients most often reflect defenses against paranoid anxieties. In this context, the patient's recognition that the therapist has been helpful or that the therapist has something meaningful to offer may make the therapist seem "too powerful" in the patient's eyes. As a result, the therapist's help can stimulate feelings of inferiority, envy, or hostility, as well as fears of being exploited or controlled, accompanied by impulses to undo whatever gains have been made. Negative therapeutic reactions as a result of paranoid anxieties associated with envy are especially common in low-BPO patients, and also in narcissistic patients across the spectrum of severity. (In the words of one patient, "I will always cut off my nose to spite my face.")

Negative therapeutic reactions as a result of paranoid anxieties can also be seen, but less commonly, in patients with higher level personality pathology. Patients with higher level personality pathology and prominent narcissistic conflicts are especially prone to negative therapeutic reactions as a result of envy.

To illustrate the two forms of negative therapeutic reaction and how they can present in TFP-E, we return to Ms. F, the patient described earlier in this chapter who was so critical and devaluating in the opening phase of her treatment, while struggling with an underlying object relation of someone fortunate, superior, and triumphant in relation to another who was envious and defeated.

Clinical Illustration 3 (*continued*): Negative Therapeutic Reaction and Working Through Paranoid and Depressive Conflicts

In a session in the early portion of the middle phase of Ms. F's treatment, the patient complained that she had been feeling down; she was no less depressed, and was perhaps even worse, than when she had started treatment. She wondered out loud whether a different therapist or a different kind of treatment might be more efficient. She wondered whether she had accomplished anything at all. As the session progressed, Ms. F began to feel suspicious of Dr. A; she wondered why he had not raised the possibility of a change in the treatment, and also why he had not responded directly to her comments about making a change.

It was only in the last minutes of the session, with Dr. A still trying to understand this recent development, that Ms. F shared that her husband had told her that he had noted a change in her: she seemed to be handling interactions with her daughter much more constructively, and her husband felt she was being kinder to him as well. In response, Dr. A pointed out the apparent contradiction between Ms. F's current attitude toward her therapist and treatment, on the one hand, and the positive feedback from her husband, on the other. It seemed that the treatment was helping her with the difficulties for which she had come for help, yet at exactly this moment, she found herself especially dissatisfied.

Dr. A went on to suggest that, perhaps paradoxically, Ms. F was not entirely happy to find that the therapy *had* been able to help. When Ms. F remained silent, Dr. A went on to suggest that perhaps the situation left her feeling that Dr. A, as her therapist, was "too powerful," as if he now had everything. Perhaps, he proposed, if her therapy was helpful, Ms. F would think that it signified yet another success for Dr. A; he got what he wanted—to feel even better about himself—while Ms. F's daughter remained ill and Ms. F continued to suffer the misery of having a chronically ill child. Maybe, Dr. A suggested, she imagined he was secretly thinking of this situation as yet another feather in his cap. Ms. F acknowledged that although it made no sense, the possibility that Dr. A *was* able to help left her feeling worse instead of better, even more frustrated and demoralized by her situation.

Later in the middle phase of the treatment, Ms. F once again received positive feedback, now in the form of extremely loving and laudatory toasts from her family and friends, including her daughter, at a birthday celebration for Ms. F. The previous 6 months of the treatment had been devoted to understanding and working through Ms. F's sadness, frustration, and anger in relation to her daughter's illness. In making a toast, her daughter had commented on how grateful she was that her mother had recently been a great source of support, and that the daughter believed her health was better as a result.

The next day, Ms. F came into her session to share the good news, but also to say that she was suddenly feeling depressed—at least as depressed as she had been on first coming to treatment. She wondered once again if the treatment was really helping, and toward the end of the session, she announced that she had decided to end the treatment. After all, it might be that she had accomplished all she could.

Once again, Dr. A linked Ms. F's current depressed mood and nihilistic attitude to favorable developments in her relationships with family members, especially her daughter. Dr. A pointed out Ms. F's paradoxical position: just when she was beginning to reap the rewards of treatment, it seemed she felt demoralized and wanted to discontinue it. Dr. A went on to suggest that perhaps Ms. F was now feeling depressed and wanting to end her treatment because, out of her awareness, she felt guilty about or undeserving of the help she was receiving, especially because nothing could ever make her daughter completely well.

Ms. F immediately commented that she had been able to enjoy the evening with her family and her daughter's encouraging words for only a brief time; quickly, she had started to focus on the many years her daughter had been suffering from her illness, and to worry about what would happen to her daughter in the future—as if, Ms. F noted, she needed to undo her own happiness. Simultaneously, for the first time, it occurred to her that Dr. A might himself have a chronically ill child—how awful if she had spent all this time speaking about her own child, inadvertently rubbing salt in Dr. A's own wounds.

Markers of Change and Transition to the Advanced Phase of Treatment

The transition from the middle to the advanced phase of treatment is a gradual one that marks the incipient ending of the therapy. By the transition to the advanced phase, BPO patients demonstrate at least some degree of identity consolidation, whereas NPO patients demonstrate decreased personality rigidity in circumscribed areas of conflict.

Borderline Level of Personality Organization

In the treatment of BPO patients, identity consolidation and resolution of splitting are the structural hallmarks of transition to the advanced phase of treatment. As BPO patients make this transition, the therapist sees a resolution of maladaptive or frankly contradictory behavioral patterns that may have been ego-syntonic and outside the patient's awareness at the beginning of treatment.

The transition to the advanced phase of treatment is further marked by a shift in the patient's affective experience, such that affects are better modulated and the patient demonstrates an increased capacity to contain and reflect on emotional states and associated object relations. The patient's relationships, both with the therapist and in interpersonal life, acquire greater depth and complexity, and the therapist will notice evidence of increased empathy and perspective taking on the part of the patient. These shifts will be clearly reflected in the patient's descriptions of her interactions with the people in her world, present and past, which acquire a sharper and more realistic quality and allow the patient's significant others to come to life in the therapist's imagination.

By the time of transition to the advanced phase of treatment, the patient will demonstrate openness to the therapist's interventions, along with a fully developed capacity to reflect on and deepen the therapist's contributions. Outside the treatment, the patient will be making use of self-observation and reflection to manage internal and interpersonal stresses and associated affect states, and to limit acting out in daily life. The impulse to act out or provoke does not necessarily disappear (although it does in some cases); more typically, as a result of the treatment, destructive impulses are toned down and the patient develops an enhanced capacity for "top-down control"—that is, the ability to notice her impulses, as well as to contain and reflect on them, rather than immediately turning to action.

For example, at this point, a patient might say, "Steve criticized me yesterday. As always, I wanted to retaliate and lash out. But I caught myself—I know myself now. And I reminded myself that he does this when he is feeling badly about *himself*. That helped. So, rather than starting a fight, I took a deep breath; then I got all supportive and nice, and asked him to tell me about his day. In the end, we had a nice evening."

As we have emphasized, the process of integration is a dynamic one, and shifts are especially marked in BPO patients. Even as patients attain progressively stable identity consolidation and capacity for self-awareness and reflection, the therapist continues to see the transient return of less-well-integrated mental states. What characterizes the transition to the advanced phase with BPO patients is the relative brevity of these episodes, along with patients' developing capacity to relatively quickly identify and reflect on such shifts or "regressions," often righting themselves without intervention from the therapist, to return to a more highly integrated level of experience.

For example, at this point, a patient might say, "After I left on Friday, I was sure you were laughing at me. For a moment, I felt so humiliated and angry, but even then I knew it wasn't true. I know I'm having trouble with your having canceled our session next week." The repeated working through of the shift between integration and short-lived "microregressions" in the transition to the advanced phase of treatment contributes to a gradual decrease in the patient's vulnerability to regression.

By the time the BPO patient is transitioning to the advanced phase of treatment, the clinical process will begin to resemble that of the treatment of NPO patients; as repression-based defenses replace splitting, the therapist hears the emergence of free associations, and the patient may also spontaneously share daydreams or fantasies as part of the clinical discourse. The therapist now has the opportunity and freedom to focus with the patient on the narrative embedded in the patient's verbal communications, deepening and enriching her level of self-understanding. Interpretations made in the here and now, characteristic of the early and middle phases of treatment, can at this point be productively linked to the patient's history with significant objects from the past, connections that often arise naturally in the patient's associations. The patient's capacity to associate also opens up the possibility of doing conventional dream analysis, in which the patient's associations to the dream can be linked to dominant issues in the treatment and in the transference. The patient may begin to make spontaneous links between her life inside and outside the sessions, going back and forth between the two while linking her behavior with the therapist to recent behavior with significant others. For example, one patient remarked, "I can't believe how badly I used to behave in relation to my supervisor at work—crying when I didn't get my way, with no awareness of how annoying and inappropriate that was.... I guess I did the same thing here; I behaved like such an awful, tyrannical baby."

Neurotic Level of Personality Organization

In the treatment of NPO patients, progression to the advanced phase of treatment is marked by the gradual emergence of greater flexibility in the patient's day-to-day functioning and in her behavior and communications in session. Greater flexibility will also be reflected in enrichment of the patient's affective experience of self and others in areas of conflict. As a result of focusing on the treatment goals during the process of working through, the presenting complaints should be resolving, typically in association with resolution of the anxiety and/or depressive states that were part of the patient's initial presentation, with a shift toward more positive affect dispositions. These changes reflect a developing capacity on the part of the NPO patient to consciously tolerate and manage conflictual aspects of experience.

As the NPO patient moves into the advanced phase of treatment, the therapist sees an increase in the patient's capacity to independently observe, reflect on, and work through conflicts that are activated, often with little need for the therapist to intervene. Outside the treatment hours, the patient will use the self-analytical skills developed during treatment to manage conflict and painful internal states. This is illustrated by the patient who says, "I felt my mood sinking yesterday, and I caught myself getting all self-critical. But rather than just going with it, I tried to think about what was happening and why. I think it was because Joe was unhappy before he went to work; I always feel guilty about enjoying things when he is feeling low, even though I know that's unreasonable. The point is that I was able to see it and think about what was happening.... I thought of our conversations, and my mood slowly lifted."

Advanced Phase of Treatment and Ending

The central tasks of the advanced phase of treatment are to consolidate gains that have been made over the course of the therapy, to mourn losses and disappointment, to facilitate ongoing change after treatment ends, and to leave the door open for the patient to return in the future if need be. All these objectives are facilitated by facing and working through the inevitable disappointments that come with ending a successful treatment.

Topics central to discussion of the advanced phase of treatment and ending include the following:

- Indications for ending treatment
- Analysis of separations
- Ambivalence in the advanced phase of treatment
- Maintaining the treatment frame through ending
- Therapist's reactions to ending treatment
- Premature endings
- Patient-therapist contact after treatment ends

Regardless of the nature of the ending of treatment, be it "ideal" or far from it, the major tasks of the advanced phase of treatment are the same. In the ideal case, treatment ends after patient and therapist agree that goals have been sufficiently met; a date for ending the treatment is then set in advance, and the patient uses the final months of the treatment to explore and work through the anxieties, disappointments, and satisfactions associated with ending treatment.

In practice, however, in the treatment of personality disorders, ideal endings are far from universal. It is not uncommon for the patient's motivation to flag, or for her to become frustrated with the investment of time, effort, or money that therapy entails and to unilaterally decide to end treatment. It is also common for the patient's life circumstances to change, as job opportunities or new relationships—sometimes born of gains made in treatment—demand relocation or reprioritization of schedules and commitments.

If possible, setting an ending date approximately 2–3 months in advance of the last session is recommended. Less than 2 months is often not enough time to optimally consolidate gains and work through the issues stimulated by ending treatment. On the other hand, if a date is set too far in advance, the prospect of ending becomes so distant that the patient cannot realistically focus on ending. Many, if not most, patients become transiently symptomatic at some point in the final months of treatment and may appear to lose many of the gains that they have made. This apparent backsliding should be managed as a relatively routine aspect of the working through of the termination phase, and is not necessarily an indication to reconsider ending the treatment.

For patients across the spectrum of severity, the manner in which separations, losses, disappointments, and successes are experienced will predict reactions to the advanced phase of treatment. Further, the manner in which these reactions are addressed during the course of treatment will have impact on the degree of preparedness with which the patient faces the challenges presented by the advanced phase and ending of treatment. In addition, throughout the course of treatment, even in the earliest months, the therapist will be preparing the patient for the ultimate ending by noting gains and marking progress toward attaining the treatment goals, helping the patient maintain awareness that treatment will indeed end and that the goals of the treatment are finite. These reminders are especially important for BPO patients, who may lose track of time and goals during the course of an intensive therapy, and who often have difficulty with separations and interruptions.

Indications for Ending Treatment

In the ideal situation, when the treatment goals have been attained or approximated sufficiently to meet the patient's satisfaction, and when the patient's gains are stable, it is time to consider ending the treatment. Symptomatic and behavioral improvement as a result of treatment should correspond with personality change—that is, with increased levels of integration, along with decreased personality rigidity in areas of functioning linked to the patient's presenting complaints. Using these structural criteria in conjunction with the treatment goals as indications for ending the treatment will distinguish personality change from symptomatic improvement that is more superficial, contingent on ongoing contact with the therapist. In contrast, gains reflecting personality change are relatively stable and will be sustained, and may even continue to develop after treatment ends (de Maat et al. 2013; Leichsenring and Rabung 2008; Shedler 2010).

Either the patient or the therapist may introduce a discussion of ending the treatment. Some patients raise this topic throughout the course of treatment. When they do so prematurely, their comments typically reflect reactions to object relations activated in the transference. The patient's premature suggestion to end the treatment can be explored as the therapist would any other clinical material.

In contrast, in the latter portions of the middle phase, when treatment goals have been met to a significant degree, it becomes appropriate to discuss termination in realistic terms. It is important that the TFP-E therapist keep in mind that regardless of whether the patient or the therapist has raised the topic, and even if the patient is comfortable with ending treatment, discussion of ending as a real possibility will stir up reactions in the patient. Before moving ahead and setting a date for ending, patient and therapist will do well to explore what it means to the patient to end treatment, with particular attention to the transference fantasies linked to this discussion.

Analysis of Separations During Treatment

The patient's responses to separations from the therapist during weekends, vacations, and illnesses over the course of treatment will predict, to some degree, the patient's reactions to ending therapy. Patients' responses to separation from the therapist can be described as falling along a spectrum of degree of integration: normal to depressive to paranoid. Normal reactions to separation from the therapist include sadness, a sense of loss, and mourning. Depending on the circumstances, a normal reaction to separation may also include a sense of freedom, a sense of well-being, and an orientation toward the future.

Depressive reactions to separation are dominated by intense sadness and idealization of the therapist, often in conjunction with feelings of guilt and unworthiness, and a tendency to cling to the relationship. Fantasies of being responsible for having driven away the therapist or having worn him out are common.

In contrast, paranoid responses to separation from the therapist are marked by severe separation anxiety such that instead of sadness, the patient experiences intense anxiety and fear of abandonment, often with underlying hostility. There is a tendency to see the therapist as a "bad" object who is purposefully abandoning, rejecting, attacking, or frustrating the patient.

Over the course of treatment, most patients will experience a combination of paranoid, depressive, and normal reactions to separations and interruptions in treatment. At those times when the patient presents with a mix of paranoid and depressive reactions to separation, paranoid reactions should be analyzed before depressive ones; as discussed earlier in this chapter (see the subsection "Exploring Paranoid and Depressive Anxieties Interfering With Integrative Processes"), analysis of paranoid object relations will facilitate more complete and successful working through of depressive conflicts. Repetitive analysis of reactions to separation, as the patient achieves increasing levels of structural integration while working through paranoid and depressive anxieties, will help move the patient from a more paranoid or depressive reaction toward a normal one, and will prepare her for ending the treatment.

Clinical Illustration 10: Anxieties Stimulated by Separation and Ending in a High-BPO Patient

Ms. C, a chronically depressed and self-critical young woman, organized at a high borderline level, presented with complaints of severe sexual inhibitions and feelings of self-loathing in the setting of a mild identity disturbance. The patient functioned relatively well professionally and socially. In the early months of treatment, conflicts around competitive sexual and aggressive themes were salient. In this setting, the therapist, Dr. D, focused on Ms. C's constant need to devalue herself, which he suggested reflected an effort to ward off retaliatory attacks for competitive triumphs, both imagined and actual.

Ten months into the treatment, Dr. D took a planned 4-week vacation. During the break, Ms. C became acutely paranoid in relation to her husband. She experienced him as selfish and callous, someone who exploited her and had no concern for her welfare. She found herself enraged. She was aware that these feelings were different from anything she had experienced during 5 years of a relatively happy marriage; she had maintained a relatively stable, idealized image of her husband throughout their marriage.

Upon Dr. D's return, it became possible to explore the object relation of a callous, powerful, and self-serving but needed maternal figure in relation to a hateful, dependent child. This paranoid object relation was seen as underlying Ms. C's conflicts around competition and her need to devalue herself; in her psychology, success or positive self-valuation activated an object relation of a diminished, dependent self in relation to a powerful, hostile, and callous maternal figure. This paranoid object relation had been dormant in the treatment, split off from the transference and from the patient's awareness in general, until it was activated by prolonged separation from the therapist.

Working through the paranoid concerns in relation to dependency that had been activated by Dr. D's absence facilitated subsequent successful working through of oedipal conflicts in relation to competition. This episode was the first of several similar ones, all of which foreshadowed a stormy period in the final months of treatment, during which Ms. C experienced the therapist as callous and as "throwing me out." This last flurry of paranoid anxieties provided opportunity for yet another working through—a final and highly successful one—of Ms. C's paranoid and then depressive anxieties during the final months of her treatment.

Clinical Illustration 11: Normal Reaction to Separation From Treatment

Mr. N began talking about ending the treatment several months before his therapist, Dr. Q, was due to begin his summer vacation. A date for ending had not yet been set, but the patient continued to feel that he wanted to wrap things up. On the eve of Dr. Q's vacation, Mr. N noted that although he anticipated missing the therapist and the treatment as he had done during interruptions of the treatment in the past, he felt less fearful and less needy about the situation. In some ways, he was looking forward to the opportunity to experience what it felt like not to have Dr. Q to lean on. Also, because he had been seeing his therapist early in the morning, Mr. N was pleasurably anticipating more leisurely mornings in bed with his girlfriend.

In contrast, during Dr. Q's vacation the previous summer, Mr. N had been aware of feeling needy before the therapist left, and he had thought that Dr. Q might be looking forward to a welcome break from Mr. N's "whining." Over that break, Mr. N had felt depressed and self-critical, and was convinced that he was doing a bad job at his work. The connection between these affects and the therapist's absence had not been evident to him until Dr. Q pointed it out upon his return.

Analysis of Separation at the End of Treatment

By the time the end of treatment is approaching, therapist and patient will have had many opportunities to analyze the patient's responses to separations from the therapist. The relative mix of paranoid, depressive, and normal reactions to ending the treatment will vary from patient to patient, depending in part on the severity and nature of the patient's pathology, on the relative success of treatment, and on the patient's level of satisfaction with the outcome. Transient paranoid reactions around ending are common in BPO and some NPO patients, and depressive reactions can be seen in both groups. A transient return of some of the presenting complaints and symptoms is also common across the range of severity.

All these developments provide a final opportunity to work through anxieties that have been addressed during the course of the treatment. If paranoid reactions to ending treatment prove persistent for BPO patients, it may be advisable to postpone the ending, to allow for further working through during ongoing treatment before ending.

Typical depressive reactions to ending treatment involve not only the experience of loss, but also reactions to success. It is common for patients ending successful treatments to entertain at least fleeting concerns that they are somehow hurting the therapist by leaving. A patient may imagine that the therapist will feel lonely or left behind in the patient's absence, or that the therapist is dependent on income from the patient and will be financially burdened by the patient's successful move onward. Analyzing these fantasies during the advanced phase of treatment provides a final opportunity to work through depressive conflicts in the transference and will help consolidate gains made in treatment.

Ambivalence in the Advanced Phase of Treatment

In addition to noting and consolidating gains, patients in the process of ending treatment must also consider what has not been accomplished in the treatment. They acknowledge and mourn not only the loss of the therapist, but also the loss of an ideal view of what they hoped would be accomplished in treatment. Even when treatment goals are successfully met, the patient is confronted with the reality that her personality and her behavior remain less than perfect. The capacity to work through both the disappointments and the gains of a successful TFP-E treatment implies that the patient has attained a comfortably integrated sense of self.

Working through disappointments also involves facing disappointment in the therapist and in the treatment. The capacity to entertain a generally positive view of the therapist, while maintaining awareness of his limitations, implies an ambivalent attitude on the part of the patient toward the therapist. In a successful termination, feelings of disappointment and resentment can be contained within an overall positive view of the therapeutic relationship, characterized by a sense of genuine appreciation for the therapist's skill and gratitude for the help the therapist has provided.

Maintaining the Treatment Frame Through Termination

Wishes on the part of the patient and/or the therapist to taper sessions, or to "wean" the patient from treatment, are common and typically reflect the desire to mitigate anxieties stimulated in the patient by ending treatment and separating from the therapist. Whereas tapering is often optimal in supportive therapies in order to mitigate anxieties resulting from separation, in TFP-E, the intent of tapering sessions is to allow these anxieties to emerge so that they can be explored and worked through while the treatment is ongoing. This process makes it easier for the patient to function well without the therapist in the posttermination phase, provides an important opportunity to consolidate treatment gains, and may facilitate the patient's ongoing growth and development after treatment ends.

We recommend maintaining the therapeutic relationship, without grossly changing the way in which therapist and patient interact, as the treatment comes to an end. Doing so provides the best opportunity for the patient to work through her feelings toward the therapist, especially feelings of disappointment or anger that may be activated around ending. Maintaining the usual style of interaction also makes it easier for the patient to return in the future, should she choose to do so. Having said this, we add that it is inevitable that the relationship between patient and therapist will take on a more realistic quality as treatment comes to an end and transferences are worked through. However, beyond this natural evolution in the therapeutic relationship, it is not recommended that the therapist change his role or assume a more socially friendly or openly supportive stance in relation to the patient during the final weeks of treatment. In the concluding sessions, it is appropriate for the therapist to mark the gains that have been made and to communicate whatever positive feelings he has about having worked with the patient.

Therapist's Reactions to Patient Ending Treatment

It is natural for the therapist to experience a mourning reaction at the ending of a TFP-E treatment, particularly one that has been especially long and/or rewarding. In addition, depressive concerns on the therapist's part are not uncommon at termination. As patients voice and work through their disappointment in the treatment, it is not uncommon for therapists to feel guilty. Feelings of regret or self-criticism—perhaps that the therapist could have done a better job, or that another therapist might have had better results with the patient—are particularly common among inexperienced therapists. Like the patient, the therapist must come to terms with what was not accomplished in the treatment.

Premature Endings

It is not uncommon for patients with personality disorders to consider ending treatment before treatment goals have been attained. When a patient verbalizes such a desire, the therapist should do the following: 1) explore the patient's motivations for leaving and link them to anxieties currently being activated in the treatment, paying special attention to the transference; and 2) seriously consider any developments in the patient's life that may preclude continuing the treatment. If the patient persists in wanting to leave, the therapist should share a realistic assessment of what has been accomplished, what has not been accomplished, and what could be expected from further work.

If the patient continues to insist on ending the treatment prematurely, the therapist should avoid engaging in a power struggle. It is appropriate for the therapist to frankly share his reservations about ending therapy at this time, and then to establish a mutually agreed-upon date to stop meeting, ideally at least a month in advance. The therapist can explain to the patient that it is helpful to allow this time period for wrapping things up and consolidating gains. The therapist should also explain that "the door is open," should the patient feel that she would like to pursue treatment at some point in the future.

Patient-Therapist Contact After Treatment Ends

If the patient does not raise the question of future contact between therapist and patient after treatment ends, it is appropriate for the therapist to do so. It is not uncommon for patients to believe that they are "not supposed to" or "not allowed to" contact the therapist in the future, or that doing so would indicate a failure of the treatment. The therapist should communicate that he is available to the patient and would be happy to hear from her in the future, should the need arise. A significant proportion of patients come for "tune-ups" over the course of years, often in the setting of a life event, such as the birth of a child, a medical illness, or the loss of a parent or spouse, whereas others return for brief courses of treatment as life developments unearth new psychological challenges. Some patients will ask about getting together with the therapist socially after treatment has ended—for example, meeting for lunch. We strongly recommend that the TFP-E therapist avoid engaging in social relationships with patients after treatment ends.

Key Clinical Concepts

- The therapeutic consultation comprises assessment, sharing of the diagnostic impression, determination of treatment goals, discussion of treatment options, and helping the patient make an informed treatment selection.

- TFP-E treatments can be seen as having early, middle, and advanced phases.

- The major tasks of the early phase are to stabilize the treatment frame, support the development of a therapeutic alliance, address early anxieties stimulated by beginning treatment, and minimize risk of the patient's dropping out of treatment before she has the opportunity to become fully engaged.

- By the transition to the middle phase, patient and therapist will be familiar with core conflictual object relations organizing the patient's experience both inside and outside the therapy.

- The major task of the middle phase is to explore and work through the paranoid and depressive conflicts linked to core object relations, which may be expressed in the form of negative therapeutic reactions.

- As conflicts are worked through in the middle phase, the therapist will focus on the treatment goals, make links to the developmental antecedents of conflictual object relations, and remain attentive to the patient's functioning outside the treatment.

- By the transition to the advanced phase, BPO patients demonstrate at least some degree of identity consolidation, whereas NPO patients demonstrate decreased personality rigidity in circumscribed areas of conflict.

- Structural changes accompanying transition to the advanced phase of treatment correspond with improved self and interpersonal functioning and attainment of treatment goals.

- The major tasks of the final phase of treatment are to consolidate gains, to mourn losses and disappointment, to facilitate ongoing change after treatment ends, and to leave the door open for the patient to return in the future, should the need arise.

References

Auchincloss AL, Samberg E (eds): Psychoanalytic Terms and Concepts. New Haven, CT, Yale University Press, 2012

Bender DS: Therapeutic alliance, in The American Psychiatric Publishing Textbook of Personality Disorders. Edited by Oldham JM, Skodol AE, Bender DS. Washington, DC, American Psychiatric Publishing, 2005, pp 405–420

Bordin ES: The generalizability of the psychoanalytic concept of the working alliance. Psychotherapy (Chic) 16:252–260, 1979

Caligor E, Kernberg OF, Clarkin JF: Handbook of Dynamic Psychotherapy for Higher Level Personality Pathology. Washington, DC, American Psychiatric Publishing, 2007

Crits-Christoph P, Gibbons MBC, Mukherjee D: Psychotherapy process-outcome research, in Bergin and Garfield's Handbook of Psychotherapy and Behavior Change, 6th Edition. Edited by Lambert MJ. Hoboken, NJ, Wiley, 2013, pp 298–340

de Maat S, de Jonghe F, de Kraker R, et al: The current state of the empirical evidence for psychoanalysis: a meta-analytic approach. Harv Rev Psychiatry 21(3):107–137, 2013 23660968

Freud S: The interpretation of dreams (1900), in The Standard Edition of the Complete Psychological Works of Sigmund Freud, Vols 4–5. Edited and translated by Strachey J. London, Hogarth Press, 1964, pp 1–626

Hilsenroth MJ, Cromer TD: Clinician interventions related to alliance during the initial interview and psychological assessment. Psychotherapy (Chic) 44(2):205–218, 2007 22122211

Hinshelwood RD: A Dictionary of Kleinian Thought. Northvale, NJ, Jason Aronson, 1991

Horvath A, Bedi RP: The alliance, in Psychotherapy Relationships That Work. Edited by Norcross JC. New York, Oxford University Press, 2002, pp 37–70

Joseph B: Projective identification, some clinical aspects (1987), in Melanie Klein Today, Vol 1. Edited by Spillius EB. London, Routledge, 1988, pp 138–150

Klein M: A contribution to the psychogenesis of manic-depressive states (1935), in Love, Guilt and Reparation and Other Works, 1921–1945. London, Hogarth Press, 1975, pp 262–289

Leichsenring F, Rabung S: Effectiveness of long-term psychodynamic psychotherapy: a meta-analysis. JAMA 300(13):1551–1565, 2008 18827212

Levy SR, Hilsenroth MJ, Owen JJ: Relationship between interpretation, alliance, and outcome in psychodynamic psychotherapy: control of therapist effects and assessment of moderator variable impact. J Nerv Ment Dis 203(6):418–424, 2015 25988432

Patrick C: Antisocial personality disorder and psychopathy, in Personality Disorders: Toward the DSM-V. Edited by O'Donohue W, Fowler K, Lilienfeld S. Thousand Oaks, CA, Sage, 2007, pp 109–166

Sandler J, Dare C, Holder H: The Patient and the Analyst, 2nd Edition. Madison, CT, International Universities Press, 1992

Shedler J: The efficacy of psychodynamic psychotherapy. Am Psychol 65(2):98–109, 2010 20141265

Steiner J: Psychic Retreats: Pathological Organizations in Psychotic, Neurotic and Borderline Patients. London, Routledge, 1993

Steiner J: The aim of psychoanalysis in theory and in practice. Int J Psychoanal 77 (Pt 6):1073–1083, 1996 9119577

Tindle K: Negative therapeutic reaction. Br J Psychother 23:99–116, 2006

Yeomans F, Clarkin JF, Kernberg OF: Transference-Focused Psychotherapy for Borderline Personality Disorder: A Clinical Guide. Washington, DC, American Psychiatric Publishing, 2015

Afterword

IN WRITING THIS BOOK, WE HAD A SERIES
of objectives in mind: 1) to describe a psychodynamically based model of
personality and personality pathology that focuses on self and interpersonal functioning; 2) to present a clinically near approach to classification
and assessment of personality pathology, one that carries direct implications for treatment; 3) to offer clinicians an integrated, psychodynamically
based treatment model for personality disorders that combines structure
and limit-setting with psychological exploration; and 4) to outline general
clinical principles that apply to treatment across the spectrum of personality pathology, coupled with 5) an understanding of specific modifications
of technique that tailor treatment to the individual patient, based on the
severity and nature of his pathology, and his moment-to-moment psychological functioning.

Even before we began, we already had much with which to work. This
book integrates a series of earlier contributions, born of many years of
productive collaboration. We have drawn most actively on the following:
1) *Transference-Focused Psychotherapy for Borderline Personality Disorder* (Yeomans et al. 2015), and the many years of clinical and research experience invested in the development of this treatment model for patients
with severe personality disorders; 2) *Handbook of Dynamic Psychotherapy for Higher Level Personality Pathology* (Caligor et al. 2007), an extension of the transference-focused psychotherapy model to the treatment
of patients with mild and subsyndromal personality disorders; 3) contemporary object relations theory as developed by Kernberg (Kernberg and
Caligor 2005), especially in its conceptualization of self and interpersonal
functioning in the normal personality and personality disorders; 4) structural diagnosis, or levels of personality organization, a model of classification and assessment of personality pathology originally conceived by
Kernberg (1975, 1984) and further developed by our group (Clarkin et
al. 2016; Horz et al. 2012); and 5) a series of recent conceptual and empirical developments in the field of personality disorders that converge

with our perspective, in particular a new emphasis on self and other functioning and levels of severity of pathology, as formalized in the Alternative Model for Personality Disorders in DSM-5 Section III (American Psychiatric Association 2013) and the *Psychodynamic Diagnostic Manual*, 2nd Edition (Lingiardi and McWilliams, 2017).

Flexible and Pragmatic Implementation

We have covered a fair amount of ground in these pages, and we hope we have met the objectives outlined in the first paragraph of this Afterword. We expect that different readers will approach this book with individual expectations and objectives. We hope that whatever readers take away will inform or enhance their work with patients with personality disorders.

At the core of this project is a model of long-term psychodynamic treatment. Rather than focusing on a specific disorder, symptom cluster, or group of maladaptive behaviors, our treatment targets underlying structural pathology that is broadly common to all personality disorders yet, with a finer lens, different in each individual patient. From this perspective, we have organized a principle-guided description of treatment, with the objective of enabling therapists to treat patients who present with a range of personality pathology, while tailoring intervention to the specific patient and clinical moment.

Although we describe an approach to long-term psychodynamic treatment, we understand that many readers may not be practitioners of long-term psychodynamic therapy. This awareness provides another rationale for our emphasis on clinical principles, organized as strategies, tactics, and techniques, that can be employed by clinicians of different orientations in a wide variety of clinical settings. We aim to be clear that many of the basic elements of transference-focused psychotherapy—extended employed in long-term treatment are directly translatable to other settings and easily combined with other forms of treatment (Choi-Kain et al. 2016; Hersh et al. 2016; Zerbo et al. 2013). The interested clinician need not be practicing long-term psychodynamic therapy to make use of structured assessment of personality pathology or careful contracting before the start of treatment. The clinician also need not be a psychodynamic psychotherapist to benefit from developing strategies for countertransference management or judicious limit-setting.

Training

Last, we offer readers a suggestion about training. In our experience, the model of pathology, assessment, and treatment described here is of great interest and utility to trainees. The conceptual clarity of the model overall, and the continuity between object relations theory, levels of personality organization, differential treatment planning, and clinical technique provides an optimal setting for clinical learning.

Of course, the therapist cannot develop clinical skills by reading a book. Ongoing clinical work under the supervision of a more senior clinician is generally needed if a trainee is to develop clinical competence, in this or any other treatment model. Study of videotaped therapy sessions in supervision is a cornerstone of our approach to training. Observing and discussing videotaped sessions brings to light the interplay of the patient's verbal and nonverbal communications and the therapist's countertransference in a manner that cannot be replicated by therapist notes or even audio recordings. Videotaping is especially central in training and in supervising the treatment of BPO patients, where sessions may be fast moving and affectively charged, often making it difficult for therapists-in-training to capture in real time the patient's various and often dissociated communications.

We have found group supervision, making use of videotaped clinical material, to be particularly productive. This format optimizes the time of our senior clinicians while exposing trainees to a broad array of patients. In addition, the group process provides a congenial learning environment that supports containment of countertransference.

This training model has also been of great benefit to us. Our many combined years of teaching and working with trainees with different levels of experience have greatly stimulated our own learning and profoundly influenced the contents of this book.

References

American Psychiatric Association: Diagnostic and Statistical Manual of Mental Disorders, 5th Edition. Arlington, VA, American Psychiatric Association, 2013

Caligor E, Kernberg OF, Clarkin JF: Handbook of Dynamic Psychotherapy for Higher Level Personality Pathology. Washington, DC, American Psychiatric Publishing, 2007

Choi-Kain LW, Albert EB, Gunderson JG: Evidence-based treatments for border-line personality disorder: implementation, integration, and stepped care. Harv Rev Psychiatry 24(5):342–356, 2016 27603742

Clarkin JF, Caligor E, Stern BL, Kernberg OF: Structured Interview of Personality Organization—Revised (STIPO-R), 2016. Available at: www.borderlinedisorders.com. Accessed August 21, 2017.

Hersh RG, Caligor E, Yeomans FE: Fundamentals of Transference-Focused Psychotherapy: Applications in Psychiatric and Medical Settings. Cham, Switzerland, Springer, 2016

Horz S, Clarkin JF, Stern B, Caligor E: The Structured Interview of Personality Organization (STIPO): an instrument to assess severity and change of personality pathology, in Psychodynamic Psychotherapy Research: Evidence-Based Practice and Practice-Based Evidence. Edited by Levy RA, Ablon JS, Kachele H. New York, Humana, 2012, pp 571–592

Kernberg OF: Object Relations Theory and Clinical Psychoanalysis. New York, Jason Aronson, 1975

Kernberg OF: Severe Personality Disorders: Psychotherapeutic Strategies. New Haven, CT, Yale University Press, 1984

Kernberg OF, Caligor E: A psychoanalytic theory of personality disorders, in Major Theories of Personality Disorder, 2nd Edition. Edited by Lenzenweger MF, Clarkin JF. New York, Guilford, 2005, pp 114–156

Lingiardi V, McWilliams N (eds): Psychodynamic Diagnostic Manual, 2nd Edition. New York, Guilford, 2017

Yeomans F, Clarkin JF, Kernberg OF: Transference-Focused Psychotherapy for Borderline Personality Disorder: A Clinical Guide. Washington, DC, American Psychiatric Publishing, 2015

Zerbo E, Cohen S, Bielska W, Caligor E: Transference-focused psychotherapy in the general psychiatry residency: a useful and applicable model for residents in acute clinical settings. Psychodyn Psychiatry 41(1):163–181, 2013 23480166

Appendix

Helpful Resources

Contents

STIPO-R Clinical Anchors for Personality Organization: Identity, Object Relations, Defenses, Aggression, and Moral Values Across the Range of Severity[1]

The Structured Interview of Personality Organization—Revised (STIPO-R) anchors are intended to serve as general guidelines for clinicians and researchers assessing personality organization. The following anchors have been adapted to benefit clinical use. For an in-depth evaluation using these anchors for research use, see the full STIPO-R interview and score sheet available at www.borderlinedisorders.com.

For each 1–5 rating, a series of descriptors is provided for each anchor, in which 1=normal and 5=most severe pathology. It is expected that some, but not all, descriptors will apply to a particular patient.

Identity

1. **Consolidated identity**—Sense of self and others is well integrated, with in-depth investment in work/school and recreation.
2. **Consolidated identity, but with some areas of slight deficit**—Sense of self and others* is well integrated for the most part, but with mild superficiality, instability, or distortion, and/or with some difficulty in investment in work/school or recreation.
3. **Mild identity pathology**—Sense of self and/or others is somewhat poorly integrated (evident superficiality or incoherence and instability, at times contradictory and distorted),* with clear impairment in ca-

---

[1]Adapted with permission from Clarkin JF, Caligor E, Stern BL, Kernberg OF: Structured Interview of Personality Organization—Revised (STIPO-R): Score Form. Personality Disorders Institute, Weill Medical College of Cornell University, March 2016. Available at: http://www.borderlinedisorders.com/assets/STIPO-R_Score_Form_March_2016%20.pdf. Accessed December 8, 2017.

Note. Narcissistic pathology is suggested by the presence of a marked discrepancy between 1) instability or superficiality in the individual's sense of others and 2) relative stability or specificity in the individual's sense of self.

pacity to invest in work/school and/or recreation; or individual invests largely to meet narcissistic needs.
4. **Moderate identity pathology**—Sense of self and others is poorly integrated (significant superficiality or incoherence; markedly unstable, contradictory, and distorted),* with little capacity to invest in work/school or recreation.
5. **Severe identity pathology**—Sense of self and others is extremely superficial, incoherent, and chaotic (grossly contradictory and extremely distorted),* with no significant investments in work/school or recreation.

Object Relations

1. **Attachments are strong**, durable, realistic, nuanced, satisfying, and sustained over time; relationships are not seen in terms of need fulfillment; capacity for interdependence and empathy is fully developed; the individual is able to combine sexuality and intimacy.
2. **Attachments are generally strong**, durable, realistic, nuanced, and sustained over time, with some conflict or incomplete satisfaction; relationships are not seen in terms of need fulfillment; capacity for interdependence and empathy is fully developed; there is some degree of impairment or conflict in intimate/sexual relationships.
3. **Attachments are present but are superficial**, brittle, and marked by conflict and lack of satisfaction; relationships tend to be viewed in terms of need fulfillment; there is some capacity for concern for the other or some degree of empathy; sexual relationships have limited intimacy.
4. **Attachments are few and highly superficial**; relationships are consistently viewed in terms of need fulfillment; there is little capacity for empathy; despite any demonstrated efforts to seek intimacy, few to no intimate relationships have developed.
5. **No true relationships exist** (may have acquaintances); the individual may be severely isolated, lacking even acquaintances; any relations that exist are based exclusively on need fulfillment; there is no demonstrated capacity for empathy; no capacity for intimacy and/or no attempts at intimacy are evident.

Defenses

1. **Flexible, adaptive coping is used**; no evidence is seen that lower-level (splitting-based) defenses are employed; stress resilience is evident in most areas; a variety of adaptive coping strategies are consistently used.

2. Adaptive coping strategies are used with less consistency or efficacy, or in some areas but not others, with general resilience to stress. Some lower-level defenses are endorsed (may be limited to idealization and/ or devaluation), but these are clearly not the predominant defensive style of the respondent; limited or no impairment in functioning is seen from use of lower-level defenses.

3. Lower-level defenses have a mixed pattern of endorsement; shifts in perception of self and others are present. Some impairment in functioning is seen from use of lower-level defenses.

4. Lower-level defenses are consistently endorsed; shifts in perception of self and others are relatively severe and pervasive. Clear evidence of impairment in respondent's life is seen from use of lower-level defenses.

5. Lower-level defenses are used pervasively across situations. Severe, radical shifts in perception of self and others are to a degree that grossly interferes with functioning, with multiple examples of instability and distortion.

Aggression

1. Control of aggression—any episodes of anger and verbal aggression appear to be appropriate to the situation.

2. Relatively good control of aggression—maladaptive expressions of aggression are limited to inhibitions (failure to express aggression), minor self-destructive behaviors or neglect, a controlling interpersonal style, or occasional verbal outbursts.

3. Moderately poor control of aggression—maladaptive expressions of aggression include significant self-destructive or higher-risk behaviors, self-neglect or noncompliance, and/or frequent tantrums or outbursts of hateful verbal aggression, chronic hostile control of others, and/or deriving sadistic pleasure from others' discomfort or misfortune.

4. Poor control of aggression—If self-directed, aggression is severe to lethal, but somewhat less pervasive, less chronic (i.e., more episodic), and/or less life-threatening than aggression in item 5. If other-directed, aggression is episodic but frequent, with hateful verbal abuse of others, frequent verbal and physical threats to hurt self or other, and/or physical intimidation that may involve physically threatening or assaulting the other, with pleasure in hurting and/or hostile control of others.

5. Little to no control of aggression—Pervasive tendency toward chronic, severe, lethal expressions of aggression is evident. Frequent

vicious, sadistic, and hateful verbal abuse and/or physical attack on others and/or self is intended to cause physical harm and pose a serious danger to the safety of others and/or self. Self and other-directed aggression involves sadistic pleasure in torture and control; self-directed aggression may involve extreme self-mutilation and/or multiple suicide attempts with intent to die.

Moral Values

1. **Internal moral compass is autonomous, consistent, and flexible;** no evidence is seen of amoral or immoral behavior; the individual demonstrates a mature and appropriate sense of concern and responsibility for potentially hurtful or unethical behavior; there is no exploitation of others for personal gain; the individual experiences guilt appropriately.

2. **Internal moral compass is autonomous and consistent, with rigidity and/or ambiguity involving questionable opportunities for personal gain;** no evidence is seen of frankly amoral or immoral behavior; the individual demonstrates some rigidity (either excessive or some laxity) in sense of concern and responsibility for potentially hurtful or unethical behavior; the individual experiences guilt, but in such a way that ruminative self-recrimination is more prevalent than proactive efforts to make amends.

3. **Some sense of internal moral standards exists, but they are excessively rigid and/or lax;** the individual may demonstrate considerable difficulty using these standards to guide behaviors, which may include some unethical or immoral behavior without confrontation of a victim (e.g., plagiarism, cheating, lying, tax evasion); the individual can be exploitative, with difficulty taking responsibility for behaviors that are hurtful to others; the individual lacks appropriate experience of guilt and concern and/or may experience "guilt" in the form of sadistic self-recrimination without true remorse.

4. **Moral values and internal standards are weak, inconsistent, and/or corrupt;** moral orientation is toward not getting caught and may include presence of aggressive antisocial behavior (e.g., robbery, forgery, blackmail); such behavior may involve confrontation of victims, but without assault, and any violence that occurs is generally not premeditated; exploitation of others is ego-syntonic and the individual freely pursues opportunities for personal gain at the expense of others; guilt or remorse is lacking.

5. **No comprehension of the notion of moral values** is evident; the presence of violent, aggressive antisocial behavior (assault, battery, premeditation) or frank psychopathy (no comprehension or notion of moral values) with or without violent behavior is evident; there is no sense of guilt or remorse.

Level of Personality Functioning Scale[2]

As noted earlier in this book, the Level of Personality Functioning Scale (LPFS) presented in DSM-5 Section III, "Emerging Measures and Models," is similar to the object relations theory–based approach to describing personality functioning and pathology used in transference-focused psychotherapy—extended (TFP-E). The LPFS characterizes personality disorders according to the severity of impairment in self and interpersonal functioning. The scale provides five levels of personality health and pathology (0 = little or no impairment; 4 = extreme impairment) that correspond quite closely with the five levels of personality organization described in the TFP-E object relations theory model (see Chapter 2, Figure 2–1). We provide the scale here for ease of clinical reference and refer readers to a full description of the scale and the alternative model for personality disorders as provided in DSM-5.

---

[2]*Source.* American Psychiatric Association: *Diagnostic and Statistical Manual of Mental Disorders,* 5th Edition. Arlington, VA, American Psychiatric Association, 2013, pp. 775–778. Copyright © 2013 American Psychiatric Association. Used with permission.

Level of Personality Functioning Scale

	SELF		INTERPERSONAL	
Level of impairment	Identity	Self-direction	Empathy	Intimacy
0—Little or no impairment	Has ongoing awareness of a unique self; maintains role-appropriate boundaries. Has consistent and self-regulated positive self-esteem, with accurate self-appraisal. Is capable of experiencing, tolerating, and regulating a full range of emotions.	Sets and aspires to reasonable goals based on a realistic assessment of personal capacities. Utilizes appropriate standards of behavior, attaining fulfillment in multiple realms. Can reflect on, and make constructive meaning of, internal experience.	Is capable of accurately understanding others' experiences and motivations in most situations. Comprehends and appreciates others' perspectives, even if disagreeing. Is aware of the effect of own actions on others.	Maintains multiple satisfying and enduring relationships in personal and community life. Desires and engages in a number of caring, close, and reciprocal relationships. Strives for cooperation and mutual benefit and flexibly responds to a range of others' ideas, emotions, and behaviors.

Level of Personality Functioning Scale (*continued*)

Level of impairment	SELF		INTERPERSONAL	
	Identity	Self-direction	Empathy	Intimacy
1—Some impairment	Has relatively intact sense of self, with some decrease in clarity of boundaries when strong emotions and mental distress are experienced. Self-esteem diminished at times, with overly critical or somewhat distorted self-appraisal. Strong emotions may be distressing, associated with a restriction in range of emotional experience.	Is excessively goal-directed, somewhat goal-inhibited, or conflicted about goals. May have an unrealistic or socially inappropriate set of personal standards, limiting some aspects of fulfillment. Is able to reflect on internal experiences, but may overemphasize a single (e.g., intellectual, emotional) type of self-knowledge.	Is somewhat compromised in ability to appreciate and understand others' experiences; may tend to see others as having unreasonable expectations or a wish for control. Although capable of considering and understanding different perspectives, resists doing so. Has inconsistent awareness of effect of own behavior on others.	Is able to establish enduring relationships in personal and community life, with some limitations on degree of depth and satisfaction. Is capable of forming and desires to form intimate and reciprocal relationships, but may be inhibited in meaningful expression and sometimes constrained if intense emotions or conflicts arise. Cooperation may be inhibited by unrealistic standards; somewhat limited in ability to respect or respond to others' ideas, emotions, and behaviors.

Level of Personality Functioning Scale (*continued*)

Level of impairment	SELF		INTERPERSONAL	
	Identity	Self-direction	Empathy	Intimacy
2—Moderate impairment	Depends excessively on others for identity definition, with compromised boundary delineation. Has vulnerable self-esteem controlled by exaggerated concern about external evaluation, with a wish for approval. Has sense of incompleteness or inferiority, with compensatory inflated, or deflated, self-appraisal. Emotional regulation depends on positive external appraisal. Threats to self-esteem may engender strong emotions such as rage or shame.	Goals are more often a means of gaining external approval than self-generated, and thus may lack coherence and/or stability. Personal standards may be unreasonably high (e.g., a need to be special or please others) or low (e.g., not consonant with prevailing social values). Fulfillment is compromised by a sense of lack of authenticity. Has impaired capacity to reflect on internal experience.	Is hyperattuned to the experience of others, but only with respect to perceived relevance to self. Is excessively self-referential; significantly compromised ability to appreciate and understand others' experiences and to consider alternative perspectives. Is generally unaware of or unconcerned about effect of own behavior on others, or unrealistic appraisal of own effect.	Is capable of forming and desires to form relationships in personal and community life, but connections may be largely superficial. Intimate relationships are predominantly based on meeting self-regulatory and self-esteem needs, with an unrealistic expectation of being perfectly understood by others. Tends not to view relationships in reciprocal terms, and cooperates predominantly for personal gain.

Level of Personality Functioning Scale (*continued*)

Level of impairment	SELF		INTERPERSONAL	
	Identity	Self-direction	Empathy	Intimacy
3—Severe impairment	Has a weak sense of autonomy/agency; experience of a lack of identity, or emptiness. Boundary definition is poor or rigid: may show overidentification with others, overemphasis on independence from others, or vacillation between these. Fragile self-esteem is easily influenced by events, and self-image lacks coherence. Self-appraisal is un-nuanced: self-loathing, self-aggrandizing, or an illogical, unrealistic combination. Emotions may be rapidly shifting or a chronic, unwavering feeling of despair.	Has difficulty establishing and/or achieving personal goals. Internal standards for behavior are unclear or contradictory. Life is experienced as meaningless or dangerous. Has significantly compromised ability to reflect on and understand own mental processes.	Ability to consider and understand the thoughts, feelings, and behavior of other people is significantly limited; may discern very specific aspects of others' experience, particularly vulnerabilities and suffering. Is generally unable to consider alternative perspectives; highly threatened by differences of opinion or alternative viewpoints. Is confused about or unaware of impact of own actions on others; often bewildered about people's thoughts and actions, with destructive motivations frequently mis-attributed to others.	Has some desire to form relationships in community and personal life, but capacity for positive and enduring connections is significantly impaired. Relationships are based on a strong belief in the absolute need for the intimate other(s), and/or expectations of abandonment or abuse. Feelings about intimate involvement with others alternate between fear/rejection and desperate desire for connection. Little mutuality: others are conceptualized primarily in terms of how they affect the self (negatively or positively); cooperative efforts are often disrupted due to the perception of slights from others.

Level of Personality Functioning Scale (continued)

	SELF		INTERPERSONAL	
Level of impairment	Identity	Self-direction	Empathy	Intimacy
4—Extreme impairment	Experience of a unique self and sense of agency/autonomy are virtually absent, or are organized around perceived external persecution. Boundaries with others are confused or lacking. Has weak or distorted self-image easily threatened by interactions with others; significant distortions and confusion around self-appraisal. Emotions not congruent with context or internal experience. Hatred and aggression may be dominant affects, although they may be disavowed and attributed to others.	Has poor differentiation of thoughts from actions, so goal-setting ability is severely compromised, with unrealistic or incoherent goals. Internal standards for behavior are virtually lacking. Genuine fulfillment is virtually inconceivable. Is profoundly unable to constructively reflect on own experience. Personal motivations may be unrecognized and/or experienced as external to self.	Has pronounced inability to consider and understand others' experience and motivation. Attention to others' perspectives is virtually absent (attention is hypervigilant, focused on need fulfillment and harm avoidance). Social interactions can be confusing and disorienting.	Desire for affiliation is limited because of profound disinterest or expectation of harm. Engagement with others is detached, disorganized, or consistently negative. Relationships are conceptualized almost exclusively in terms of their ability to provide comfort or inflict pain and suffering. Social/interpersonal behavior is not reciprocal; rather, it seeks fulfillment of basic needs or escape from pain.

Index